XFORD
IVERSITY PRESS

t Clarendon Street, Oxford OX2 6DP

rd University Press is a department of the University of Oxford.
hers the University's objective of excellence in research, scholarship,
ducation by publishing worldwide in

rd New York

and Cape Town Dar es Salaam Hong Kong Karachi
Lumpur Madrid Melbourne Mexico City Nairobi
Delhi Shanghai Taipei Toronto

offices in

tina Austria Brazil Chile Czech Republic France Greece
mala Hungary Italy Japan Poland Portugal Singapore
Korea Switzerland Thailand Turkey Ukraine Vietnam

d is a registered trade mark of Oxford University Press
UK and in certain other countries

ned in the United States
ford University Press Inc., New York

ublished 2010

ibrary Cataloguing in Publication Data
ailable

of Congress Cataloging in Publication Data
ailable

by Cepha Imaging Private Ltd., Bangalore, India
in China
free paper through
ific Offset

8–0–19–923962–7

7 6 5 4 3 2 1

University Press makes no representation, express or implied, that the drug
in this book are correct. Readers must therefore always check the product
ion and clinical procedures with the most up-to-date published produ
ion and data sheets provided by the manufacturers and the most r
conduct and safety regulations. The authors and publishers do no
bility or legal liability for any errors in the text or for the misu
of material in this work. Except where otherwise stated, dr
endations are for the non-pregnant adult who is not breas

Oxford Handbook of Women's Health Nursing

Oxford Handbook of Women's Health Nursing

Edited by

Sunanda Gupta

Consultant in Community Gynaecology,
ONEL Community Services,
Honorary Clinical Senior Lecturer,
St Bartholomew's and Royal London,
School of Medicine and Dentistry,
London, UK

Debra Holloway

Consultant Nurse, Gynaecology,
Guy's and St Thomas' NHS Foundation Trust,
Visiting Lecturer, King's College London,
London, UK

Ali Kubba

Consultant in Community Gynaecology,
Lambeth Community Services,
Honorary Clinical Senior Lecturer,
Guy's and St Thomas' NHS Foundation Trust,
London, UK

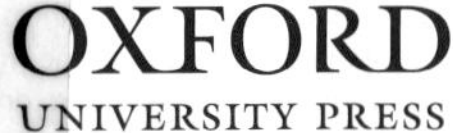

Foreword

I am delighted to provide the foreword for the *Oxford Handbook of Women's Health Nursing*.

Women's health is a major public health challenge that contributes to high morbidity and mortality rates. Globally, women bear the greatest burden of sexual and reproductive ill-health, the sequelae of which, cause a wide range of illnesses (mental and physical) and significant long-term disability. Maternal mortality alone already kills over half a million worldwide each year—with the majority of deaths being from treatable or preventable causes.

During my career I have worked with women who have faced multiple barriers in accessing healthcare, sometimes due to discrimination by healthcare staff. I have also met some who, through poor access to information, have thought using wet tissues would provide them with a barrier method to protect against pregnancy and sexually transmitted infections. Poor access to services and to health information has been a recurring theme and one which I feel passionately about.

Since 2002, I have had the honour of working on the first ever National Strategy for Sexual Health and HIV, initially leading the Department of Health Sexual Health Policy Team, and then since 2006, heading up the National Support Team for Sexual Health to support implementation of the strategy at service, commissioning, and provision levels to improve and increase access to services.

Developing the role of the workforce, including nurses, is a key aspect of the national strategy and I strongly believe that nurses have the ability to improve access to services and to provide the information needed to support women in making their own decisions in relation to their healthcare. Developing nurses' roles and their skills and competencies will improve access to skilled health practitioners and this important and timely publication will provide support to nurses and others working in the field to make a difference for women, not only in the UK but worldwide.

Jane Mezzone
Head of the National Support Team for Sexual Health
and Response to Sexual Violence
Department of Health (England)
2009

Preface

Women are the backbone of a healthy society, and ensuring that they receive good reproductive, gynaecological, and sexual healthcare is paramount.

The widening of options in women's healthcare, the shift of emphasis towards autonomy and empowerment, and the technological advances in gynaecological subspecialties have created the need for expert nursing care.

In recent years nursing roles have developed and expanded incorporating roles that were traditionally seen as exclusively medical. These changes mirrored developments in more cost effective healthcare, with ambulatory and shorter hospital stay interventions. As a consequence, nursing care has to be delivered in shorter time frames and often closer to home. Embedded within all care is clinical governance and evidence-based practice. This book provides nurses with easy to digest, up-to-date information that bridges the practice theory gap across the tiers of healthcare.

When developing this book, we have mainly approached nurses who are working within these areas to develop the text and produce content relevant to nurses of all grades. The format is of a quick and easy reference book, with both breadth and depth, that will allow nurses to dip into subjects while working with pointers in the pathology, investigations, and management of common problems. When more in-depth reading is needed, the book provides more details and directs the reader to further resources.

We are confident that this handbook will be of use to nurses and students working within women's healthcare in all settings, and hope you, the reader, will enjoy this handbook as much as we have.

Sunanda Gupta
Debra Holloway
Ali Kubba
2009

Acknowledgements

We are grateful to all the authors of the chapters who have given up their time so generously to produce work of such clarity. We have thoroughly enjoyed editing these contributions. We also remain indebted to the reviewers who have painstakingly read and reviewed the chapters. Our special thanks to the editors of the *Oxford Handbook of Cancer* Nursing for allowing us to dip in and use content for some of the oncology chapters.

We wish to acknowledge the patience and skill of the development team, in particular, the editor Jamie Hartmann-Boyce and the production team, particularly Kate Wanwimolruk at OUP for keeping the book on track. Their support has been invaluable.

Sunanda Gupta
Debra Holloway
Ali Kubba
2009

Contributors

Debbie Barber
Oxford Fertility Unit,
Oxford, UK

Dianne Crowe
Northumbria Healthcare
NHS Trust, Hexham,
Northumberland, UK

Kavita Dass
Guy's and St Thomas'
NHS Foundation Trust,
London, UK

Alice W. Denga
Guy's and St Thomas'
NHS Foundation Trust,
London, UK

Joanne Fletcher
Sheffield Teaching Hospitals
NHS Foundation Trust,
Sheffield, UK

Rosemary Gebhardt
Guy's and St Thomas'
NHS Foundation Trust,
London, UK

Alison Genge
Guy's and St Thomas'
NHS Foundation Trust,
London, UK

Aggie Jokhan
Guy's and St Thomas'
NHS Foundation Trust,
London, UK

Emma Kennedy
Lambeth PCT,
London, UK

Kaushika Kuntawala
Guy's and St Thomas'
NHS Foundation Trust,
London, UK

Chris Pearce
Great Western Hospitals,
NHS Foundation Trust,
Swindon, UK

Margaret Ramage
Partner Therapy Group,
London, UK

Viola Schulz
Lambeth PCT,
London, UK

Marie Shannon
Guy's and St Thomas'
NHS Foundation Trust,
London, UK

Ellie Stewart
Guy's and St Thomas'
NHS Foundation Trust,
London, UK

Lisa Story
Queen Charlotte's and
Chelsea Hospital,
London, UK

Laura Stretch
REACH Domestic Abuse Project,
A&E and Minor Injuries Unit,
Guy's and St Thomas'
NHS Foundation Trust,
London, UK

Claudia Tye
Guy's and St Thomas'
NHS Foundation Trust,
London, UK

Madelaine Ward
Westside Contraceptive Services,
London, UK

Contents

Symbols and abbreviations

❶	caution
🕮	cross reference
⚠	warning
🖱	website
►	important
►►	act quickly
A&E	accident & emergency
AIS	androgen insensitively syndrome
BASMT	British Association of sexual and marital therapists
BNF	British National Formulary
BRCA	breast cancer gene
BSL	British sign language
CHD	coronary heart disease
CHM	complete hydatidiform mole
CIN	cervical intra-epithelial neoplasia
COCP	combined oral contraceptive pill
COPD	chronic obstructive pulmonary disease
COSHH	control of substances hazardous to health
CPP	chronic pelvic pain
CSM	Committee of Safety of Medicines
CSWs	client support workers
CVD	cardiovascular disease
DEXA	duel energy X-ray absorptimetry
DH	Department of Health
DHEA	dehydroepiandrosterone
DHEA	dehydroepiandrostenedione
DHEAS	dehydroepiandrosterone sulphate
DMPA	depot medroxyprogesterone acetate
DO	detrusor over-activity
DSU	day surgery unit
DVT	deep vein thrombosis
EC	emergency contraception
EGUs	emergency gynaecology units
EHC	emergency hormonal contraception
EPAU	early pregnancy assessment unit

EUA	examination under anaesthesia
FGM	female genital mutilation
FIGO	International Federation of Gynaecologists and Obstetricians
FNA	fine-needle aspiration
FPA	Family Planning Association
FSD	female sexual dysfunction
FSH	follicle stimulating hormone
FSRH	Faculty of Sexual and Reproductive Health
GMC	General Medical Council
GnRH	gonadotrophin-releasing hormone
GTT	Glucose tolerance test
GUM	genito-urinary medicine
HAART	highly active anti-retroviral therapy
HBV	Hepatitis B
HCA	healthcare assistant
HCG/hCG	human chorionic gonadotrophin
HDL	high density lipoprotein
HMB	heavy menstrual bleeding
HPV	human papilloma virus
HRT	hormone replacement therapy
HSV	herpes simplex virus
HT	hormone therapy
ICSI	intra-cytoplasmic sperm injection
IDS	interval debulking surgery
ISC	intermittent self-catheterization
IUS/IUD	intrauterine system/intrauterine contraceptive device
LFTs	liver function tests
LH	luteinizing hormone
LLETZ	large loop excision of the transformation zone
LMP	last menstrual cycle
LNG	levonorgestrel
LNG-IUS	levonorgestrel intra-uterine system
LOD	laparoscopic ovarian diathermy
LPA	lasting power of attorney
LUNA	laparoscopic uterine nerve ablation
MEC	medical eligibility criteria
MHRA	Medical Health Regulatory Agency
MI	myocardial infarction
MRI	magnetic resonance imaging

MRSA	methicillin resistant staphylococcus aureus
NAAT	nucleic acid amplification test
NHS CSP	NHS cervical screening programme
NICE	National Institute for Health and Clinical Excellence
NIDDM	non-insulin dependent diabetes mellitus
NMC	Nursing and Midwifery Council
NMES	neuro-muscular electrical stimulation
NPSA	National Patient Safety Agency
NpfIT	National Programme for Information Technology
NVQ	National Vocational Qualification
OAB	overactive bladder
OR	odds ratio
OTC	over the counter
PCOS	polycystic ovarian syndrome
PCR	polymerase chain reaction
PCT	Primary Care Trust
PEP	post-exposure prophylaxis
PFE	pelvic floor exercises
PGD	patient group direction
PGE2	prostaglandin E_2 (endometrial prostaglandin)
PHM	partial hydatidiform mole
PID	pelvic inflammatory disease
POF	premature ovarian failure
POP	progesterone only pill
PSN	presacral neurectomy
PSTT	placental-site trophoblastic tumour
PVR	post-void residual urine volume
RCOG	Royal College of Obstetricians and Gynaecologists
RCT	randomized controlled trial
RMI	risk of malignancy index
RR	relative risk
RSH nurses	reproductive and sexual health nurses
SABE	sub-acute bacterial endocarditis
SABS	Safety Alert Broadcast System
SALS	surgical admission lounge
SERM	selective estrogen receptor modulators
SHBG	sex hormone binding globulin
SNRI	serotonin and noradrenaline reuptake inhibitor
SSRI	selective serotonin reuptake inhibitor

STI/HIV	sexually transmitted infections/human immunodeficiency virus
SUI	stress urinary incontinence
TAH BSO	total abdominal hysterectomy, bilateral salpingoophorectomy
TAS	transabdominal scan
TENS	transcutaneous electrical nerve stimulation
TNM	tumour node metastasis
TOP	termination of pregnancy
TOT	transobturator tape
TSH	thyroid stimulating hormone
TVS	transvaginal scan
TVT	tension-free vaginal tape
UAE	uterine artery embolization
UPSI	unprotected sexual intercourse
UTIs	urinary tract infections
VaIN	vaginal intra-epithelial neoplasia
VDU	video display unit
VIN	vulval intraepithelial neoplasia
VTE	venous thrombo-embolism
VVC	vulvovaginal candidiasis
WHI	Women's Health International

Chapter 1

Introduction

Overview: community women's health

Women require contraceptive and reproductive/sexual health care from menarche to menopause. An holistic approach to care enables women of all ages to make effective and safe choices regarding contraceptive methods, managing sexually transmitted infections/human immunodeficiency virus (STI/HIV), unplanned pregnancy care, or pregnancy care within the community and other specialist services provided by health professionals.

The multidisciplinary team comprises Consultant Community Gynaecologists (now called Consultants in Reproductive and Sexual Health), GPs, sessional doctors, nurse consultants, nurses, midwives, health visitors, pharmacists, health advisors, healthcare assistants, counsellors, client support workers (CSWs), and receptionists providing client-centred care.

Service providers are there to meet the local needs of rural and urban communities. Examples of care are:

- Contraception (and pregnancy advice): most is provided from general practice but also in specialist services, e.g. Brook Advisory Services, to increase choice and compliment general practice. For the under 25s, young persons' clinics provide targeted care, and for vulnerable young women, outreach services in their homes, colleges, or prison, among other outlets.
- Specialist sexual healthcare: investigation and treatment for STIs/HIV, hepatitis A/B/C, sexual dysfunction, victims of sexual assault, female and male sex workers.
- Screening and health promotion for cervical neoplasia, national chlamydia screening (under 25s), other STI screening, breast disease, bowel cancer, and smoking cessation.
- Management of menopausal problems (osteoporosis, hormone replacement therapy (HRT)).
- Lifestyle advice and health education—including advice on weight, smoking, and alcohol.
- Abortion services, self-referral or through GPs, within a maximum of 3 weeks from presentation to the procedure. Some Primary Care Trusts (PCTs) have arrangements with the private sector, Marie Stopes International or British Pregnancy Advisory Services, and central booking systems.
- Open-access walk-in clinics, pharmacies providing emergency hormonal contraception (EHC) and chlamydia screening.
- Voluntary sector: chlamydia screening via Terrance Higgins Trust.
- Specialist advice telephone helplines: Family Planning Association (FPA) or local clinics.

Overview: hospital setting

Women's health within the hospital setting is complex and requires varying levels of expertise and specialization.

The patient's journey starts normally with a referral to the outpatient setting for a consultation. This has changed in recent years to a place where investigations, treatments, and minor procedures can be carried out, instead of admitting patients to the ward. The traditional general gynaecology outpatients is increasingly dependent on the size of the secondary care setting, subdivided to include specialist clinics for incontinence, pain, endometriosis, colposcopy, ambulatory gynaecology, gynaecological oncology, infertility, contraception, sexual health, and menopause. Increasingly, many patients will be managed within the outpatient setting and never become an inpatient and equally may have their care entirely managed by a nurse specialist.

Some patients in gynaecology do require surgery. This can increasingly be managed within a day-surgery setting, where patients are in hospital for the minimum amount of time possible. This in itself can be a challenge for the staff to ensure that there is a seamless process through the system and that all care is individualized and meets the expectations of the patients. For more complex operations, the normal admission to a ward is still the norm. However, in recent years the move of patients from inpatient to day care and from day care to outpatients has led to a decline in the gynaecology wards. Many have been combined with surgical wards and this can lead to loss of the specialist nursing care that women with gynaecological conditions need.

Women's healthcare can also be delivered within sexual and reproductive health, maternity, and as an emergency. Women with problems in early pregnancy can often bypass A&E and be seen in an early pregnancy assessment unit. They have the benefit that they can be seen in a dedicated unit, often with access to ultrasound, and have fewer examinations and admissions when compared to the A&E department. In some instances, the model has been extended to include all gynaecology emergencies managed in dedicated emergency gynaecology units (EGUs).

Women's healthcare is provided in a number of sub-specialties. These include:

- Fertility and reproductive medicine.
- Sexual health (contraception and other reproductive health).
- Menopause.
- Menstrual dysfunction.
- Gynaecological endocrinology.
- Recurrent pregnancy loss.
- Colposcopy.
- Hysteroscopy/hysteroscopic surgery.
- Minimally invasive surgery.
- Gynaecological oncology.
- Paediatric gynaecology.
- Pelvic pain.
- Urogynaecology.
- General gynaecology.
- Emergency gynaecology.
- Early pregnancy assessment.

Within the next chapters, these will be covered in more detail and the role that nurses can play within them will be highlighted.

Chapter 2

Nurses' impact on care, role, training, and career pathway

Women's health—nurses in primary care and community

Nurses working within the community can have many roles. These can be:
- Practice nurses.
- Specialist practice nurses/nurse practitioners.
- Sexual and reproductive health nurses.
- School nurses.
- Independent prescribers.
- Nurse consultants.
- Nurse trainers.

Practice nurses

Practice nurses can have a generalist role within the community or they may have a specialist role, where they deliver care to women with specific problems. Generally, nurses will be working in GP surgeries, where they may be in teams or working independently. Practice nurses provide assessment, screening, treatment, care, and education to patients from all sections of the community. Typical work activities may include:
- providing advice, consultation, and information about a range of health conditions and minor ailments, referring to other members of the practice team, as necessary;
- performing investigatory procedures;
- setting up and running clinics for conditions such as asthma, diabetes, well-woman/man clinics;
- providing contraceptive advice, and the fitting and removing of contraceptive devices (if trained);
- taking samples, such as blood, urine, swabs, and cervical cytology, and perfoming pregnancy tests;
- performing routine procedures, such as ear syringing, eye washing, applying and removing dressings, and treating wounds, etc.;
- offering specialist information and advice in areas such as blood pressure, weight control, smoking cessation, heart conditions, diabetes, etc.;
- administering travel immunizations and offering travel healthcare advice and infant vaccinations;
- offering first aid and emergency treatment, as required;
- advising patients in respect of their continuing medical and nursing needs;
- re-stocking and maintaining clinical areas and consulting rooms;
- taking accurate and legible notes of all consultations and treatments, and maintaining clear records;
- updating/amending clinical computer systems with details of patient and treatments;
- liaising with other practice nurses, GPs, reception and office staff.

To be a practice nurse you need to be a qualified nurse, normally with about 2 years experience. Some employers may require a community specialist practitioner programme. Training will depend on the individual role that is undertaken and there are numerous courses at different educational levels to support the role. It may help to have knowledge and experience working with patients in areas such as: chronic disease management, wound dressing, childhood immunization, cervical cytology and women's health, travel immunizations, physical examinations and phlebotomy (taking blood), health promotion, and advice. Some employers may require a community specialist practitioner degree or postgraduate diploma or a specialism in general practice nursing. Courses combine theoretical study with work-based experience across a range of public health services. Some courses include training in nurse prescribing.

Practice nurses can be on a variety of grades and can move on to be more senior practice nurses or nurse practitioners, where they are managing their own case loads. Many practice nurses are also nurse prescribers—📖 see p.16.

Sexual and reproductive health nurses

Nurses have always worked in family planning and STI services where they may be employed by the hospital or the PCT. More recently the services embrace both reproductive and sexual health. Within these services, nurses provide a significant proportion of care, as stand-alone practitioners.

Nurses working in sexual and reproductive healthcare have a clinical and an educational role, and offer advice by providing HIV testing and counselling, family planning, and sexually transmitted infection services. Some clinics specialize in support and advice to young people under the age of 21, including those under 16, core contraception, and specialist contraception; many services run community gynaecology clinics. Typical work activities include:

- carrying out health assessments;
- prescribing contraception or administration under a patient group direction (PGD);
- undertaking diagnostic and screening tests;
- providing pre- and post-test counselling;
- providing information and advice about treatment;
- educating clients through health-promotion initiatives;
- undertaking outreach work in schools, colleges, youth projects, and hostels, where relevant;
- training other nurses;
- audit and research;
- child protection issues—📖 see Chapter 4, p.53;
- domiciliary contraceptive care to hard to reach and vulnerable women.

Reproductive and sexual health (RSH) nurses need to have a postgraduate qualification before they move into this specialist area and then can develop from there. Many nurses are non-medical prescribers or work via PGDs. There are a number of clinical nurse specialist roles in sexual health. There are also opportunities to move into teaching or management.

School nurses

School nurses provide a variety of services, such as providing health and sex education within schools, carrying out developmental screening, undertaking health interviews, and administering immunization programmes. School nurses can be employed either by the local health authority, Primary Care Trust, community trust, or sometimes by the school directly.

School nurses have understanding of the following areas:

- knowledge of health promotion;
- child protection;
- family planning;
- education;
- screening;
- some insight into the health needs of children and teenagers is useful.

School nurses have a key role in providing sex education and contraceptive advice.

Healthcare assistants

Healthcare assistants (HCAs) play an important role in all aspects of women's health in general practice, community (where they are called client support workers/CSWs), and hospital settings.

The traditional place for HCAs is in outpatient departments or on the gynaecology ward as a chaperone or assistant in the clinic, as a vital part of the nursing team in setting up clinics or in the delivery of care.

Generally HCAs work under the guidance of a qualified healthcare professional, but the role can vary.

HCAs are important members of the team and can, within the hospital setting, spend time with patients, helping to maintain the daily activities of living. Duties can vary from setting up equipment for procedures, undertaking observations, vene-puncture, to assisting with hygiene needs. HCAs can frequently act as chaperones within various settings (📖 see Chapter 3, p.21). In the community, HCAs undertake varying duties, such as restocking and maintaining clinical rooms, and acting as chaperones.

Training and education

Traditionally HCAs' appointments did not require formal qualifications. Previous experience in a caring role is helpful but this will depend on the role that they undertake. Once in the role, in-job training is set up, which depends on the needs of the role and past experience. However, there are opportunities to train formally on the National Vocational Qualification scheme. This can be at level 2 or 3, or even 6, and has various components and modules that relate to healthcare directly, or to customer care or to management. Generally, HCAs who have an NVQ at level 2 will have greater responsibility as the training can be linked to the role that they are in.

►The NVQ level 3 is the minimum requirement for entry on to nursing courses, and some may progress on to nursing or other health-related courses. After a year or two, HCAs can be seconded on to nurse training courses for entry on to nursing.

Hospital nurses—clinic and ward

Within women's health in a hospital setting, nurses can work within:

- outpatient clinics, such as gynaecology, genito-urinary medicine (GUM);
- early pregnancy assessment clinics/units;
- gynaecology wards;
- female surgical wards;
- day surgery or operating theatres;
- multiple settings, as nurse specialists.

The work of ward nurses is changing as care changes, and a large amount of work is now carried out in an outpatient setting. This can lead to a heavier workload in wards, as women have complex surgical and oncology surgical procedures. This can be at a variety of grades starting from a newly qualified band 5 to a ward manager, on to matrons or managers. To work as a newly qualified nurse there are generally no other qualifications needed, but a period of mentorship is required. As nurses progress through a career in women's healthcare within the hospital setting, there are many educational courses that can be undertaken, such as care of gynaecological patients, oncology, sexual health, and so on. Nurses within a ward setting undertake the care of patients admitted for gynaecological operations, and as emergencies. They need to be skilled at providing care, reassuring patients, and undertaking assessments. As they progress, they need management skills in the running of the ward and may undertake a mixture of clinical and management courses.

Nurses within clinic settings may act as chaperones, provide support for patients, oversee the organization of clinics, and may, as they become more experienced, undertake consultations, such as pre-assessment of patients. Hospitals with specialist outpatient units employ nurses to support outpatient procedures as assistants and support for the women. Nurses working in genito-urinary medical clinics will need to have specialist training, which can either be as in-house training or formal courses, to enable them to undertake nurse-run clinics and consultations.

The roles are varied and there is no one set training path for career development. Under 'agenda for change' there are core competencies that need to be achieved for each grade and area that the nurses are working within. A personal development plan ensures that knowledge and skills objectives are met in line with the service and the individual's needs.

Specialist nurses

With the change in workforce over recent years, the role of specialist nurses in women's health has grown considerably. These posts, whatever the title, have a significant impact on the care provided to women: being the reference point for women's care, seeing women in clinical situations, managing a case load of patients, and supporting women in navigating the healthcare system. These posts can be in primary and secondary care and can bridge the interface between the two. They are in all areas and all sub-specializations of women's healthcare.

Specialist nurses have many different titles:

- nurse practitioners;
- clinical nurse specialists;
- advanced practice nurses;
- nurse consultants.

None of these titles are currently regulated by educational standards or regulations and can be, with the exception of nurse consultants, initiated by Trusts or individuals. This has prompted a review by the Nursing and Midwifery Council (NMC) to define advanced practice and the educational level at which this should be set. This is currently under consultation but is likely to be at Masters level. The key components of advanced practice are highly skilled nurses who:

- take a comprehensive patient history;
- carry out physical examinations;
- use their expert knowledge and clinical judgement to identify the potential diagnosis;
- refer patients for investigations, where appropriate;
- make a final diagnosis;
- decide on, and carry out, treatment, including the prescribing of medicines, or refer patients to an appropriate specialist;
- use their extensive practice experience to plan and provide skilled and competent care to meet patients' health and social care needs, involving other members of the healthcare team, as appropriate;
- ensure the provision of continuity of care, including follow-up visits;
- assess and evaluate, with patients, the effectiveness of the treatment and care provided and make changes as needed;
- work independently, although often as part of a healthcare team;
- provide leadership; and
- make sure that each patient's treatment and care is based on best practice.

Nurse consultant posts were first established in 1999. They are central to the process of health service modernization, helping to provide patients with services that are fast and convenient. Nurse consultants spend a minimum of 50% of their time working directly with patients, ensuring that people using the NHS continue to benefit from the very best nursing skills. In addition, the nurse consultants are responsible for developing personal practice, being involved in research and evaluation, and contributing to education, training, and development. Nurse consultants are highly experienced registered nurses, who will specialize in a particular field of healthcare.

The career pathway of advanced practice nursing is varied and depends on the area of specialism. Most nurses have undergone further training and are actively involved in the training of other nurses and healthcare professionals.

Most jobs now are covered by 'agenda for change' and have a profile that, in the future, may make it more transparent as to the role being undertaken.

Nurse prescribers/supplementary prescribing/PGDs

In order for specialist roles to evolve, the question of how to give medication to patients has always been a thorny issue. The Department of Health (DH) introduced non-medical prescribing after a long consultation, with the aims of giving patients quicker access to medicines, of improving access to services, and to make better use of nurses' and other health professionals' skills.

There was a first wave of non-medical prescribers where many nurses qualified and were able to independently prescribe from a nurse's formulary, which was limited by conditions and certain medications. This was useful for some nurses, especially those working within contraceptive services. A further step came with supplementary prescribing, where nurses were able, after assessment by a doctor and in agreement with the patients, to draw up a clinical management plan that allowed review and changing of medication within the plan. This was used extensively within primary care and in some hospital settings for patients with long-term conditions.

Since 2006, the entire British National Formulary (BNF) became open to non-medical prescribers. Nurses who are non-medical prescribers have undertaken additional training and have been assessed academically and in practice to be able to prescribe medication. Nurses who are independent prescribers are able to prescribe from the BNF, with the exception of controlled drugs. In reality, this is normally limited to the area of expertise and by the controls placed by hospitals, practices, and Primary Care Trusts (PCTs). Undertaking a non-medical prescribing course has enabled nurses to work much more comprehensively as independent practitioners.

PGDs

Patient group directions (PGDs) are documents that make it legal for medicines to be given to groups of patients with an identified condition, without individual prescriptions having to be written for each patient.

A PGD is a written direction relating to the supply and/or administration of a prescription-only medicine. The direction must be signed by a doctor or dentist and by a pharmacist. The healthcare practitioners using the PGDs are individually named and are required to ensure that they follow appropriate professional relationships and codes of conduct.

PGDs are valuable in the provision of direct access, in outpatient and in certain emergency situations and in nurse-led services.

A search of the web will show many examples of PGDs, particularly in sexual and reproductive healthcare, where they have been successfully used to enhance service delivery.

Mentorship/supervision/career development

Over the last twenty years, the development of careers has undergone radical change. The days of the traditional career progression, from staff nurse to sister, have gone, with more roles (as described in the previous sections) added to complement the nursing workforce. These roles and careers may not be planned but may develop from a service need and/or the personal goals and ambitions of the nurses concerned.

Career development

This can be a major contributing factor in the advancement of the nursing profession and the health service. An appropriate career pathway has the capacity to ensure the development and maintenance of high quality delivery of care. It is essential that this is underpinned by a flexible educational programme and recognized career structures. Alongside this there should be appropriate recognition by advancement and remuneration. It is the individual nurse's responsibility to plan and develop her career through continuous self-assessment, reflection, and goal-setting, in conjunction with the mentor or line manager.

Women's health nursing, in any area or setting, can be complex. It involves dealing with fertility, sexuality, and body image, as well as the physical aspects of disease. All of this can be daunting for the novice and sometimes even the more experienced nurse. As well as being skilled in providing care and in assessing women's needs, nurses within this area also need to be aware of their own feelings and beliefs in relation to fertility, contraception, and pregnancy, so as not to influence care decisions.

Mentorship

All nurses, once they qualify, should be able to have a mentor to help them through the transition from student to qualified nurse. Some trusts/employers may have guidance on this and set objectives that nurses are expected to achieve. Mentorship can be on a formal or an informal basis. Most nurses will have worked with someone in their career whom they considered a mentor and from whom they were able to learn—this can be either a formal or informal mentorship.

As nurses extend their roles and skills, mentorship becomes more important. As a career develops, mentorship and supervision will come from peers or more experienced nurses, either within their own area or from outside. With the development of roles that were traditionally within the sphere of medics, it is becoming more commonplace to have a medical mentor, especially in areas such as non-medical prescribing. Conversely, nurses are now taking on the formal mentorship of medical staff. As important as mentorship, is the development of the theoretical knowledge that will underpin practice. This can be thorough on-the-job learning, formal courses, or one-off study days.

Clinical supervision

The NHS Management Executive defined clinical supervision in 1993 as:

> '... a formal process of professional support and learning which enables individual practitioners to develop knowledge and competence, assume responsibility for their own practice, and enhance consumer protection and safety of care in complex situations.'

It allows nurses to develop their skills and knowledge and helps them to improve patient/client care.

Clinical supervision—the key factors

- Identify solutions to problems.
- Increase understanding of professional issues.
- Improve standards of patient care.
- Further develop their skills and knowledge.
- Enhance understanding of their own practice.

Resources

www.nhscareers.nhs.uk
www.rcn.org.uk
www.nmc-uk.org

Chapter 3

The basics

Reproductive anatomy

Vulva

The vulva is the name for female external genitalia and consists of:

- mons pubis;
- labia majora;
- labia minora;
- vestibule;
- the perineum.

The vestibule is the depression between the labia minora into which open the urethra, vagina, and the ducts of the Bartholin gland. It also contains the hymen. The anterior and posterior limit of the vestibule are the clitoral prepuce and fourchette, respectively (see Fig. 3.1).

Pelvic floor

The pelvic floor consists of muscles, pelvic fascia, ovarian ligaments, round ligaments, and the ureters.

Muscles

The perineal group of muscles share a common insertion point with the levator ani into a midline raphe, called the perineal body. The levator ani muscles form a sling from the lateral pelvic walls, passing downwards and backwards to their insertion in the perineal body, coccyx, and sacrum. Levator ani muscles act as a support for the vagina, which is consequently held in an S shape. The levator ani muscles, by supporting the vagina, also support and raise the bladder neck. Below the levator ani, on each side, is the ischiorectal fossa containing fatty connective tissue.

Pelvic fascia

The pelvic fascia is connective tissue lying between and above the levator ani muscles and below the pelvic peritoneum. It condenses to form transverse cervical or cardinal ligaments, pubocervical and uterosacral ligaments. The peritoneum over the round ligament, fallopian tubes, and ovarian ligaments is the broad ligament but has no supportive function. The infundibulo-pelvic ligaments are continuations of the broad ligament to the pelvic brim.

Pelvic organs

Vagina

The vagina is a fibromuscular, distensible, 8–10cm long tube passing upwards and backwards from the introitus at the vulva and ending superiorly with its attachment to the cervix. It is held in a slight S-shape by the tone of the levator ani muscles acting through the perineal body. The hymen is a thin fold of mucous membrane across the entrance to the vagina. The urethra and bladder neck lie in front of the anterior wall of the vagina. The perineal body and rectum lie behind the posterior vaginal wall. The lateral vaginal walls are separated from levator ani muscles by pelvic fascia (see Fig. 3.2).

Uterus

This is a pear-shaped organ with variable dimensions. The cavity is shaped as an inverted triangle. It has three layers:

- peritoneum—the outer serous layer;
- myometrium—the middle muscular layer;
- endometrium—the inner mucous layer.

The longitudinal axis of the uterus is at right angles to the vagina and normally tilts forward—anteversion. The uterus is also usually flexed forward on itself at the isthmus—anteflexion.

Cervix

The cervix is cylindrical and 2.5cm long. It is divided into upper supravaginal and lower vaginal portions. At birth, the cervix is twice the length of the body of the uterus; at puberty, the uterus grows much faster and the size ratio reverses: the body becomes twice the length of the cervix; after the menopause, the uterus undergoes atrophy.

The ovary

The ovary is attached to the cornu of the uterus by the ovarian ligament. The surface of the ovary is covered by a single layer of cuboidal cells, the germinal epithelium. It has a central medulla and an outer thicker cortex. In the young adult, it is almond-shaped, solid, white in colour and 3x1.5x1cm in dimension.

The ureter, bladder, rectum, and sigmoid colon have not been discussed in the reproductive anatomy.

⚠ Be aware in practice that there may be some abnormal anatomy such as double cervix and double vagina.

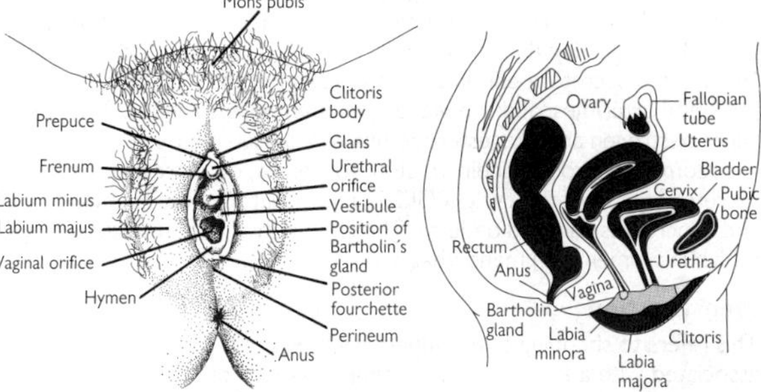

Fig. 3.1 External female genitalia. Reproduced from Collier J, Longmore M, and Brinsden M (2006) *Oxford Handbook of Clinical Specialties 7th edn*, with permission from Oxford University Press.

Fig. 3.2 Female genital anatomy. Reproduced from Pattman R, *et al.* (2005) *Oxford Handbook of Genitourinary Medicine HIV and AIDS* with permission from Oxford University Press.

The menstrual cycle

At birth the human ovaries contain 1,000,000 follicles, of which only about 400 will acquire gonadotrophin receptors and possibly ovulate.

The menstrual cycle is controlled by the hypothalamic–pituitary–ovarian axis. Pulsatile production of gonadotrophin-releasing hormones by the hypothalamus stimulates the pituitary to produce gonadotrophins: follicle stimulating hormone (FSH) and luteinizing hormone (LH). Day one of the cycle is the first day of menstruation, and cycle lengths vary with only about 12% being 28 days.

The proliferative/follicular phase

This begins at the end of the menstrual phase and ends at ovulation, day 13–14. Ovarian follicular development, growth, and oestrogen production is dependent on pituitary FSH, when oestrogen levels rise as a result of production from the developing follicle; there is suppression of pituitary FSH production by a negative-feedback system. During this phase, under the effect of oestrogen, endometrial glands proliferate. Follicular oestrogen synthesis is essential for the endometrial priming but is also part of the positive-feedback system that induces the LH surge and ovulation. (📖 See Fig. 3.3.)

The secretory/luteal phase

This starts with ovulation and ends with menstruation. The LH surge from the anterior pituitary leads to final maturation of the dominant follicle and is preceded by a rise in serum oestrogen concentration. Prostaglandin and cytokine release leads to rupture of the follicle wall and ovulation about 38h after the LH surge.

The empty follicle fills with blood, and the theca and granulosa cells of the follicle luteinize forming the corpus luteum. Progesterone is synthesised by the corpus luteum and its concentrations rise to above 25nmol/l, suggesting that the cycle is ovulatory. This phase lasts for about 14 days and secretory endometrium develops with coiling and growth of the spiral arterioles, and the glands become more tortuous. The gradual fall of oestrogen and progesterone finally results in menses.

Endometrial prostaglandin (PGE2) concentration increases during the secretory phase of the cycle. PGE2 is a vasodilator of the spiral arterioles and it increases pain and oedema. The endometrial concentration of PGE2 is high in women with menorrhagia.

Menstruation

This refers to shedding of the superficial layers of the endometrium and is associated with a fall in circulating concentrations of progesterone, which occurs due to failure of 'rescue' of the corpus luteum by an implanted early pregnancy. Endometrial repair begins as early as 36h after the onset of menstrual bleeding, while menstrual desquamation is still in progress. The amount lost in a normal cycle is up to 80ml.

Along with the changes that occur within the ovary and the endometrium, cyclical changes occur in the cervical mucous, which becomes thinner, more elastic, and more copious at the time of ovulation, to facilitate the penetration of the cervix by the sperm in the secretory phase. It becomes scanty and thick under the influence of progesterone.

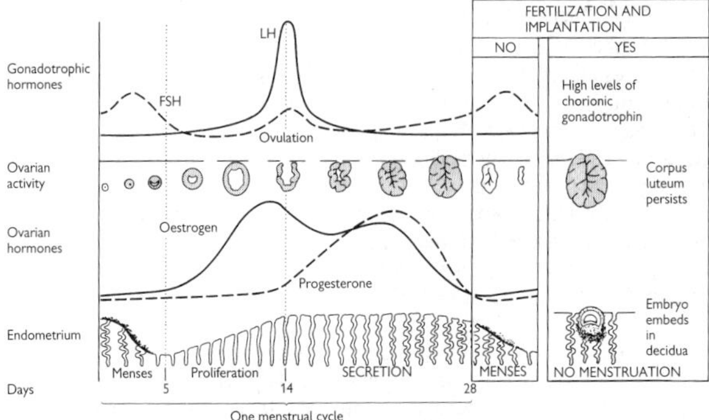

Fig. 3.3 Pituitary, ovarian, and endometrial cycle. Reproduced from Collier J, Longmore M and Brinsden M (2003). *Oxford Handbook of Clinical Specialties, 7th edn*, with permission from Oxford University Press.

Physiology of conception

For conception to occur there needs to be sexual intercourse. For a male, this requires an erection and the ejaculation of semen. For a female, lubrication comes from the vaginal walls and the movement of the penis can cause pleasure. The woman may experience an orgasm, where the uterus may contract, which may facilitate the movement of the sperm but is not necessary for conception.

The egg is released from the ovary into the fallopian tube. Fertilization normally takes place within the ampullary region of the fallopian tube. The sperm move from the uterus into the tubes, propelled by their tails. This is assisted by the contractions of the uterus and tubes. The wastage of sperm at this point is large, with several hundred million at the time of ejaculation but only a few thousand reaching the tubes.

The sperms, which mainly mature in the epididymis, complete maturation while on their journey, this maturation will allow them to penetrate the oocyte.

In general, only one sperm enters and fertilizes the oocyte. The oocyte is suitable for fertilization for up to 24h after ovulation, while sperms retain the ability to fertilize for up to 7 days.

Once the sperm head is inside the ovum, the maternal and paternal haploid chromosomes come together and the process is completed with the restoration of the diploid chromosomes. The tubes play an important role in movement of the ovum by small contractions and ciliary movement, which ensures continuation of the journey of the fertilized ovum to the uterus.

► It is at this point that damaged or blocked tubes can give rise to ectopic pregnancies.

The fertilized egg reaches the uterus in the blastocyst stage. It takes up to 2 days to start implanting and another 3 days to complete the implantation process. This is when human chorionic gonadotrophin (hCG) starts to be produced by the placental unit. Pituitary LH maintains the production of oestrogen and progesterone from the corpus luteum. HCG is detected 8 days after fertilization, increases exponentially, and peaks at 9 weeks; the placenta then takes over maintainance of the pregnancy from the corpus luteum.

History taking

With women's health, as with all specialties, taking an accurate history is of paramount importance. The art of history taking gets refined with experience. It can range from a nursing history assessment, in order to plan care, through to a full history as an advanced practitioner, in order to establish a diagnosis and plan treatment or medication. Even within advanced practice there can be variations in questions, depending on the sub-specialty area that nurses are working in, such as gynaecology, sexual health, and community services. Any additional important questions can be found within the following chapters.

The focus for history taking within any area is the woman's account of her symptoms or presenting complaint. Following this, it is a good idea to take a structured history to ensure completeness. At the end of the history taking, it is important to have an idea of differential diagnoses and then a plan of care.

Nursing history

This should include an assessment of all the systems in a logical sequence that can be used to plan care within the ward or day-surgery environment.

Advanced history

- Age.
- Presenting complaint.
- History of presenting complaint.
- Past obstetric history, including births, miscarriages, and terminations.
- Past gynaecological history.
  - Menstrual history, including age at menarche, first day of last menstrual cycle (LMP), cycle length, bleeding pattern, amount of bleeding (if light, moderate, or heavy, presence of clots, and the frequency of change of protection), menstrual pain, post-coital bleeding, and inter-menstrual bleeding.
  - Age at menopause, if appropriate, and HRT use.
  - Last smear test-date and result, and any abnormal smears in the history.
  - Any history of vaginal infections/discharge.
  - Contraceptive use and current needs in relation to fertility.
- Past medical history.
- Past surgical history.
- Medication—prescribed or over-the-counter medications.
- Allergies.
- Social history, including alcohol intake and a smoking history. The patient's domestic circumstances should also be explored, as well as occupation.
- Family history.
- A brief systems review—enquiry as to whether there are any neurological, gastrointestinal, respiratory, cardiovascular, or musculoskeletal symptoms.

What is useful is to watch others taking histories and formulate your own style. Within history taking, it is useful to be flexible, as women may not always answer questions in the order of a standard medical history.

In starting a consultation, an open-ended question (such as, What has brought you here today?) and allowing the woman to narrate will often give a good synopsis of the problem.

When using this book and the chapters on specific disorders, the basis for all history taking is within this section. It is important to remember to document the history accurately for future records and consultations.

Presenting complaints

For each of the presenting complaints or symptoms, the following should be included. The presenting complaint is often in the patient's own words and is best elaborated on with open-ended questions. Following this, you may need to delve deeper in order to make a diagnosis.

- Exact nature of the symptom.
- When and how it began.
- How often does it happen and how long does it last for?
- Is it getting worse or staying the same?
- What makes it worse and better?
- Associated symptoms.
- Medication tried and the outcome.

Following a history there should always be an impression or a provisional diagnosis. Alongside this, there needs to be a plan of care, whether it is nursing or an advanced history.

Physical examination 1

The physical examination in gynaecology is an intimate procedure that should always be undertaken based on relevant history and as an aid to reaching a diagnosis. It should never be an automatic part of the consultation. Nurses within women's health all have a part to play in physical examinations, as either a chaperone or a practitioner undertaking the examination. The examination may be part of an assessment to aid diagnosis, for screening, or as part of a treatment programme. Throughout the whole examination process, it is important to let the woman know what you are doing.

There will also be women who find the examination process difficult due to past experiences and these may need more time and discussion and possibly multiple visits before the examination is conducted.

Special groups

- Under 16 years old.
- Women with learning/physical disabilities or mental health problems.
- Women with limited understanding of English.
- Women with a history of sexual or physical abuse in the past.
- Women who have never had an examination in the past.

One should also stop the examination if the woman becomes upset, finds it painful, or gains sexual stimulation during the examination.

The full examination should include abdominal, pelvic, and bi-manual examination, followed by a speculum examination in order to inspect the cervix and vagina. In certain situations, e.g. cervical cytology, a speculum examination may be all that is needed. However, on presentation of acute pain, all of the above would be indicated.

It is of paramount importance that all nurses undertaking an extended role should have had adequate training and be competent in that role. You should ask why you are going to examine the woman, what will the information that you gain add to the woman's care, and if you are competent to carry out the examination. For this, you need to understand the basic anatomy and physiology, and have been trained adequately.

The setting

Physical examinations should take place in a private room, where there is an area that allows women to undress in privacy. Women should be encouraged to empty their bladder prior to the examination and then to undress from the waist down, ensuring dignity is maintained with a disposable cover. Access to a couch and good lighting is crucial.

Prior to examination, explain fully the procedure and gain the woman's consent. Check for any allergies such as latex.

Abdominal examination

Undertake a visual inspection of the abdominal skin, looking for scars and any hair distribution.

Palpate the abdomen, working from the umbilicus down to the pubic bone or away from the site of pain to the site of pain. Make a note of the uterus, size, position, and tenderness, general pain and guarding.

The abdomen can be divided into four quadrants (📖 see Fig. 3.4).

The abdomen is characteristically examined in quadrants. In describing the abdomen in this way, other sites, apart from the uterus, are also important in gynaecology, e.g. the liver in Fitz Hugh Curtis syndrome. Describing it in this manner allows for accurate localization of pain, i.e. right-lower quadrant, right-upper quadrant. Percussion may also be useful in looking for size and shape of enlarged organs or masses, and eliciting rebound tenderness.

► Nurses undertaking pre-assessment should refer to the *Oxford Handbook of Clinical Examination and Practical Skills* for chapters on examination of the cardiovascular system.

Vaginal inspection and palpation

The labia, clitoris, and urethral and vaginal openings should be inspected for:

- discharge;
- redness;
- swelling;
- ulcers;
- atrophy;
- scarring;
- hair distribution;
- pelvic organ prolapse;
- sexual maturity.

The labia should be palpated for any cysts—particularly around the Bartholin's area.

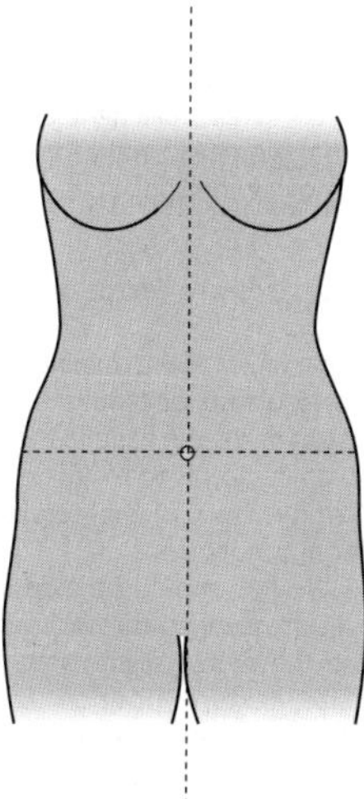

Fig. 3.4 The four quadrants of the abdomen.

Physical examination 2

Speculum examination

There are two types of speculums that are used: most common is the Cusco speculum, the other is the Sim's speculum that is used for women with prolapse and in the operating theatre for gynaecological surgery. Both speculums come in different sizes. Cusco's are more commonly available in plastic now, for single-use items. The aim of speculum examination is to be able to visualize the vagina and cervix and to take smears or swabs.

You will need to ensure that the correct size is selected and that it is lubricated with gel or water. With the blades closed, insert at an oblique angle and slowly rotate, and insert until it is flush with the perineum. It is important to ensure that you continually check the woman's level of comfort during the procedure. The speculum can then be opened to visualize the cervix.

Practice note

The cervix may not be immediately obvious and you may need the woman to cough, place her hands under her bottom, or press on her tummy, dependent on the position of the cervix. It may be necessary to remove the speculum and try and locate the cervix with a digital examination. Once the cervix is seen, fix the speculum open and observe the cervix. Note:

- size;
- position;
- discharge;
- appearance of the cervix;
- presence of an ectropion;
- presence of any nabothian cysts or follicles;
- presence of any cervical polyps;
- evidence of any previous treatment to the cervix.

Release the speculum and carefully remove it. Assess the vaginal walls as the speculum is being removed, making a careful note of any vaginal atrophy in post-menopausal women. Take care not to trap the cervix or the vaginal walls when removing the speculum.

Bimanual

During a bimanual, the vagina, cervix, uterus, and adenexae can be examined. First inspect the vulva.

Insert the index and middle finger of the dominant hand into the vagina and assess the vaginal tone, any prolapse, or tenderness. The other hand will be on the abdomen and press towards the hand in the vagina (📖 see Fig. 3.6).

The first part of the examination is to examine the cervix. In doing this you are looking for the movement of the cervix—if it is free or fixed, indicating possible infection or adhesions.

Next, the surface and the feel should be assessed and any discomfort recorded. By applying light pressure to the back of the cervix, the internal hand will be able to raise the uterus slightly into the abdomen. This can then be examined for size, texture, position, and any tenderness. The last part of the examination is to examine the adenexae. The fingers are moved to either the left or right side in the vagina (into the lateral fornix), while the abdominal hand should also move to the same side. The fallopian tubes should not be palpable or tender. The ovaries are between 2–4cm in length, smooth and firm. Any discomfort on palpation should be recorded.

After the examination, provide privacy for the woman to get dressed, ensuring that there are tissues and pads, if needed. The examination should be recorded in full and discussed with the patient.

Chaperones

All women who have an examination, have the right to have a chaperone present. As nurses extend their roles, there may be times when the nurse who is chaperoning is better qualified to undertake the examination. This can cause some problems with the traditional power-balance and needs skilful negotiation.

The role of the chaperone is multi-faceted and needs skill and experience to ensure that they fulfill all aspects of the role. Some of these aspects are listed below:

- Accompanying women and staff.
- Supporting patients and staff.
- Comforting.
- Giving reassurance.
- Providing advocacy.
- Assisting doctors/nurses.
- Ensuring appropriate examination.
- Ensuring/maintaining privacy and dignity.
- Information giving.
- Acting as a witness.
- Acting as a protector.

It is essential to have some knowledge of the procedure that is being carried out in order to reassure the patient and also to ensure that the room is correctly prepared, so that the examination is seamless.

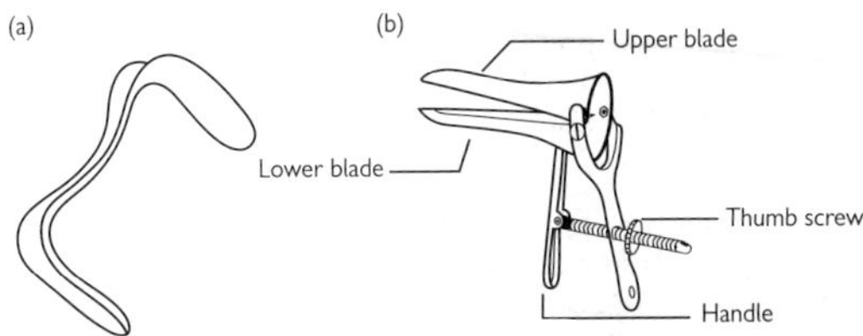

Fig. 3.5 (a) Sim's speculum—used mainly in the examination of women with vaginal prolapse (b) Cusco's speculum. Reproduced from Thomas J and Monaghan T (2007) *Oxford Handbook of Clinical Examination and Practical Skills*, with permission from Oxford University Press.

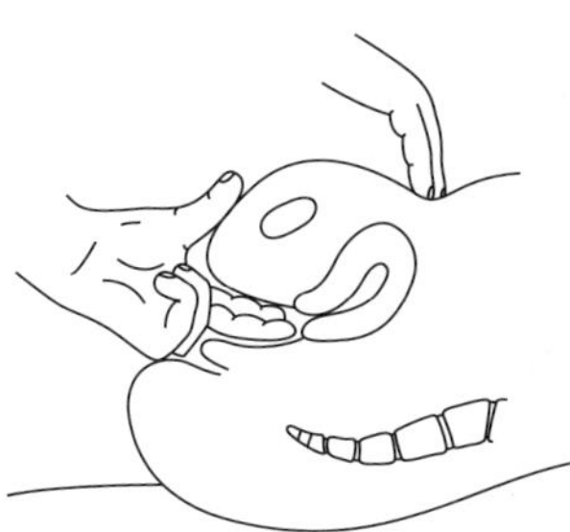

Fig. 3.6 Bimanual examination of the uterus. Reproduced from Thomas J and Monaghan T (2007) *Oxford Handbook of Clinical Examination and Practical Skills*, with permission from Oxford University Press.

Diagnostic tests in gynaecology

Haematological tests

- Haemoglobin—to diagnose anaemia and ferritin.
- White cell count—this rises in systemic infections.
- Blood group prior to surgery, where more than average blood loss is expected and where the woman's rhesus group needs to be checked, e.g. for problems of early pregnancy.
- Coagulation screen, where indicated by the history, e.g. if the patient is on warfarin or suffers from liver disease.
- Thrombophilia screen—if needed, in relation to risks of venous thromboembolism (VTE) and hormones.

Biochemical tests

- Urea and electrolytes pre-operatively in major surgery, also in monitoring women with post-operative paralytic ileus/intestinal obstruction.
- Liver function tests (LFTs) in gynaecological malignancy and to monitor ovarian hyperstimulation syndrome.
- Serum alpha fetoprotein levels, as they may be raised in germ-cell ovarian tumours.
- Ca125 estimation in investigating ovarian masses and as a non-specfic way of monitoring response to chemotherapy; this is also raised in endometriosis.
- hCG—for diagnosis of pregnancy and the monitoring of ectopic pregnancies, gestational trophoblastic disease, and as a marker for germ-cell ovarian tumours.

Endocrine tests

- A timed serum progesterone is measured around 7 days prior to menses. High levels suggest ovulation.
- LH:FSH ratio >2:1 in PCOS (📖 see Polycystric ovarian syndrome, p.110).
- In menopause, premature ovarian failure, and resistant ovary syndrome, the follicle stimulating hormone (FSH) is high and the luteinizing hormone (LH) is normal. In hypothalamic and weight-related amenorrhoea, FSH tends to be low.
- In molar pregnancy, the LH is very high and the FSH is low.
- Testosterone is elevated in polycystic ovarian syndrome (PCOS) and in androgen-secreting tumours of the adrenal and ovary.
- Testing for prolactin is indicated in galactorrhoea, amenorrhoea, and oligoamenorrhoea.
- Estradiol is tested to measure ovarian response in subfertile women and in establishing menopause and response to some HRT treatments.
- Thyroid function tests in *some* women with menstrual problems.

Pregnancy testing

This can be as a urine hCG test, which picks up levels low enough to be positive prior to the onset of menstruation, or an even more sensitive serum hCG assay, to determine outcome in early pregnancy. (📖 See Chapter 15, p.415.)

Bacteriological investigations

📖 See Chapter 8, p.167.

Cytology

Including: cervical cytology, cytology of fluid from ovarian cysts, peritoneal washings at laparotomy for ovarian cancer, cytology of catheter specimen of urine for cervical cancer staging, fine-needle aspiration (FNA) of solid neoplasms.

Imaging

Transabdominal and transvaginal scanning

Ultrasound is indicated in:

- the differential diagnosis of pelvic masses (cysts, tumours);
- investigations for pelvic pain;
- investigation of abnormal bleeding and uterine pathology;
- as a baseline investigation in infertility;
- follicle tracking for ovulation induction;
- for location of intra-uterine devices/systems and implants in sexual and reproductive health;
- in urogynaecology to measure residual volume and confirm renal lesions;
- as part of the investigation of ectopic pregnancy, early pregnancy, abnormal pregnancy, and molar pregnancy;
- ovarian cancer screening in high risk groups;
- the evaluation of post-menopausal bleeding and bleeding on HRT.

Conventional X-rays

Chest X-ray may be indicated pre-operatively in gynaecological surgery and in women with ovarian cancer. An abdominal X-ray may be used to assess the location of an intra-uterine system/intra-uterine contraceptive device (IUS/IUD) not seen in the uterus, to rule out an extra uterine location.

CT scanning

Limited role in detection of small-volume disease but used to measure the size of brain and liver metastases. There is limitation in assessment of peritoneal deposits. CT can be used to assess the extent of disease in ovarian cancer, but it is of limited value in stage I and II disease.

MRI

Magnetic resonance imaging is a form of scan that does not use ionizing radiation, but instead utilizes a static magnetic field and radio frequency pulses, which alter the alignment of hydrogen ions within body tissue. When the radiofrequency pulse stops, the ions return to their original energy state. It is this change in energy that is detected by the receiver cell and is used to create the image. It is of little value in visualizing peritoneal surface tumours, but superior to CT in assessing small-volume disease and in oncology.

Hysterosalpingography

Involves instilling contrast media into the uterine cavity through the cervix in the post-menstrual phase. It is indicated when checking for uterine abnormalities and for assessment of tubal patency.

Consent

Consent is a patient's agreement to receive healthcare. The Department of Health has set up the 'Good Practice in Consent' initiative. Consent can be verbal, written, implied, and informed.

Valid consent

The cornerstone of valid consent is making a decision on the basis of comprehensive and sufficient information. The patient must be competent to agree to the treatment.

National standards of consent

The Royal College of Obstetricians and Gynaecologists and the Faculty of Sexual and Reproductive Healthcare have produced advice on taking consent and this follows the structure of the Department of Health Standard Consent Forms and Policy (2004). This consent policy has now been revised to incorporate provision of the Mental Capacity Act. The RCOG produces standard patient information leaflets and the Family Planning association produces sexual health pamphlets.

Choice

Choice in treatment is important, but consent should be valid if an unscheduled procedure becomes necessary.

New procedures

NICE advises on new interventional procedures, where benefits and risks are uncertain. Special care needs to be exercised to make sure that the patient agrees to the procedure in the knowledge that the outcome is uncertain.

Mental Capacity Act

The Mental Capacity Act was implemented on 1 October 2007. Problems in consent can arise from requests to carry out operations which take away a woman's ability to reproduce, e.g. sterilization or hysterectomy, in adults who lack capacity. The official guidance states that, if a sterilization is necessary for therapeutic reasons, as opposed to contraceptive reasons, then there may be no need for an application to the courts, but, if the case is anywhere near the boundary, other colleagues need to be involved and the case should be referred to the courts, where a solicitor (lasting power of attorney/LPA) will represent the adult who lacks capacity to consent.

Under 16s

Young people over 16 are deemed to have the competence to consent for themselves. For those under 16, the Department of Health guidance confirms that Fraser criteria should be followed in contraceptive advice and treatment. This includes:

- Encouraging the girl to involve her parents or a responsible person.
- Ensuring that he/she has the capacity to understand the treatment, the risks and benefits, and the consequences, if not treated.
- Assessing competence.

- Offering advice and treatment without parental consent, only if it is in their best interests.
- If a competent child consents to treatment, a parent cannot override the decision.

The Sexual Offences Act became law in 2004 and enables the prosecution of abusive and exploitative sexual activity but recognizes that teenagers may engage in mutually agreed non-coercive sexual intercourse. The Act does not prevent the provision of sexual health advice and treatment to young people under 16, including 13 and under. However, a child under 13 does not have legal capacity to consent to sexual intercourse, and health professionals should individualize each case, and consider reporting to area child protection officers/social service, as indicated or appropriate. They should exercise professional discretion.

Unlicensed drugs

The patient must be made aware of unlicensed drugs and her agreement to receive unlicensed drugs must be fully documented in the clinical record, e.g. misoprostol for early medical termination of pregnancy, post-coital copper IUD, levonelle up to 120h after sexual intercourse and 4% prilocaine for cervical local analgesia.

Clinical governance and audit

Consent is part of clinical governance and high quality healthcare.

Resources

Department of Health (2004) Consent. *What you have a right to expect.* 🖰 www.dh.gov.uk (Accessed January 2009.)

Department of Health (2004) *Best practice for doctors and other healthcare professionals in the provision of advice and treatment for young people under sixteen on contraception, sexual and reproductive health.* 🖰 www.dh.gov.uk (Accessed January 2009.)

Confidentiality

Confidentiality is a duty for all healthcare workers, but is extremely complex. Patient confidentiality underpins the trust between patient and health professionals. Patient information in any healthcare setting is held under legal and ethical obligations of confidentiality. Information held in confidence should not be disclosed in an identifiable form, without explicit consent, with the following exceptions:

- Information sharing protocols between organizations, teams within the NHS and/or non-NHS bodies—clinical governance, research, and audit.
- Health and Social Care Act (2001)—Section 60 of the act allows sharing patient identifiable information in an anonymized way, such as for clinical audit, record validation, and research. This can be used without consent.
- Public interest—protecting health of the patient and public if third party is put at harm. It is permissible to overrule a patient's desire for anonymity where the life of another healthcare professional or patient is endangered or where a disclosure may assist in the prevention or detection of a serious crime.
- Staff dealing with minors need to be able to weigh up the conflicting priorities of the need for confidentiality and the possibility of sexual exploitation (📖 see Consent p.36).
- Social care—within this, patients also need to understand their rights to access information held about them

Disclosure without consent should always be discussed with other senior colleagues, General Medical Council (GMC), or Medical Defence Union, and only carried out if there is a clear indication.

The main areas of law that relate to disclosure of confidential information are:

- Common Law of Confidentiality.
- Data Protection Act (1998)—includes processing information, e.g. holding, obtaining, recording, using, and disclosing information; the Act applies to all forms of media.
- Human Rights Act (1998) Article 8 establishes a right to respect for private and family life.
- NHS Confidentiality Code of Practice (2003) is a requirement for those who work within or under contract to NHS organizations, concerning confidentiality.
- NHS Venereal Disease Act (1977).
- NHS Trust and PCT directions (2000).

Caldicott guardians are senior staff appointed to protect patient information in the NHS.

Caldicott prinicples

- Justify the purpose of using confidential information.
- Only use it when absolutely necessary.
- Use the minimum that is required.
- Access should be on a need-to-know basis.
- Everyone must understand his or her responsibilities.
- Understand and comply with the law.

National Programme for Information Technology (NPfIT)

Modern computer systems are due to be introduced into the NHS nationally to integrate patient care. Patient confidentiality is a concern with access to electronic health records, but efficient systems can allow access only to authorized healthcare professionals. In practical issues relating to children and young people, NHS planning, and payment by results, there is need for robust information governance.

The NHS Care Records Guarantee sets out the rules that will govern information held in the NHS Care records service.

Resources

Department of Health (November 2003) *Confidentiality NHS Code of Practice*. www.dh.gov.uk

NHS connecting for health programmes for information technology (IT). www.connectingforhealth.nhs.uk (Accessed April 2008).

Record-keeping

'Absence of proof is not proof of absence'. However, in the absence of accurate contemporaneous notes, it may be difficult to recall one's actions and decisions or justify them, if required to do so (perhaps in a court of law). It is, therefore, good practice to maintain such records. They are also an essential means of communication between healthcare professionals in promoting continuity of care. This acts as a mechanism for demonstrating the quality and complexity of nursing with evidence of clinical reasoning.

Record

A permanent form of data regarding a patient/client either on paper or stored electronically.

Principles

- Legible.
- The date and time the information was recorded.
- Write in permanent black ink (for reproducibility).
- Contemporaneous.
- Clear, comprehensive but concise, and focused on the factual, accurate, relevant information relating to the patient's/client's needs, diagnoses, treatment, and care.
- Written in collaboration with the patient/client.
- Signed (and dated) by the health professional/trainee.
- Only use abbreviations that are generally or locally agreed.
- Indicate nature and identity of any interpretive services.

Records should not include anything that one would not say or reveal to the patient/client. They should not be altered, except to make corrections to inaccurate information: Any alterations must be clearly indicated, signed, and dated.

Details to include

- Reason for attendance/presence (from the patient/client or relative/friend, if unconscious).
- Relevant information on past medical history, medications, family and social history.
- Observations.
- Test results or special examination findings.
- If chaperone offered and accepted or declined; name and role of chaperone, if present.
- Record consent, where appropriate.
- Impressions of current situation/priorities of care or treatment.
- Problems/needs for which decisions have been taken.
- Action plan discussed with the patient/client, e.g. investigations required, referrals made, prescriptions given.
- Follow-up care/next appointment.
- Decisions shared, advice, concerns/worries.
- Essential communications with other health professionals.
- Written information leaflets/booklets/websites.

Records of prescribing and issuing of drugs or devices

Record and sign all drugs or devices that are supplied, recording batch numbers, expiry date, and whether the manufacturer's product patient information leaflet given.

Complete proformas according to local protocols for patient group directions and record actions observed/completed.

Adverse reactions should be recorded, (including any reactions with 'black triangle' drugs) and sent to the Medicines and Healthcare Products Regulatory Agency (MHRA) as a yellow card or via their website.

Storage of records

When not required, all records should be stored securely (including laptops and personal digital assistants). Should notes be required/held, tracer cards should be used to track them.

Electronic records

- Terminals should not be left unattended when signed-in, or a password-protected screensaver should be used.
- Never share passwords.
- Passwords should be changed regularly.
- Clear the screen between each patient/client.

Manual records

- Store files/notes in a logical order.
- Use a tracking system to monitor the order of the filing system.
- Return files/notes to storage venue when they are no longer needed.

Infection control

Infection control within women's health nursing is no different from any other branch of nursing and relies on the principles that have been taught within training as a nurse or in National vocational qualification (NVQ) or in-house inductions.

Approximately 10% of patients will acquire an infection as a result of a healthcare intervention. It is, therefore, essential that all staff have an understanding of the epidemiology of infections and what places patients at risk.

The risk of infections to patients from hospital settings has already been recognized. The current focus within the hospital setting is on methicillin resistant staphylococcus aureus (MRSA) and *clostridium difficile*. These two infections are responsible for many of the complications that can arise for patients within a hospital setting who are already vulnerable, due to illness or disease. Many organizations are undertaking stringent measures to decrease the rates of both of them. The measures that are being taken include:

- Use of laundered uniforms.
- Removal of jewellery.
- Hand washing.
- Removal of wrist watches by all staff in clinical practice.
- Having no sleeves that are below the elbows.
- The use of protective clothing, e.g. theatre scrubs, aprons, gloves.
- Cleaning of the ward environment.
- MRSA screening of patients prior to routine admission.
- Deep cleaning of rooms where there has been MRSA.
- Accurate record-keeping of intravenous cannulae, catheters.
- Stringent decontamination of medical equipment.
- Use of disposal curtains.
- Safe disposable of waste.
- Accurate decontamination and sterilization of equipment, and the ability to trace equipment through the process. There are three levels of decontamination:
  - cleaning—to remove physical dirt and micro-organisms;
  - disinfection—this kills micro-organisms but not spores; and
  - sterilization, which kills micro-organisms and spores.
- Reducing risk with the use of single use equipment.

Infection control is also to protect the staff. All staff should assess any interaction or contact that they are having with patients and wear the most appropriate clothing.

Interactions can be no risk of body fluids, such as consultation, where no protective clothing is worn; contact with fluids, but no risk of splashing of body fluids, such as bed-bathing, which requires gloves and apron; full protective clothing, including, mask, sterile gloves, and hat, in the theatre setting.

As well as protective clothing, such as gloves, there is no substitute for hand washing, before and after contact with patients, to reduce the risk of infections within all healthcare settings.

Resources

Prevention of healthcare associated infection in primary and community care. www.nice.org.uk (Accessed March 2008)

Summary of guidance for infection control in healthcare settings (April 2008). www.dh.gov.uk and www.infectioncontrol.nhs.uk (Accessed March 2009)

Health and safety and control of substances hazardous to health (COSHH)

The Health and Safety at Work Act (1974) sets out the general duties that employers have towards employees and members of the public, and that employees have to themselves and to each other.

The Health and Safety at Work legislation explains the specifics of what is required by employers. This legislation requires:

- An assessment of risk.
- Controls put in place, as identified by risk assessment.
- Arrangements implemented as agreed.
- Provision of clear information and training to employees.
- Repeated risk assessment after putting controls in place and provision of training.
- Deletion of the risk from the risk register, if actions have been completed and there is now no further risk.

Health safety and welfare regulation 1992 covers a wide range of issues like ventilation, heating, lighting, workstation seating, and welfare facilities.

There are further requirements if working with video display units (VDUs). These are provided by the Health and Safety Display Screen Equipment Regulations (1992).

Provision and Use of Work Equipment Regulations (1998) requires employers to ensure that all equipment, including electricals, are serviced and safe, e.g. defibrillators, cryotherapy equipment, Valleylab, ultrasound machines, and so on.

Manual Handling Operations Regulations (1992) cover moving of objects by hand.

RIDDOR is the Reporting of Injuries, Diseases, and Dangerous Occurrences Regulations (1995) and requires employers to notify certain occupational injuries, diseases, and dangerous events.

COSHH regulations (2000) and (2002)

This requires employers to assess the risk from hazardous substances and to take appropriate precautions and controls for their employees. The COSHH website covers lists of chemicals—if not listed, seek advice on 0845 345 0055. Substances can be identified by their warning labels.

Workers Gas Safety Installation and Use Regulations (1994) covers:

- Safe installation, maintenance, and use of gas systems in premises, e.g. exposure to bacteria in an air-conditioning system that is not properly maintained.
- O_2 for resuscitation.
- Cryotherapy for treatment of genital warts.

- The CO_2 workplace exposure limit is 15,000ppm over a 15-minute reference period.
- Dealing with spills immediately.
- COSHH also applies to use of bleach at the work place.
- Substances produced in chemical processes, e.g. Gram staining.
- Any kind of dust, if its average concentration exceeds the levels specified in COSHH.
- Immersion oil, crystal violet, and acetone.

Resources

Control of substances hazardous to health. www.hse.govt.uk (Accessed March 2008.)

Disability

The Disability Discrimination Act (1995) defines a disabled person as someone who has a physical or mental impairment that has a long-term adverse effect on their ability to carry out day-to-day activities. Disability is an important public health problem in England and Wales, and could be congenital or acquired. Healthcare professionals should be well-informed in addressing the needs of this group, particularly in making services available for them.

Assessment

- History should be accurate and careful.
- Communication aids, charts and pictures, electronic voice output devices, partial sight low-vision aids, hearing aids, and hand-held magnifiers can help in history taking and examination.
- Particular attention to co-existing conditions.
- History of medication.
- Individualized approach is important.
- Gynaecological, obstetrical, and contraception history.
- If a pelvic examination is required for a woman with limited movement (spinal cord injury, multiple sclerosis), be gentle in manner, bladder should be empty, couch at 45-degree angle with padding to the table may prevent autonomic dysreflexia (dangerous elevation in blood pressure).
- Use a warm speculum.

Role of nurse

This is paramount in providing sensitive care to women with disabilities, empowering them to lead their lives to the fullest potential by listening to them and helping them to acquire skills. Community nurses can work closely with the women, their GP, hospital, and local social services, and can provide help and advice on a wide range of health issues.

Speech and language therapists can assist with communication difficulties, occupational therapists can work with women with learning disabilities or physical disabilities, and enable them to lead as independent a life as possible. Personal mobility aids, including wheelchairs, walking sticks, zimmer frames, and crutches can be useful.

Women with sensory/visual impairment

- Braille signage should be available in healthcare settings.
- Speak low and clearly.
- Face clients if they can lip read.
- Identify the need for an interpreter.
- Ensure adequate light without glare.
- British Sign Language (BSL) is a primary language and English is a secondary language.

Seizure disorders

Some medications may interfere with contraceptives or other drugs—caution is required. Learning disability may be profound and issues around informed consent are important.

Developmental delay

Informed consent issues are also relevant here. Women may be vulnerable to sexual abuse, parents and carers may ask for sterilization, but sometimes less restrictive choices may be more appropriate and clinicians should inform, educate, and make these available.

Disability needs to be taken into account in relation to the disorder and consideration of appropriate contraception or medication, e.g:

- If decreased level of sensation, women may not feel symptoms of pelvic pain or uterine perforation and an IUD may not be appropriate.
- Depo-Provera® is popular.
- Diaphragms are associated with an increase in urinary tract infections.
- Women may have difficulty swallowing pills for contraception or other conditions, immobility can increase the risk of VTE.

Resources

UK based charity for disabled people: www.dppi.org.uk (Accessed January 2009)
Disability Discrimination Act www.directgov.uk (Accessed April 2009)

Domestic abuse

The Inter-Ministerial Group on Domestic Violence defines domestic abuse as: 'any incident of threatening behaviour, violence or abuse (psychological, physical, sexual, financial, or emotional) between adults who are or have been intimate partners or family members, regardless of gender or sexuality'. In addition, we have to be careful to include such issues as female genital mutilation, lesbian and transgenders being forcibly 'outed' by their partners or ex-partners, elderly persons being maltreated by their caregivers, stalking and harassment, forced marriages, and so called 'honour killings'.

Whilst the majority of incidents of domestic abuse/violence are hidden and take place behind closed doors, dealing with the effects and consequences affects us all. A quarter of all reported violent crime is domestic-related[1] and the cost to the National Health Service of dealing with physical injuries alone is £1.2 billion a year. It is widely recognized that 90% of domestic violence cases are committed by men against women and their children. However, abuse also occurs in same-sex relationships, therefore our response and commitment to dealing with this issue should be the same regardless of the gender of the woman's partner.

The Royal Colleges and other health professional governing bodies have issued position papers or guidelines advising on the need to provide changed responses to those experiencing domestic abuse. Despite these documents, the health service response to domestic abuse has been poor. Many survivors describe how they desperately wanted NHS staff to ask them what was happening at home.

Domestic abuse will not only affect women who access health services, health staff may also be victims or survivors and may need help and support in dealing with any issues that occur as a result of providing healthcare to abused women.

Domestic abuse and sexual assault

Rape is an offence that is almost always carried out by men, mainly against women and girls, and whilst this crime is portrayed in the media as predominately an attack that is committed by someone who is either a stranger or someone she has been on a date with, the reality is that 54% of UK rapes are committed by a woman's current or former partner. In the past 5 years, the number of recorded rapes has nearly doubled from 8,593 in 2001 to 14,409 in 2005–06. Many women still believe that because they are married they do not have the right to say no. It is easy to see why this is still believed when we consider that it has only been since 1991 that the concept of rape within marriage has been recognized in UK Law.

Domestic abuse and pregnancy

Contrary to popular belief, pregnancy does not provide a respite or reprieve from abuse. In fact more than 30% of cases of domestic violence start during pregnancy and more than 14% of maternal deaths occur in women who have told their health professional they are in an abusive relationship.[2] In addition, 40–60% of women experiencing domestic violence are abused while pregnant.[3]

Professionals also have to consider the impact of domestic violence on children who are living in an environment where domestic abuse is taking place. The Department of Health paper on Working Together to Safeguard Children (1999) states that: 'everyone working together with women and children should be alert to the frequent inter-relationship between domestic violence and the abuse and neglect of children'.[4]

The introduction of routine enquiry, where all women accessing health services are asked questions in relation to abuse, increases the likelihood of women disclosing and seeking help in preventing further abuse. However, staff should be properly trained in how to use enquiry tools and interview techniques, as well as responding appropriately and ensuring that confidentiality and information-sharing protocols are adhered to.

Supervision and support should also be available, as should support services for those staff who face reminders or triggers of their personal abuse due to them working with women and children who have been abused.

In addition, Primary Care Trusts have had a statutory duty since April 2004 to work with other local agencies to reduce crime. By the health practitioner recognizing and working with victims and their children to alleviate the pain of domestic violence, the health organization is able to fulfill its statutory responsibilities.

Resources

British Medical Association (1998) *Domestic violence a healthcare issue.*

Department of Health (2005) *Responding to domestic abuse: a handbook for health professionals.* Department of Health, London.

Home Office (2003) *Safety and justice.* Home Office, London.

Department of Health (2005) *Responding to domestic violence: a handbook for professionals.* Department of Health, London.

Walby, S and Allen, J (2004) *Home Office Research Study 276: domestic violence, sexual assault and stalking.* Findings from the British Crime Survey.

1 Women's Aid (2007) *What is domestic violence?*

2 Lewis, G and Drife, J (2001) *Why mothers die. Report from the confidential enquiries into maternal deaths in the UK.*

3 McWilliams M and McKlamans (1993) Bringing it out in the open. HMSO Belfast.

4 Department of Health (1999) *Working together to safeguard children.* Department of Health, London.

Risk management in women's health

Risk management is a process of preventing harm to patients, staff, visitors, and hospital property and of reducing the incidence of near misses by promoting a safe healthcare environment. It refers to the culture, processes, and structures that are directed towards:

- realizing potential opportunities, while managing adverse events;
- need for an organizational and departmental risk-management strategy; clinical improvement groups/risk management groups are designed to oversee the implementation of the organization's risk-management strategy;
- units or departments should have trigger lists for incident reporting in gynaecology/women's health;
- trusts' need to maintain an electronic risk register identifying risks and measures to control them.

Risk management includes:

- Identification of risk, analysis, assessment of risk, treatment of risk, ongoing monitoring, and control.
- Addressing risks flagged up by complaints, incidents, and medico-legal claims or by National Patient Safety Agency (NPSA), national confidential enquiries, by Safety Alert Broadcast System (SABS) alerts, and Medical Health Regulatory Agency (MHRA) reports.
- Risk assessment of clinical areas, outpatient clinics, and minor outpatient theatres should be conducted, and risks identified, managed, and disseminated to the wider multidisciplinary team.
- System analysis reports should include learning points and an action plan that reflects a commitment to learning and sharing from incidents.
- Staff training, supervision, appraisal, and personal development plans should be part of the local risk-management framework.
- When things go wrong, openness with the patient is essential.
- Full, clear, and reasonable explanations should be given.

In gynaecology, sexual health, and family planning, identification of risk is important, e.g.

- Identifying risk factors for venous thromboembolism, myocardial infarction, smoking, body mass index, and family history of early onset heart disease, before prescribing the combined oral contraceptive pill. The bottom line is safe medical prescribing. Consider all contraindications before prescribing a drug or a device.
- Issues around consent, contraceptive and abortion provision to minors and those who lack capacity are some of the key areas where clear precise guidelines are required.

Resources

National Patient Safety Agency: www.npsa.nhs.uk (Accessed December 2008)

Royal College of Obstetricians and Gynaecologists (RCOG) Risk Management: www.rcog.org.uk (Accessed January 2009)

Clinical governance

Clinical governance is the mechanism by which the public can be reassured that the organizations have robust systems in place with teams/forums. Clinical governance framework systems are developed throughout the UK, in each NHS healthcare organization. Within the UK, each region has specific guidance on implementation. Every organization has statutory and mandatory responsibilities to provide resources and to provide a robust framework of clinical governance. The frameworks are intended to improve the quality of care for patients/clients wherever healthcare is being given/performed. Each organization has a clinical professional lead to support a yearly clinical governance plan and report. In addition, individual department leads are responsible for ensuring clinical governance is implemented within their micro-departments, they remain accountable to the trust clinical governance committees.

Key themes of clinical governance

- Patient and public involvement.
- Health community partnerships.
- Planning services for the needs of the local population.
- Leadership and performance review.
- Supporting staff and staff management.
- Team working.
- Education, training, and continuing professional development.
- Quality improvement.
- Risk-management and assessment.
- Incident reporting and learning from incidents.
- Learning from complaints.
- Research and clinical effectiveness.
- Clinical audit.
- Placing the patient at the heart of healthcare.
- Environment care.
- Health and safety.
- Support from other agencies.
- Child protection.
- Use of information.

External drivers are nationally available, e.g. clinical guidelines (NICE) and national set quality and service targets (National Service Frameworks) and NHS performance indicators.

Patient surveys are often also used to measure performance and plans for improvement both for staff development and service changes.

Chapter 4

Paediatric and adolescent gynaecology

Puberty: normal and abnormal features

Definition

Puberty is the reproductive phase during which the functionality of the genito-reproductive processes is established. Menarche is the age of 1st menstrual period. Coitarche is the age of the start of sexual activity.

Several milestones define the various endocrine and morphological changes:

- Breast growth—starts at 8–9 years but can be as late as 13, and takes on average 4 years to complete.
- Growth in height starts around the same age and peaks at around age 12, when there is a height spurt of 9cm per year compared to 5cm prepubertally.
- Pubic followed by axillary hair grow later in the pubertal age.
- Menarche can predate hair growth but usually occurs after, with the average age being 12–13. The age of menarche is decreasing in developed countries, where child nutrition is improving significantly.

The parallel changes in the reproductive organs include the establishment of ovarian follicular activity, and uterine growth.

Precocious puberty

This is defined as menses occurring before age 10 or breast growth before age 8; it could be physiological. Causes include: encephalitis, meningitis and intracranial lesions, oestrogen-secreting ovarian tumours, the rare Albright syndrome characterized by the café-au lait skin features.

Delayed puberty

This occurs when puberty is later than average age, approximately 13.4 years in girls. History should be taken with reference to pubic hair development, breast development, chronic diseases, and any growth spurts. It is important to be aware of the emotional impact on the teenager. Menses delayed up to age 16 does not require investigation; however, if accompanied by absence of secondary sexual characters, it should be looked into by age 14. If this needs to be investigated, then the following should be undertaken, preferably in specialist units with expert support and experience in breaking bad news.

- FSH/LH/oestrogen.
- Karyotyping.
- Ultrasound.

📖 **For causes of delayed puberty** 📖 see Chapter 6, Primary amenorrhoea.

Menstruation, conception, and reproduction

The pubertal ovary contains up to 600,000 primordial follicles. Under the effect of pituitary FSH, several follicles mature each cycle and a dominant/graafian follicle, which contains the egg, would reach a size of up to 3cm before it ruptures at ovulation. The egg survives for up to 36h, during which it is fertilizable. The spermatozoa, however, survive in the female genital tract for an average of 5 days and a maximum of 7 days. If fertilization occurs in the outer-third of the fallopian tube, the fertilized egg takes

3 days to reach the uterine cavity in the morula stage. It takes another 2 days to start implanting and another 3 days to complete implantation. The 1st biochemical evidence of pregnancy is then detected through measurement of serum βhCG. Post-ovulation, the granulosa cells, under the influence of LH, transform into the theca leutein cells of the corpus luteum. The ovary secretes progesterone, as well as oestrogen. If pregnancy does not occur, the corpus luteum atrophies, the hormone levels drop, and menstruation ensues.

The average chance of pregnancy from a single act of intercourse any time in the cycle is 4%. Intercourse in mid-cycle carries a pregnancy risk of 25–30%.

Labial development and clinical presentation

The labia minora grow considerably in puberty, often asymmetrically with one side developing up to 2 years after the other side. Parents and/or adolescents may present with concerns about asymmetry. They can be reassured with a simple explanation of the development milestones.

Labial adhesions are another common cause of concern. This tends to rectify with gentle finger separation.

Resources

Boraei S, Clark C and Frith L (2008) Labioplasty in girls under 18 years of age: an unethical procedure? *Clinical Ethics* **3**: 37—41.

Congenital abnormalities

Definition

A congenital abnormality may present any time from birth and often presents in adolescence. The aetiology is polygenic and there is association with renal tract abnormalities.

Classification, presentation, and management

- Agenesis and hypoplasia—characterized by absence of the uterus and/or vagina, with rudimentary, blind, lower vaginal pouch. The chromosome compliment is either XY with androgen insensitivity or XX presenting with primary amenorrhoea. Management is vaginal dilatation, psychological support, hormone replacement therapy (HRT), and excision of testicular tissue in androgen insensitivity.
- Fusion and non-canalization abnormalities include uterine and vaginal septae, double uterus with 1 or 2 cervical os, bicornuate uterus, and unilateral atresia with rudimentary horn. These may be discovered incidentally, but can present as menstrual abnormalities, infertility, early pregnancy complications, or recurrent miscarriage. Diagnosis is with ultrasound or dye studies. Treatment is surgical but should be undertaken after careful counselling.
- Cervical atresia is another fusion and canalization anomaly that can lead to haematometra (blood within the uterus) and pelvic mass formation. Management is difficult and failure of corrective surgery is common.
- Imperforate hymen is another manifestation of fusion or canalization failure. It presents with amenorrhoea and cyclical abdominal pain and haematocolpos or haematometra with pressure on pelvic organs, if long-standing. Treatment is surgical with restoration of function.

Many of the above anomalies may be associated with renal anomalies such as absent kidney. An intravenous urogram (IVU) may be indicated. Chromosome studies/karyotyping may be required. Referral to a paediatric urologist is indicated.

Delayed sexuality disorder (DSD)

Aetiology

- Chromosomal causes include Turner's syndrome, XXX female, XXY female, and Klinefelter's syndrome.
- Gonadal causes include gonadal dysgenesis (XY female with uterus but no testosterone or functional testosterone deficiency, due to lack of the converting enzyme 5 alpha reductase); androgen insensitivity, which may present with ambiguous genitalia at birth; and true hermaphrodites.
- Genitalia/end organ causes include congenital adrenal hyperplasia.

In all cases expert advice and counselling is required to determine sex, taking into account the suitability of external genitalia.

Examination and investigations

This should be performed by an expert clinician and should include:

- Assessment of size of clitoris/phallus.
- Assessment of inguinal canals for masses.

- Identifying the urethra, vaginal, and cervix.
- Ultrasound for any masses.
- Blood tests as detailed below.

Turner's syndrome

Ovarian dysgenesis is the other term used. Although this is not strictly speaking intersex, it comes into the differential diagnosis. Presentation is with primary amenorrhoea and short stature. Treatment is with growth hormone and oestrogen replacement therapy to start with, and combined hormone therapy once bleeding occurs in response to oestrogen withdrawal. Support to the patient and her family is essential.

Congenital adrenal hyperplasia (CAH)

An autosomal recessive defect of cortisol synthesis, in 95% of cases this is 21 hydroxylase deficiency, leading to androgenization of male and virilization of female foetus (ambiguous genitalia). There is loss of salt and water, which can be life-threatening, if severe. Diagnosis is biochemical + by taking a family history. Treatment with cortisol reverses the genitalia changes by suppressing hyperplasia and over-production of androgens. Other presentations of CAH include: precocious puberty, delayed puberty, hirsutism/virilization, menstrual irregularities, subfertility (📖 see Chapter 17, p.447), or congenital abnormalities (📖 see Table 4.1).

A subsequent pregnancy in a couple with a CAH child has a 1:4 chance of being affected.

Table 4.1 Congenital adrenal hyperplasia

Deficiency	Clinical presentation	Age of presentation
Severe 21 hydroxylase deficiency	Vomiting and dehydration	Infants
	Ambiguous genitalia	
	Female infants virilization	
Moderate 21 hydroxylase	Virilization	Pre-pubertal children
Mild 21 hydroxylase	Androgenization	
Infertility		Young and adult women

Resources

Hughes, IA, Houk, C, Ahmed, SF, and Lee, PA (2006) LWPES Consensus Group: ESPE Consensus Group. Consensus statement on management of intersex disorders. *Archives of diseases of children* **91**(7): 56–62.

Vaginal bleeding

Definition

Oligoamenorrhoea, menorrhagia, menometrorrhagia, and polymenorrhoea can all occur soon after menarche due to anovulation, unopposed oestrogen stimulation of the endometrium leading to heavy and irregular bleeding. At the other end of the spectrum, poor oestrogen production can lead to intermenstrual bleeding (IMB), which tends to be light.

Causes

- Anovulation accounts for over 40% of abnormal adolescent bleeding, especially in the early post-menarchal years.
- Coagulopathies/haematological problems account for 1/5 cases. Conditions such as thrombocytopenic purpura, von Willebrands and, less commonly, leukaemia.
- Complications of pregnancy—sudden unexpected bleeding with pain should raise the suspicion of miscarriage, ectopic pregnancy, or an adverse effect of a contraceptive.
- STIs cause menorrhagia and IMB, and all young women should be offered testing/screening for chlamydia.
- Miscellaneous causes include: trauma, foreign body, neoplasia, and other endocrine conditions, such as thyroid disease.
- Vaginal bleeding in the neonate is uncommon and transient. If it persists, it needs investigating.

Diagnosis

The diagnostic work-up should include:

- Medical, gynaecological, and drug history.
- The type of sexual activity (vaginal, oral, etc.).
- General physical examination.
- Gynaecological examination—consider rectal examination if virgo intacto, check LMP.
- FBC and coagulopathy screening.
- Pregnancy test.
- STI screen, as appropriate.
- Thyroid functions.
- Pelvic ultrasound.

Treatment

The teenager and her family need an explanation and when a physiological cause is most likely, reassurance.

- Menstrual charting signposts when treatment is best initiated.
- Anaemia should be corrected.
- If menstruation is painful as well as heavy, treatment should include mefenamic acid. Simple analgesics, such as paracetamol, have no effect on bleeding.
- Haemostatic doses of oestrogen and progestogens are used to arrest major menstrual haemorrhage.

- Maintenance treatment is with the combined pill or cyclical progestogens.
- Follow-up should be frequent, initially 2–3 months, to ensure adherence to treatment.

For amenorrhoea 📖 see Chapter 6, p.99.

Resources

For heavy menstrual bleeding guideline 44 or National Institute for Health and Clinical Excellence: www.NICE.org.uk (Accessed January 2008)

Vaginal discharge

Prepubertal vaginal discharge

This is the commonest gynaecological presentation in this age group. It is distressing to the child and concerning to the parents. Its association with poor hygiene, sexual abuse, and/or infection makes careful counselling and management essential. It can present as yellow/green discharge, purities, or inflammation.

Causes

- Foreign body—it may cause an offensive blood-stained discharge.
- Lichen sclerosis —self-limiting childhood condition that is not related to malignancies and does not often recur after childhood.
- Warts—general transmission from the hands of carers and self-limiting.
- Vaginitis.
  - Mixed bacterial infection—non-specific and non-sexually transmitted.
  - Streptococcal.
  - Candida—not common in this age group.
  - Associated with systemic viral infections such as varicella.
- Vulval dermatosis.
  - Chemical due to urine, sandpit material, and other irritants.
  - Contact due to soaps and other bath preparations.
  - Skin conditions such as eczema and psoriasis.
  - Nappy rash.
- STIs—associated with sexual abuse, which is a child-protection issue (📖 see Child protection, p.67).
- Non-genital causes.
  - Threadworm infection.
  - Often toddlers may present with labial abrasions, which are due to chronic inflammation and asymptomatic.

Management

The diagnostic work-up should include:

- Medical and drug history, with bath hygiene an essential part.
- General physical examination.
- Gynaecological examination, done with the child in her mother's lap or in the frog-leg position.
- Inspection of the vulva with separation of the labia.
- Urethral swab size sampler is used to sample pool of discharge in posterior lower vaginal area.
- General anaesthetic (GA) may be necessary if more extensive examination is required.

Treatment

Related to the cause and can include treatment of any organisms with antibiotics, hygiene, clothing, and avoidance of constipation.

Removal of foreign bodies is often performed under a GA.

Vaginal discharge in teenagers

- Is managed as for adults with Fraser and child-protection rules applied (see Chapter 8, p.167).

Resources

Department of Health (2005) *Competencies for providing more specialised sexually transmitted infection services within Primary Care Gateway*. Ref 5503. (Accessed January 2009)

Contraceptive choices for teenagers

For in depth information on the contraceptive range, 📖 see Emergency contraception, p.366. This chapter will deal with the aspects of contraception as they apply to teenagers:

- Emergency hormonal contraception (EHC)—awarness of EHC is high among teenagers but they do not seek it every time they have unprotected sex, as they underestimate the risk of pregnancy (e.g. you cannot fall pregnant if there is no full penetration). The method is nearly without contraindications, can be used more than once in a cycle, and the request offers an opportunity to put the teenager on a regular contraceptive and screen her for STIs.
- The combined pill—a popular choice among young women but open to default and failure. Some link it to subfertility, a myth that needs dispelling. Teaching use is essential with emphasis on *aide-mémoires* to taking the daily pill on time, such as setting up a reminder on their mobile phone. Everyday versions may have an advantage for those who forget when to start a new packet. Warn about early cycles breakthrough bleeding and choose a less androgenic pill to ensure no androgenic side-effects occur. Highlight the gynaecological advantages of the pill for teenagers in making menstruation lighter, shorter, less painful, and more predictable. Arrange follow-up at shorter intervals and give a helpline phone number for emergencies.
- The contraceptive patch—ideal for those who forget pills, as it needs changing once a week. It is visible and may not be appropriate for young women who wish to keep their contraceptive 'secret'. Warn the user that oestrogenic side-effects are more common in the first two cycles.
- Progestogen-only pills—this method is more open to failure in non-compliant users and, therefore, is not ideal. Cerazette®, a desogestrel POP that inhibits ovulation, has a profile similar to the combined pill and is appropriate where an oral method is required and there are contraindications to oestrogen.
- Barrier methods—these should be promoted as methods to prevent STIs and to be used with a systemic or intra-uterine contraceptive. Emphasize the importance of lubrication and the danger of oil-based lubricants and body piercing to the integrity of the condom. Caps and diaphragms are likely to be problematic for this age group.
- Injectable progestogens—Depo-Provera® is effective and popular among young women. The advice from NICE is that it could be a choice for teenagers, provided all other methods have been considered. The issue of short-term bone loss should be discussed with emphasis on healthy lifestyle.
- Subdermal implants—Implanon® is extremely effective. Counselling should highlight the associated irregular bleeding in first 6 months.
- IUD/IUS—contrary to popular belief, these are options for young women. There is no long-term effect on fertility. Screening for STIs is essential.

Adolescent health: pregnancy, sexual health

Adolescence is a phase of learning, maturing, experimentation, and, at times, risk taking. Sexuality is expressed in a multitude of ways, including sexual activity. Unplanned sexual activity, especially where the participants are under the influence of alcohol or drugs, tends to be unprotected. The inevitable consequences are unplanned pregnancies and sexually transmitted infections. The UK has the highest teenage conception and abortion rates in Western Europe. The cause is multi-factorial: social deprivation, aspirations for independence, alcohol and drug misuse, poor access to contraceptive information and services, and the lack of effective sex education.

- In England, the government set a target to reduce the rate of <18 conceptions by 50% from the 1998 rate of 46.6/1000.
- In 2007 the rate is just 10% down.
- The percentage of teenage conceptions ending in termination of pregnancy is rising from 42.4% in 1998 to nearly 50% in 2007.

Where can teenagers access contraception and sexual health advice?

Information is available in written leaflets at surgeries and social venues and many other places. An emerging source of information is the web. Useful websites include:

🖱 www.brook.org.uk
🖱 www.fpa.org.uk
🖱 www.ruthinking.co.uk

The following are mainstream services:

- GP surgery—young people attend their doctor for many health-related reasons. These encounters are ideal for the opportunistic raising of sexual health issues, whilst re-emphasizing the right to confidentiality. A healthcare provider who lacks expertise or training or has ethical restrictions should refer the young person on.
- Community contraception and sexual health services—these provide comprehensive one-stop care and many manage STIs too. Some have young people sessions and many offer outreach services to school and other non-NHS venues.
- Brook centres—specialist centres for young people. A special feature is availability of trained counsellors.
- Pharmacies—selected pharmacies have an extended role to provide emergency contraception through PGDs, pregnancy tests, chlamydia screening, and condoms.

Principles of young people-friendly services

- Confidentiality. The most consistent worry for young people is lack of confidentiality. Services should have visible evidence/a display/posters assuring that all consultations are confidential. Breach of confidentiality could be a disciplinary matter.
- See Children's, Bureau Publication (2008) *Are you getting it right?* which deals with young people's perspectives on sexuality and relationships.

- Friendly clinic environment with magazines, comfortable furniture, drinks machines, and pods for accessing the web make it more likely that the young person will return to the facility.
- All staff should undergo training in dealing with young people and have child-protection training.
- The young person's autonomy should be respected. The healthcare provider should introduce her/himself and identify their role to the client.
- If a young girl attends with her mother, it is appropriate to ask to see the girl without the mother.
- Child-protection rules dictate that, for all teenagers, but especially for <14s, the nature of the sexual activity must be ascertained and, if there is suspicion of coercion or abuse, the child-protection team/social services must be involved.

Assessment of Fraser competence

When seeing an <16-year-old without parental consent, a health professional must follow the Fraser guidelines to assess the young person's competence to understand and receive treatment:

- Encourage them to seek parental support.
- Is the young woman sexually active or about to be?
- Would withholding contraceptive advice be detrimental to the physical/mental health of the woman?
- Is she mature enough to understand the advice given?
- Is giving contraception/advice without parental consent in the best interests of the young woman?

Partnership working

Practitioners need to be aware of the role of school nurses and know who delivers sex and relationship education in the local school. Teenage pregnancy co-ordinators in the local PCT should be able to provide this information.

Resources

Are you getting it right: a toolkit for consulting young people on sex and relationships education (2008) ☞ www.ukyouthparliament.org.uk. (Accessed January 2009.)

Eating disorders

Anorexia nervosa is primarily a psychiatric disorder. Up to 90% of those affected are female. It affects 0.3% of women but the incidence is higher in adolescents. Sufferers have an exaggerated concern about shape and weight, and can tolerate food restriction, excessive exercising, and use purging routines, including self-induced vomiting.

Criteria for diagnosis

Five criteria are used to define the illness—they all need to be present:
- BMI <17.5 or poor pubertal growth spurt.
- Self-induced weight loss through dieting, purging, over exercising, and abuse of diuretics and/or appetite suppressants.
- Fear of being fat and negative attitude to current body image.
- Endocrine pathology of amenorrhoea (sometimes masked by intake of oral contraception) + high cortisol or growth hormone + abnormal insulin patterns.
- If onset prepubertal, then a delay in the puberty milestones is experienced.

Management

A multidisciplinary approach recognizing a slow progress and tendency to relapse is essential. Those in charge of treatment must ensure clear policies on follow-up and fail-safe.
- Care in the community is preferable to hospitalization.
- Hospitalization is required if there is nutritional decompensation that threatens the life of the patient.
- Psychotherapy is the main stay of treatment.
  - Cognitive behaviour therapy.
  - Motivational enhancement techniques work best.
  - Group therapy.
  - Family therapy—support and encourage assertive care by relatives.
  - A combination of the above.
- Managing substance misuse—alcohol, overdosing, and insulin abuse.

Prognosis

- Prognosis tends to be poor.
- Mortality is the highest for any psychiatric disorder.
- No drug therapy has emerged as effective.
- Secondary depression is common.

Child protection

All nurses within any practice should be able to identify child-protection issues.

Definition—all children or young persons who are at risk of harm or being abused or neglected.

Following on from Victoria Climbie, who was injured and came into contact with many healthcare professionals with little intervention, an enquiry was set up that made recommendations to put in place policies, procedures, and training.

The policy needs to have the following for effective protection:

- Good communication.
- Effective sharing of information by healthcare professionals and other interested parties, i.e. social workers.
- Adequate training.
- Listening to children.
- Each employer is responsible for checking the criminal records of staff.

Child abuse and neglect can take many different forms, which staff need to be able to recognize. For this, Trusts and PCTs have child-protection courses. These range from level one, which is for all staff, with or without professional qualifications, to level 3 for staff working with children or young people. Training involves an understanding of different types of abuse:

- Physical abuse—such as hitting, burning, shaking, throwing, and drowning.
- Emotional abuse—persistent ill-treatment that affects the development of the child, such as being in constant fear, being told they are worthless.
- Sexual abuse.
- Neglect—failing to meet basic needs, such as food, clothes, and shelter; this includes emotional needs.

Some of these may manifest with external signs, such as bruises, or repeated attendance at health clinics or disclosures from the child.

Nurses have a professional duty to be aware of child-protection issues, with guidance from the NMC, RCN, and employers. They must be able to recognize abuse or neglect, and be able to discuss, and know where to pass the information on to, such as the child protection lead for the organization.

Resources

www.everychildmatters.gov.uk (Accessed January 2009.)

Chapter 5

Menstrual and bleeding disorders

Heavy menstrual bleeding/menorrhagia: definition, assessment, and diagnosis

Definition

Menorrhagia or heavy menstrual bleeding (HMB) is a common debilitating condition defined as excessive menstrual blood loss of more than 80ml per cycle. This occurs in women with regular cycles.

For clinical purposes, HMB is defined subjectively as excessive blood loss leading to interference with physical, emotional, and social quality of life. This can occur alone or with other symptoms.

Prevalence

Menorrhagia occurs most commonly in women over the age of 35 years, although it can occur in young adolescents. One in three women experience the problem at some stage in their lives. HMB has been shown to have a major impact on a woman's quality of life. In almost half of women complaining of menorrhagia, objective assessment is likely to reveal normal menstrual loss. However, in practice, women seeking treatment for HMB can often reflect a woman's perception, and hence tolerance, of her menstrual loss.

Assessment

History

The aim of history taking is to ascertain the nature of menstrual blood loss (MBL), determine its impact on the sufferer, and identify symptoms that may indicate significant pathology. A comprehensive history should be obtained, including: menstrual, contraceptive, sexual, obstetric, medical, family, and social history. An effort should be made to evaluate the extent of MBL. Some features of the menstrual history may help to assess the severity of the condition, such as the duration of the bleeding, simultaneous use of pads and tampons, and frequent change of sanitary protection. Flooding, clots, and frequent soiling of clothing and bed sheets may also correlate with the degree of MBL. A useful practical tool is the pictorial assessment chart that examines the appearance of the sanitary towels.

⚠ Inter-menstrual bleeding and post-coital bleeding may indicate underlying problems, such as sexually transmitted infections or be one of the first symptoms of gynaecological cancer, and indicates the need for a pelvic examination (📖 see Physical examination 1, p.30).

Assessment of HMB

- Cycle length and number of bleeding days—regular, irregular, or absent cycle.
- Amount of bleeding, including flooding and clots, if prolonged.
- Any pain.
- Frequency of change of sanitary wear.
- Social accidents, soiling clothes and bedding.
- Impact on life: social, occupational, and relationships.
- General health: lethargy, bruising, breathlessness.

For assessment of bleeding disorders—📖 see Examination, p.71

Examination

- A general examination may reveal signs of thyroid disease, anaemia, or clotting disorders.
- An abdominal and pelvic examination should be performed when there is alteration in the menstrual cycle.
- Speculum examination is undertaken to visualize the cervix and vagina to exclude any local cause.
- A bimanual examination is performed to check for uterine enlargement (fibroids), uterine mobility, and adnexal masses; a tender fixed uterus is suggestive of pelvic inflammatory disease or endometriosis.
- Around 20% of women with menorrhagia have an inherited bleeding disorder, most commonly von Willebrand disease. Questions should include: bruising tendency, excessive bleeding after surgery and teeth extractions, family history of bleeding disorders.

► In the absence of any suspicious features in the patient's history (cyclic HMB is the only complaint in a woman who is not at risk for endometrial cancer or infections), oral medical treatment can be commenced without the need to undertake a physical examination or other investigations.

Diagnosis

Investigations

- A full blood count should be performed so that oral iron therapy can be commenced, if anaemia is diagnosed. The prevalence of anaemia in women complaining of menorrhagia is thought to be 11–17%.
- Thyroid function tests and other endocrine investigations and/or a coagulation screen should be performed only if clinically indicated.
- A cervical smear is not routinely performed and should be obtained only in accordance with the national screening programme.
- Pregnancy should be excluded, if this is suspected.
- A transvaginal ultrasound scan can be used as a diagnostic tool for identifying structural pathology such as fibroids (📖 see Vaginal discharge: investigations and treatment p.178).
- If the ultrasound scan results are inconclusive or focal pathology (fibroids, polyps, and endometrial disease) is suspected, a hysteroscopy is indicated to assess the nature and location of any intra-uterine pathology, in particular fibroids that impinge into the uterine cavity (submucous).
- An endometrial biopsy to exclude endometrial cancer or atypical hyperplasia is mandatory in women with historical risk factors, women who have persistent inter-menstrual bleeding, and those aged 45 and over who have declined adequate medical treatment or where such treatment has been ineffective.
- STI screening if indicated in history.

Menorrhagia: causes

About two-thirds of sufferers will have no obvious underlying pathology, with the abnormal bleeding being labelled as 'dysfunctional uterine bleeding' (DUB). Examination may reveal evidence of local pathology in some women. Systemic disease may account for a small proportion of cases.

Dysfunctional uterine bleeding

This is a diagnosis by exclusion where careful assessment has shown neither an organic pathology nor a systemic disease. It accounts for approximately 60% of cases. HMB is thought to be related to disruption of local haemostatic mechanisms within the endometrium. Components of the local fibrinolytic system and prostaglandins are implicated in the pathogenesis of menorrhagia. DUB is divided into ovulatory (80–90%) and anovulatory (10–20%) cycles. Anovulatory cycles are more common in women at the extremes of reproductive ages (young adolescents and peri-menopausal).

Local pelvic pathology

- Accounts for approximately 35% of cases.
- Fibroids are the commonest cause of HMB and occur in 25% of women over 40. Fibroids are benign, oestrogen-dependent tumours composed of fibrous and muscular tissue. One-third of women with fibroids which complain of menorrhagia. It is believed that fibroids that distort the uterine cavity (submucous) are likely to cause HMB.
- Heavier and longer menstrual bleeding is common during the first 3–6 months of copper-bearing IUD use. Bleeding usually becomes lighter over time.
- Adenomyosis: up to 40% of women with adenomyosis may have HMB.
- Endometriosis: a significant number of women sufferers will present with increased MBL.
- Polycystic ovarian disease can be associated with anovulatory dysfunctional bleeding, with infrequent but heavy, prolonged menses.
- 19% of peri-menopausal women with abnormal bleeding can have pre-malignant (hyperplasia) or malignant (cervical or endometrial) lesions of the endometrium. This is a rare cause of menorrhagia.
- Oestrogen-producing ovarian tumours are rare causes of menorrhagia.
- Endometrial polyps can, on occasions, cause excessive bleeding, although not a common cause. A fibroid 'polyp' causes erratic heavy bleeding.
- Infections: cervicitis, endometritis, salpingitis.
- Trauma: lacerations, abrasion, foreign body, IUD.
- Endocrine: PCOS, sex steroid secreting ovarian neoplasm.

Systemic disorders

These may account for less than 5% of cases of menorrhagia. Coagulation defects such as von Willebrand disease, idiopathic thrombocytopaenia, or, rarely, leukaemia, may present with excessive menstrual loss. It is suggested that a quarter of adolescents with HMB and anaemia (haemoglobin <10g/dl) have an associated coagulation disorder. Other rare systemic causes are hypothyroidism, chronic liver failure, and systemic lupus erythematosus.

Common causes of menorrhagia

Dysfunctional uterine bleeding (diagnosis by exclusion):

- Ovular cycle.
    - Usually regular, heavy periods, often painful.
    - May be due to inadequate production of progesterone by the corpus luteum.
- Anovular.
    - Tends to occur at the extremes of reproductive age.
    - Can result in endometrial hyperplasia.
    - Pain is not normally a feature.
- Fibroids.
    - Mainly submucous fibroids that impinge into the uterine cavity.

Menorrhagia: medical treatment

Women should be encouraged to try medical therapy as first line, as this is relatively safe, inexpensive, and effective.

Non-hormonal treatments

Tranexamic acid

This is an anti-fibrinolytic agent, which reduces MBL by 46%. It can cause gastrointestinal side-effects and is contraindicated in women with a history of thromboembolic disorders.

Mefenamic acid

This is an anti-prostaglandin, which reduces MBL by 30%. It is beneficial in relieving dysmenorrhoea. It is contraindicated in women with a history of peptic ulcer.

MA and TA are taken on days of heavy menstrual loss and should be stopped if they do not improve HMB within three menstrual cycles. They can be used together.

Hormonal treatment

Levonorgestrel-releasing intra-uterine system (LNG-IUS)

This is a long-acting, reversible, progestogen-only intra-uterine device (IUD) or system licensed for contraception for 5 years and for treatment of HMB (5-year license). The effects are local, including suppression of endometrial proliferation and thickening of cervical mucus. There is a 71–96% reduction in MBL. LNG-IUS should be offered as a first-line treatment for HMB sufferers. It matches, or even surpasses, the efficacy of ablative therapies (📖 see Fig. 5.1).

Norethisterone (oral progestogen)

Cyclic oral norethisterone (5mg tds from day 5 to 26 of cycle) has been shown to reduce MBL by 83%. Compliance is a problem due to relatively high rate of side-effects.

Long-acting progestogens

There have been no trials to support the role of Depo-Provera® (injectable progestogen) as a treatment for HMB. However, evidence suggests that in 45–50% of users, amenorrhoea develops after 1 year of use.

Combined oral contraceptive pill (COCP)

Low-dose COCP reduces MBL by 43% and improves dysmenorrhoea. Contraindicated in smokers over 35 years.

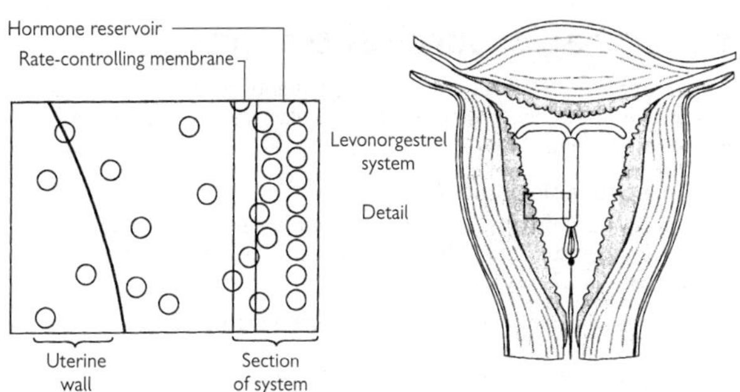

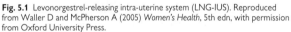

Fig. 5.1 Levonorgestrel-releasing intra-uterine system (LNG-IUS). Reproduced from Waller D and McPherson A (2005) *Women's Health*, 5th edn, with permission from Oxford University Press.

Menorrhagia: surgical treatment

Surgical treatment is usually reserved for patients in whom medical treatments have failed. Hysterectomy, in particular, should not be used as a first-line treatment.

Endometrial ablation (EA)

Endometrial ablation aims to destroy the endometrium, thereby reducing or stopping menstruation. MBL is significantly reduced to an acceptable level in most women.

► Endometrial ablation is indicated in women with dysfunctional uterine bleeding who have completed their family, who choose not to have medical treatment, and/or where medical treatment has failed.

There are various ablative modalities available:

- The 'first-generation' hysteroscopic method, or transcervical resection of the endometrium, is performed under direct vision, using a gynaecological resectoscope. This has been shown to be an effective, minimally invasive alternative to hysterectomy. However, this modality requires expert hysteroscopic surgical skills to minimize the risk of complications and optimize treatment results. It offers better outcomes in the presence of uterine pathology, such as small submucous fibroids and polyps.
- The 'second-generation' devices that negate the need for hysteroscopic skills but achieve deep endometrial destruction. Many of these new ablative methods are being performed in an outpatient setting using local anaesthetic, with or without intravenous sedation.

All endometrial ablative techniques appear to be equivalent in terms of clinical outcome. Approximately 75% of women obtain a satisfactory improvement in their symptoms and up to 40% develop secondary amenorrhoea (absence of periods) at 1 year. Thermachoice EA, Microwave EA and NovaSure EA have equivalent clinical outcomes to the first-generation endometrial resection procedure.

Hysterectomy

Hysterectomy provides a definitive cure for menorrhagia. The procedure can be performed abdominally, vaginally, or laparoscopically. The decision upon which route to choose depends on various factors: age, parity, history of pelvic surgery, presence of pelvic disease, and desire for preservation of the ovaries. In addition, the size and mobility of the uterus, and the size and location of fibroids, influences this decision. Although hysterectomy is an effective treatment for HMB, it is invasive, costly, and can be associated with substantial morbidity. However, in a systematic review of hysterectomy against endometrial ablation, patient satisfaction favoured hysterectomy at 12 months.[1]

Women who opt for hysterectomy should have a full discussion of the psychosexual impact, fertility implications, bladder function, need for further treatment, surgical complications, the woman's expectations, alternative options, and psychological distress.

1. NICE. Heavy menstrual bleeding. National collaborating centre for women's and children's health (2007) ↗ www.nice.org.uk (Accessed April 2009.)

Dysmenorrhoea: definition and assessment

Definition

This is the pain that occurs with menstruation. It can be in the pelvis or lower abdomen, with radiation into the lower back, groin, and sometimes upper thighs. The pain can be just prior to and/or with menstruation. It is cyclical in nature.

- Dysmenorrhoea in the absence of any structural pathology is defined as primary dysmenorrhoea.
- Secondary dysmenorrhoea is associated with identifiable disease.

Painful periods can occur in isolation in primary dysmenorrhoea but may also occur with other pathology such as menorrhagia (📖 see Heavy menstrual bleeding/menorrhagia: definition, assessment, diagnosis, p.70) and pelvic or abdominal pain in secondary dysmenorrhoea.

Assessment

The assessment process involves a general history (📖 see Chapter 3, p.21) and then more detailed history taking and assessment.

Menstrual history that focuses on:

- Onset of dysmenorrhoea. This can sometimes by relieved by the flow of menstrual blood. Dysmenorrhoea that is relieved once the bleeding starts is normally not associated with pathological or organic causes. This is most likely to be in nulliparous women once they start ovulatory cycles. Secondary dysmenorrhoea may occur at any time after menarche but tends to be late onset and may occur after years of pain-free periods.
- Length of cycle.
- Number of days of bleeding.
- Days of pain.
- Location and intensity of the pain.
- Variability of the cycle. Is it predictable? Is the pain always there?
- Amount of bleeding.
- What relieves the pain?
- What makes it worse?
- Analgesia used.
- Associated factors, such as headaches, nausea, diarrhoea.
- Assessment of urinary symptoms—pain on urination, relief of pain on micturition.
- Assessment of bowel symptoms—painful defecation or relief of pain on defecation, any change in bowel habits.
- Risk factors for pelvic inflammatory disease (PID) (📖 see Chapter 8, p.192).
- Risk factors for adhesions—previous surgery, PID.
- Symptoms that may relate to organic pathology, such as inter-menstrual bleeding, post-coital bleeding, other pelvic pain, dyspareunia, back or thigh pain, vaginal discharge.
- Contraception used.
- Elicit family history, e.g. endometriosis in a first-degree relative may suggest causation.

Examine the abdomen looking for tenderness or masses

Vaginal examination (bimanual and also speculum) indicated:

- if the history suggests secondary dysmenorrhoea;
- if previous drug treatments have been unsuccessful;
- for adolescents, who are unlikely to have underlying pelvic pathology and so do not generally require a pelvic examination;
- if the woman is sexually active (see Physical examination, p.30).

Within the examination, look especially for fibroids and restricted mobility of the uterus, which may indicate adhesions/endometriosis.

Dependent on the results of the examination an ultrasound may be indicated.

When is referral indicated (laparoscopy may be needed)

- Pain outside of the menstrual cycle.
- Pain-management problems with disruption to daily living.
- Abnormal bleeding, dyspareunia.
- Non-response to treatment—oral contraceptives and NSAIDs.
- Abnormal findings of examination and investigations.
- Pelvic congestion syndrome.

Diagnosis

In cases of primary dysmenorrhoea, diagnosis can be made from the presenting symptoms. In cases of secondary dysmenorrhoea, further investigations will be needed, as above, to rule out pathology as a cause. Other potential differential diagnoses can be:

- Congenital malformations of the reproductive organs.
- Ovarian cysts.
- Endometriosis.
- Irritable bowel syndrome.
- Inflammatory bowel disease.

Diagnosis of the causes of pain may only be able to be made after the woman has had ultrasound, hysteroscopy, and/or laparoscopy.

Dysmenorrhoea: causes

Primary dysmenorrhoea is idiopathic. As menstruation starts, endometrial cells release prostaglandins, which can stimulate myometrial contractions and cause dysmenorrhoea. The severity of dysmenorrhoea depends on the levels of prostaglandins.

Abnormally high levels can be associated with severe dysmenorrhoea and other symptoms, such as vomiting, diarrhoea, and feeling weak due to hypotension.

In secondary dysmenorrhoea, in addition to the pelvic disease process, prostaglandins are also implicated.

The nine main causes of secondary dysmenorrhoea are given below.

Fibroids

All types of fibroids can be associated with painful periods.
📖 See Fig. 7.1, p.129 for types of fibroids.

Adenoymosis

The presence of endometrial tissue within the muscle of the uterine wall can be responsible for pain and related heavy periods. It normally occurs in women between 40 and 50 years old, and can be responsible for the late onset of dysmenorrhoea. Ultrasound would show expanded uterine volume.

Endometrial polyps

Polyps within the uterine cavity may be responsible for pain and IMB, and require ultrasound or hysteroscopy to establish a diagnosis (📖 see Fig. 5.2).

Endometriosis

The presence of endometrial tissue outside of the uterus, normally within the pelvic cavity (📖 see p.136).

Endometriosis can cause painful periods and typically the pain can start prior to menstruation and be relieved once the period starts. Laparoscopy is the gold standard diagnostic test.

Pelvic inflammatory disease

This is an infection and inflammation of the upper genital tract, uterus, fallopian tubes, or ovaries that is normally caused from ascending or, rarely, intra-abdominal infections. (📖 See Pelvic inflammatory disease (PID): treatment, p.194).

Ovarian tumours

📖 See Benign ovarian tumours: pathology and assessment, p.152.

Previous pelvic or abdominal surgery

Previous surgery can lead to scar tissues, which can alter the anatomy within the pelvis and may cause adhesions, which fix the uterus into position and cause pain. Dyspareunia can be elicited on bimanual examination.

Functional pain/psychological problems including sexual abuse

There can be psychological issues that can manifest themselves as problems. This always needs to be remembered when undertaking consultations, and appropriate and sensitive questions used. If this is suspected, then appropriate referral to a specialist service is recommended.

Intra-uterine contraceptive device (IUD)

The use of copper IUDs can be related to painful periods and this needs to be excluded as a cause. Although correctly placed IUDs can cause pain, it is important to exclude misplaced IUD/IUS.

Women who stop the COCP may also complain of dysmenorrhoea as the COCP would have given them pain-free menses.

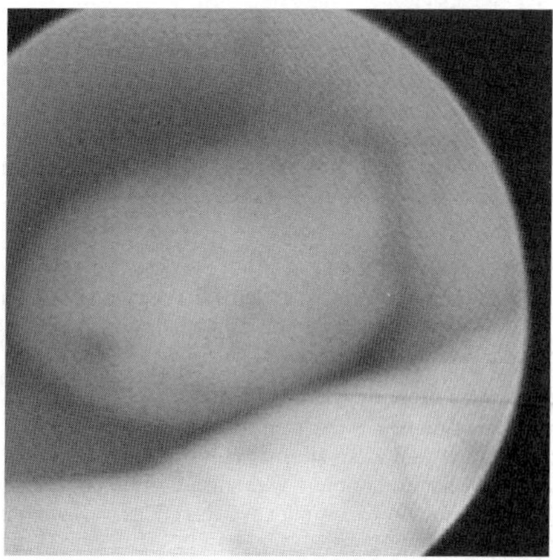

Fig. 5.2 Endometrial polyp.

Dysmenorrhoea: treatment

Primary dysmenorrhoea

As primary dysmenorrhoea is not associated with organic pathology, the following medical treatments aim to alleviate pain.

Pharmacological intervention

Simple analgesics

Paracetamol can be helpful if the pain is mild or if there is a contraindication to NSAIDs.

Non-steroidal anti-inflammatory medications (NSAIDs)

NSAIDs are more effective compared to simple analgesics and relieve symptoms in up to 70% of women. NSAIDs work by inhibiting or reducing prostaglandin synthesis. Different formulations of NSAIDs provide similar relief. Alternatives should be considered in women with a history of gastroduodenal ulceration, as gastrointestinal side-effects can occur with NSAIDs.

Combined oral contraceptive pills (COCP)

These are widely used for period problems that include painful and heavy periods, especially when contraception is needed. Also used in secondary dysmenorrhoea, due to endometriosis.

Levonorgestrel intra-uterine system (LNG-IUS)

The IUS may be of benefit if the pain is associated with heavy bleeding. The IUS can also be used as an alternative if there is IUD-associated pain and the patient wishes to continue with intra-uterine contraception. The IUS has also been shown to be effective in reducing dysmenorrhoea in women with endometriosis.

Lifestyle advice

There is some evidence that stopping smoking can help relieve pain. Obesity has also been linked with period pain and having a low-fat diet and reducing weight can relieve pain. This may be linked to the decrease of oestrogen found by reducing adipose tissue. Physical exercise may reduce dysmenorrhoea; however, current studies have methodological flaws.

Alternative therapies

Some women will try self-help measures to relieve the pain.

- Vitamin B1.
- Vitamin E.
- Heat pads.
- Transcutaneous electrical nerve stimulation, which involves stimulation of the skin current at variable frequencies and intensities to provide pain relief. However, Cochrane systematic review found little evidence that TENS can reduce pain.
- Acupuncture.

Surgical treatments

If treatment in primary care fails, then women should be referred to secondary care for further investigations and sometimes surgical treatment, in the form of presacral neurectomy and uterine nerve ablation. The idea is to interrupt the sensory nerve fibres and reduce the uterine pain, but the evidence-base for efficacy is unsubstantiated.

Secondary dysmenorrhoea

- Treatment depends on the cause.
- The treatments listed above can still be used, even if there are pathological causes found for the pain.
- Sometimes abolishing the menstrual cycle with medication can alleviate the pain. This can be achieved with gonadotrophin-releasing hormone (GnRH) analogues, with add-back oestrogens to limit adverse effects.
- Otherwise the treatment will depend on the cause.
  - Fibroids—(see Fibroids: definition, assessment, diagnosis, p.128) can be removed by hysteroscopic resection, myomectomy, uterine artery embolization, or a hysterectomy may be required.
  - Adenomyosis—can be difficult to treat and may respond to medical treatment, as above, IUS, or surgery such as hysterectomy.
  - Endometriosis (see Endometriosis risk factors, p.136).
  - PID (see Chapter 8, p.194).
- Hysterectomy is indicated only when there is complete failure of other treatments and the problem is interfering with quality of life, and fertility is not an issue.
- IUD—this can be removed and replaced with IUS, if needed. This is an uncommon cause of pain.
- Ovarian neoplasms (see PID, p.156).
- Adhesions—these may be treated surgically with division of adhesions, thereby restoring the normal pelvic anatomy. There is a chance that further surgery can lead to more adhesions. Measures can be taken at surgery to introduce solutions into the pelvis that help to minimize adhesion reformation. Dependent on the severity of the adhesions, surgery may be undertaken with general surgeons and urologists. If surgery is not indicated, then referral to a pain team may be required.

Resources

Department of Health. *Prodigy patient information leaflet:* www.prodigy.nhs.uk (Accessed January 2009.)

PMS: definition, assessment, diagnosis, and principles of management

Definition

The recent RCOG guideline defines PMS as a condition that manifests with distressing physical, behavioural, and psychological symptoms, in the absence of organic or underlying psychiatric disease. PMS regularly recurs during the luteal phase of each menstrual (ovarian) cycle and disappears, or significantly regresses, by the end of menstruation. The degree and type of symptoms can vary significantly from woman to woman. Symptoms of PMS are distinguished from normal physiological premenstrual symptoms because they cause significant impairment of daily activity (📖 for typical symptoms, see Table 5.1).

Within the spectrum of PMS the following categories are defined:

- Mild PMS—symptoms do not interfere with personal/social and professional life.
- Moderate PMS—interferes with life but able to function, though suboptimally.
- Severe—unable to interact.
- Premenstrual exaggeration—where background psychopathology and other conditions flare up premenstrually, with incomplete relief of symptoms when menstruation ends.
- Premenstrual dysphoric disorder—this condition is recognized in the United States only. It defines severe PMS, which accounts for 3% of the spectrum.

Causes and prevalence

There is no consensus on the precise aetiology of PMS. However, the association with cyclical ovarian activity and the effect of the levels of oestrogen and progesterone on serotonin uptake, is recognized as a key factor in the symptomology of PMS. The prevalence of clinical PMS is as high as 30%, but severe PMS is thought to affect 3–5% of PMS presentation.

Establishing the diagnosis is essential. Symptoms should be recorded prospectively over 2–3 cycles, using a symptom diary/menstrual chart.

Assessment and diagnosis

History and prospective symptom charting is the basis for establishing a diagnosis. History should include enquiry into lifestyle, such as diet, exercise, smoking, alcohol, and drug habits. Menstrual, sexual, and obstetric histories are essential. PMS is more common in women who have had post-natal depression.

Principles of management

- The consultation should focus on explaining the condition, acknowledging that it is a recognized entity, and establishing what are the problems with the most impact on quality of life.
- The patient is instructed in using a symptom chart.

- Lifestyle advice should be the 1st component of treatment highlighting:
  - Avoidance of smoking, alcohol, and caffeine, ensuring a balanced diet including magnesium rich food, potassium rich food (banana), and drinking plenty of water.
  - Exercise and relaxation strategies.
  - Some recommend a dietary regimen of small frequent complex carbohydrate meals (pasta, rice, and rich tea biscuits) to ensure a steady blood sugar, reduce tendency to overeating, and ensure regular bowel habit.
- Depending on the outcome of the assessment, referral may be considered to a psychologist for cognitive therapy, a dietician if there is a problem with obesity, smoking cessation advice or appropriate services if there is an element of dependence.
- The role of complementary therapies:
  - The evidence on efficacy is poor and limited.
  - Biological activity of some remedies is unknown.
  - There is evidence for the efficacy of magnesium, and Agnus castus, but not for evening primrose oil, vitamin B6 and St John's Wort.

Table 5.1 Typical PMS symptoms

Psychological symptoms	Physical symptoms	Behavioural changes
Irritability	Headache	Reduced cognitive ability
Mood swings	Bloating	Increased risk of accidents
Depression	Breast tenderness	Poor concentration
Aggression	Swelling of the limbs or fingers	Irrational thoughts

Resources

RCOG *Green-top Guideline No. 48* (December 2007). Available from RCOG website: www.rcog.org.uk (Accessed January 2009)

PMS: treatment

Types of treatment available

Symptomatic treatment such as:

- SSRIs/SNRIs are seen as first-line treatment, where the main feature of PMS is psychological symptoms, though physical symptoms improve too. Low-dose SSRI (selective serotonin reuptake inhibitor), such as 20mg fluoxetine, or SNRI (serotonin and noradrenaline reuptake inhibitors) used either continuously or from mid-cycle to menstruation—so-called luteal phase treatment. This cyclical use reassures the user that these are not habit forming.

► Discontinuation of treatment should be gradual where these agents are used continuously. The counselling and selection of patients is as recommended for psychiatric use but there have been no reports of suicide when SSRIs are used for PMS.

- Analgesia for breast pain.
- NSAID for dysmenorrhea.

Hormonal manipulation of the ovarian cycle with the aim to inhibit ovulation or over-ride the ovarian cycle. The options are:

- COCP—ideally this should be used in an extended regimen omitting the hormone-free interval. This will eventually achieve amenorrhoea for the majority but it does have a higher risk of breakthrough bleeding in the early cycles.

  ► Oestrogen dominant pills perform better. Yasmin®, a combined pill containing 3mg of the spironolactone-derived progestogen drospirenone, which has anti-mineralocorticoid and anti-androgenic properties, with ethinylestradiol 30μg is likely to pose less risk of water retention. A 20μg ethinylestradiol/3mg drospirenone preparation has FDA approval for PMDD.
- The progestogen-only pill Cerazette® (75μg desogestrel)—this inhibits ovulation but is oestrogen-free. There have been several anecdotal reports that Cerazette® works in selected cases, where the patient is intolerant of oestrogen.
- HRT in the form of high-dose oestrogen as a patch (100–200μg patches), or implant (100mg), combined with short courses of cyclical progestogen (1–5mg norethisterone for 7 days).
- The Mirena® hormone-delivery intra-uterine system (IUS) reduces the production of prostaglandins, which some attribute PMS to. So it may reduce PMS symptoms on its own.

► More importantly it provides endometrial protection when a woman takes unopposed oestrogen. The IUS allows a further combination of high-dose oestrogen and local progestogen.

- GnRH analogues—these inhibit ovarian activity, produce amenorrhoea, and eliminate PMS. However, because hypo-oestrogenism may affect bone health, add back hormone therapy is recommended, either as a continuous combined oestrogen/progestogen preparation or tibolone. GnRH analogues should be reserved for severe cases as second-line options.

Surgery

This is reserved for intractable cases and should only be done after very careful counselling and assessment. Simple hysterectomy is not enough for PMS. Bilateral oophorectomy is required, which means that young women will require oestrogen only replacement therapy till age 50.

Summary of treatments

- SSRI.
- Analgesia.
- COCP.
- POP.
- Mirena®.
- IUS.
- GnRH analogues.
- Surgery.

Inter-menstrual bleeding: definition, assessment, and diagnosis

Inter-menstrual bleeding (IMB) is common in women and can occur regularly or intermittently. It is rarely a sign of sinister pathology in the under-40 years age group but it is important to exclude malignancy. The investigation and management of these symptoms can be undertaken in a one-stop clinic.

Definition

Inter-menstrual bleeding (IMB) is defined as bleeding that occurs outside of expected menstrual bleeding.

Assessment

With appropriate management in general practice, gynaecology referrals should be limited to women with repeated episodes of IMB. Once these patients have been referred, they should ideally be seen within the one-stop diagnostic and treatment clinic. The clinic should have the facility to undertake ultrasound and/or hysteroscopy.

History

- A full gynaecological history should be taken.
- A contraceptive history and sexual history.
- Menstrual history should include normal or abnormal bleeding pattern, and last menstrual period. Identify the duration, amount, type, and timing of bleeding.
- Important to explore relationship of bleeding to normal menses and sexual intercourse.
- Elicit history of hormone intake, associated vaginal discharge, trauma to the genital tract.
- History of bleeding disorder.

Examination

- General examination.
- Abdominal palpation.
- Inspection of vulva.
- Cuscoe's speculum examination.
- Bimanual pelvic examination.

Investigations

Should be performed as indicated from history and symptoms:

- High vaginal swab for culture and endocervical swab for gonorrhoea culture and chlamydia analysis.
- Cervical smear, if indicated, due to abnormality on examination.
- Pregnancy test if possibility of pregnancy.

- Transvaginal ultrasound.
- A hysteroscopy and endometrial biopsy should be performed if the scan is abnormal or if the woman is over 40, to exclude endometrial pathology.
- Platelet count, coagulation screen if suspicion of bleeding disorder.
- Serum Ca125 if ovarian tumour suspected. Referral may be indicated.

The main role of outpatient procedures is diagnostic but, with advancements in technology, there is an increasing role for treatment procedures, such as endometrial polypectomy and submucosal fibroids under 2cm at the time of making a diagnosis in the outpatient clinic.

Inter-menstrual bleeding: causes

Physiological causes

The physiological causes are related to the normal fluctuations of oestrogen and progesterone in the menstrual cycle. A large rise in oestrogen in the follicular phase, followed by an excessive post-ovulation fall, can give rise to the endometrial shedding, leading to regular mid-cycle IMB.

Hormonal contraception

IMB and IBTB are not unusual within the first few cycles after starting the pill and resolve spontaneously. Some women do not absorb the combined oral contraceptive pill well. This leads to reports of inter-menstrual bleeding. Irregular bleeding can occur with progestogen-only contraceptives, particular during the first few months. Compliance with the pill can be a likely cause, such as missed pills or poor concurrent intake of interacting drugs.

Interacting drugs

Women who are epileptic or who have been on antibiotics whilst taking the combined oral contraceptive pill commonly get IMB or breakthrough bleeding and need a higher dose pill and/or additional contraception until the drug course has stopped.

Endometritis/PID

Chlamydial or gonorrhoeal cervicitis may cause IMB or PCB, being the number one cause of IMB in young women. Intra-uterine infections, secondary to sexually transmitted infections, including gonorrhoea and chlamydia, can result in IMB or post-coital bleeding (PCB). Evacuation of retained products of conception can lead to inter-menstrual bleeding and PCB, if cervicitis is present or endometritis develops.

Pregnancy-related bleeding

Includes threatened, incomplete, or missed miscarriage, and needs exclusion (see Chapter 15, p.415).

Benign endometrial or cervical pathology

Cervical polyps, including endocervical polyps, may give rise to IMB and PCB. Submucosal fibroids, endometrial polyps, fibroid polyps, and endometrial hyperplasia, may all be associated with IMB.

Cervical ectopy and ectropion

The cervix is composed of two types of epithelium: the columnar epithelium is usually inside the cervical canal, while the squamous epithelium is visible and is over the outer part of the cervix. These two epithelia meet at the squamo-columnar junction (SCJ), which moves into and out of the cervical canal in response to hormonal changes.

An ectropion occurs when the SCJ moves on to the surface of the cervix. The columnar epithelium that becomes visible appears reddened and inflamed. This epithelium is fragile and can bleed easily on contact, especially after intercourse. This may sometimes be interpreted as IMB. An ectropion can be the cause of a persistent vaginal discharge that may be blood-stained if there is associated cervicitis.

(📖 See Colposcopy, p.494.)

Malignant causes

The malignancies to consider are: cervix, endometrium, and rarely, vagina, vulva, fallopian tube, or ovary. Women with cervical cancer often present with IMB and/or PCB. Endometrial cancer is rare in women under 40 years but 25% of cases occur before menopause. Ovarian tumours of germ cell or sex cord stromal tumours may present with IMB if oestrogen-producing.

Vaginal/vulval causes

Includes vulvitis due to *Candida* or *Trichomonas vaginalis* and dermatological conditions—psoriasis, impetigo, lichen planus, and scabies. These may rarely present with bleeding interpreted as IMB.

Bleeding abnormalities

Von Willebrand's disease and idiopathic thrombocytopenia (ITP) may result in IMB/PCB. Women on warfarin or long-term anticoagulants are also more prone to IMB.

Inter-menstrual bleeding: treatment

The treatment of IMB is dependent on the cause, if known.

Physiological

For physiological causes, reassurance that all is normal is all that is needed. This can sometimes be backed by a menstrual calendar to explore and show when in the cycle this happens.

Hormonal contraception

If the problem is related to combined oral contraceptive pills, once chlamydia is excluded, then changing to a higher dose progestogen or a more potent progestogen may resolve the problem

Bleeding related to progestogen-only contraceptive can be managed with a short course of combined oral contraceptive pill, a change of the brand of progestogen-only pill, or use of an alternative contraception method.

Breakthrough bleeding related to drugs that interact with the pill, need a higher dose of combined oral contraceptive pill and/or an alternative method of contraception (📖 see Chapter 13, p.359).

Endometritis/PID

This will require specific therapy (📖 see PID, p.192).

Benign endometrial or cervical pathology

Cervical polyp

Cervical polyps can be removed, checking if there are any further endometrial polyps, which may compound the problem.

Submucosal fibroid

Submucous myoma <2cm in size can be removed or resected hysteroscopically.

Endometrial hyperplasia

Diagnosis of endometrial hyperplasia with no atypia can be treated with long courses of high dose progestogens. If atypia is present, referral to gynaecological oncologist is indicated.

Cervical ectropion

There is no need to treat a cervical ectropion if the smear is normal unless the woman considers the symptoms to be a problem. Treatment is cryocautery or diathermy.

Malignant lesions

If cervical cancer is suspected consider early referral for colposcopy or gynaecological oncologist—📖 see Chapter 11, p.293.

Bleeding disorders
Referral to a haematologist if bleeding disorders are suspected.

Vaginal/vulval lesions
Vulvitis can be treated with prescription of antifungal or antibacterial medication as appropriate.

For specific skin conditions, refer to a dermatologist or a specialist vulva clinic.

Post-coital bleeding

Definition

Post-coital bleeding is the term used to describe vaginal bleeeding related to intercourse. Although this is a significant symptom with regard to cervical neoplasia, the majority of cases are not malignant. Women who present with this require appropriate assessment and referral for colposcopy, if cancer is suspected, or to gynaecology clinics in the presence of a normal cervial smear.

Assessment and diagnosis

Relevant history should be taken to elicit the symptoms:

- When did this start?
- How much bleeding? Just with sex or after as well? Associated with pain? Is it related to a particular time in the cycle?
- Is it fresh red or dark brown?
- Is there any co-existing inter-menstrual bleeding (IMB)? (📖 see IMB p.90.)
- Risk assessment for sexually transmitted infections (STI)—has there been a change in partner recently, any history of vaginal discharge?

Ensure that a full examination is undertaken and that cervical screening is up-to-date:

- Examination of the cervix is mandatory to exclude visible signs of cancer, such as a tumour, or to make a diagnosis of cervical polyps or overt cervicitis.
- Examination of the external genitalia to check any lesions or areas on the vulva.
- If history or examination in women under 25 suggests cervical or other genital tract infection, take chlamydia and gonorrhoea swabs and/or referral to a genito-urinary medicine clinic should be considered.[1]

Investigations

These may include:

- Genital swabs—high vaginal swab (HVS), endocervical swab for aerobes/anerobes, and for chlamydia.
- Pelvic ultrasound—if associated menstrual problems.

Causes

- Cervicitis.
- Cervical ectropion.
- Cervical polyps.
- Chlamydia infection.
- Coital trauma.
- Cervical intraepithelial neoplasia (CIN)/cervical cancer.
- Cervical fibroids.
- Endometrial polyps/fibroids.

- Misplaced IUD—particularly within the cervical canal.
- Vulval problems—lichen sclerosis, vulvitis, severe atrophy.
- Decrease in the amount of vaginal secretions, e.g. atrophic vaginitis, bleeding, and pain can occur with sexual intercourse.
- Rarely—vaginal cancer.

Management

- Treat underlying infection and/or refer to genito-urinary medicine.
- Women who are over 40 years presenting with this symptom should be referred for gynaecological examination and onward referral for colposcopy, if neoplasia is suspected.[1]
- Cauterization to cervical ectopy in the absence of cervical neoplasia and infection may be necessary if persistent, troublesome, post-coital bleeding. If polyps are found, these can be removed (see Cervical polyps, p.506).

For the management of fibroids see p.128.

Resources

CKS. Patient information leaflet on bleeding after sex: www.cks.library.nhs.uk (Accessed January 2009.)

1. Luesley, D and Leeson, S (2004) Colposcopy and programme management guidelines for the NHS. Cervical Screening Programme **4**(10): 13.

Post-menopausal bleeding (PMB)

Definition

PMB is unscheduled bleeding that occurs a year after the last natural menstrual period. It can also occur when on hormone replacement therapy (see Chapter 9, p.221) or tamoxifen. 10% of women with PMB will have endometrial cancer.

Assessment

Women who present with PMB should be referred to a gynaecology department as a 2-week wait patient, to exclude cancer as a cause for the bleeding.

Bleeding on HRT is covered in Chapter 9.

All women should have a history taken, including the following:

- Last cervical smear, with results and any abnormalities in the past.
- Amount and type of bleeding.
- Last natural menstrual period.
- Intake of exogenous hormones.
- Risk factors for endometrial cancer (see box).

Risk factors for endometrial cancer

- Unopposed oestrogen.
- Oestrogen-secreting tumours.
- Obesity.
- Nullip.
- Late menopause.
- Diabetes.
- Previous hyperplasia.
- PCOS.

Investigations

Women with PMB should have the following:

- Speculum examination with cervical screening and swabs, if indicated. If the cervical screening result is abnormal, then a biopsy should be considered with colposcopy.
- Ultrasound—the management will depend on the endometrial thickness and outline of the endometrium. A general cut-off is 4–5mm as normal for post-menopausal women.
- Bimanual examination.
- Hysteroscopy and biopsy, if indicated from ultrasound. If the endometrium is 5mm or more, or the endometrium is irregular in its outline.

PMB—causes and treatments

There can be many causes of PMB. Once investigated with hysteroscopy and biopsy, there may be no cause found, but negative histology is reassuring and patients can then be discharged. Other causes and their treatment are listed in 📖 Table 5.2.

📖 Where the cause is cancer, refer to Chapter 11.

Table 5.2 PMB—causes and treatment

Pathology site	Treatment
Endometrial pathology	
Polyps	Removal
Fibroids	Removal if sub-mucosal and bleeding is an on-going problem
Cancer	Referral to gynaecological oncologist
Atrophic endometrium	Reassurance
Hyperplasia—simple, complex, focal, and atypical	Simple—consider progestogens or IUS. Referral? TAH BSO
Adenomyosis	Reassurance
Endometritis	Reassurance
Cervical pathology	
Polyps	Removal
CIN	Referral colposcopy
Cancer	Referral to gynaecological oncologist
Ectropion	Reassurance ? 📖 see Chapter 18 for treatment
Ovarian pathology	
Tumours	US, tumour markers? Further imaging and referral to gynaecology oncology
Vaginal and vulval pathology	
VIN	Monitoring and treatment dependent on stage (📖 see VIN, p.163)
Cancer	Referral to gynaecological oncologist
Atrophic vaginitis	Consider vaginal oestrogens
Hormonal such as HRT, endogenous cycles	Check if post-menopausal, consider FSH/LH. Check compliance with HRT (📖 see Chapter 9)

Chapter 6

Hormone and endocrine disorders

Primary amenorrhoea: definition, assessment, and diagnosis

Definition

Amenorrhoea is the absence of menstruation or uterine bleeding for 6 months in the absence of pregnancy.

Primary amenorrhoea is the failure to establish menstruation. This is generally thought to be by the age of 14 in girls who have no secondary sexual characteristics or 16 in girls who have. This affects about 0.3% of women who fail to menstruate.

Failure to menstruate when peers are can place considerable stress on women. The thought that there may be something wrong and the implications for future fertility can make this a difficult time for the girl and her parents.

Assessment

- Full history.
- Age of the woman.
- Age of menarche of older sisters and mother.
- Family history of genetic abnormalities.
- Sexual history.
- Any cyclical symptoms, such as abdominal pain.
- Symptoms of hypothyroidism.
- Symptoms related to chronic illnesses.
- Recent emotional turmoil.
- Changes in body weight.
- History of anorexia.
- Excessive exercise.
- Medication history.
- General health, including: vasomotor symptoms, increasing body hair, greasy skin, galactorrhoea, headaches, palpitations, and visual field disturbances.

Physical examination

- With particular reference to secondary sexual characteristics, the development of breast buds, and pubic hair.
- Height and weight to calculate the BMI.
- Signs of thyroid disease.
- Signs of excessive androgens—facial hair and spots.
- Galactorrhoea.
- Features of Turner's syndrome (📖 see box, Features of Turner's syndrome, p.101).
- Appearance of external genitalia—enlarged clitoris indicating virilization, or bulging membrane at the labia indicating haematocolpos.

Features of Turner's syndrome

- Short stature.
- Web neck.
- Shield chest.
- Widely spaced nipples.
- Wide carrying angle.
- Scoliosis.
- Slow at school.
- Poor growth.

Investigations

Specialists normally carry out investigations. However, these can be started in primary care.

- Pregnancy test, if indicated.
- Blood tests, which include: thyroid stimulating hormone (TSH), prolactin, testosterone, FSH, LH.
- Pelvic ultrasound.

Also, depending on these results, maybe karyotyping, CT or MRI scanning, and sometimes a laparoscopy.

Primary amenorrhoea: causes and treatment

Physiological causes

Pregnancy is the commonest cause followed by constitutional delay. A regular menstrual cycle is unlikely to occur if a BMI is under 19.

Pathological causes if secondary sexual characteristics are present

- Androgen insensitivity syndrome (AIS)—complete or partial deletion in the androgen receptor gene on the Y chromosome. This leads to regression of the mullerian system, so that there is no upper two-thirds of the vagina, uterus, and fallopian tubes. The testes are normally in the inguinal canal but can be present in the labia or abdomen. The external genitalia are normally female and the karyotype is XY. This diagnosis is generally made in early childhood.
- Anatomical abnormality of the vagina/genito-urinary tract—imperforate hymen through to absent vagina, vaginal septum, rudimentary uterine horn development.
- Resistant ovary syndrome.
- Acquired problems due to early infections leading to gonadal dysgenesis.
- Chemotherapy/radiotherapy in childhood.

Pathological causes if secondary sexual characteristics are absent

- Gonadotrophin deficiency.
- Gonadal failure, e.g. Turner's, where there is ovarian dysgenesis secondary to the absence of one X chromosome, karyotype 45 XO, agenesis, POF.
- Hydrocephalus.
- Hyperprolactinaemia—increased amount of prolactin acts on the hypothalamus and reduces the amount of gonadotrophin-releasing hormone (GnRH). This is normally caused by prolactinoma. Other causes can be non-functioning pituitary adenoma that presses on the pituitary gland and disrupts prolactin secretion, stress, dopaminergic antagonist drugs, and primary hypothyroidism.
- Hypopituitarism.
- Hypothalamic dysfunction—there is a disruption to the gonadotrophin-releasing hormone pulsatility, which results in impaired levels of hormones and low levels of oestrogen. Dysfunction can result from chronic illness, anorexia, and exercise.
- Hypothyroidism.
- Tumours of the hypothalamus or pituitary.
- Delayed puberty—constitutional delay.

📖 See Table 6.1.

Treatment

The treatment of amenorrhoea depends on the needs of the woman and the causes.

If abnormal TSH is found, suggesting hypothyroidism, levothyroxine would correct the abnormality.

In young girls where there is a suspicion of anorexia, referral for treatment is indicated.

Where there are genetic problems, these need to be investigated within a multi-professional team, including Geneticists.

Of importance here is access to a counsellor and the ability to obtain advice in relation to fertility.

In some cases, fertility is possible; otherwise the options are limited to egg donation or surrogacy (see Chapter 17, p. 447).

If there is a surgical defect, such as an imperforate hymen, surgery is required, and once this is performed, then the problem will be corrected.

However, some genital tract abnormalities co-exist with renal abnormalities and these women will be best managed within a specialist centre.

Many women will require hormone replacement therapy. This will be of paramount importance in the prevention of osteoporosis, as these women would not have reached peak bone mass. See section on Premature ovarian failure (POF). In addition, some women may need testosterone replacement, in addition to oestrogens.

Table 6.1 Establishing a cause from results of investigations

Diagnosis	LH	FSH	Testosterone	Oestradiol	Karyotype
Turner's	High	High	Normal	Low	45XO or mosaic
AIS	High	High to normal	Male range or low	Low	46XY
Hypothalamic anomaly	Low	Low	Low/normal	Low	Normal
Resistant ovary	High	High	Low/normal	Low	

Secondary amenorrhoea: definition, assessment, and diagnosis

Definition

Amenorrhoea is the absence of menstruation. It can be physiological, due to pregnancy or menopause; or secondary, due to a disorder, disease, or contraception. It is defined as the absence of menstruation for 6 consecutive months in a woman who has previously had regular periods. It is estimated to affect 3% of women, with higher prevalence in students and competitive athletes and dancers.

With most women, the primary anxiety when they have stopped having a period is the concern for their future fertility.

Assessment

A full history is needed (📖 see Chapter 3, p.21). Assessment needs to focus on the following:

- Could the woman be pregnant, as this is the most common cause of secondary amenorrhoea?
- Has the woman been recently pregnant?
- Is she breastfeeding?
- History of post-partum haemorrhage with shock (think of Sheehan's syndrome), and dilatation and curettage (consider Asherman's syndrome). Rarely seen.
- Is there a recent history of weight loss?
- How much exercise is she taking?
- Are there any vasomotor symptoms, hot flushes, night sweats, dry vagina?
- Any signs of excessive androgen production—greasy skin, increased hair growth on face (📖 see Hirsutism: overview, p.116).
- Any galactorrhoea?
- What method of contraception is the woman using now and in the last 6 months?
- Past medical history, especially in relation to chemotherapy and radiotherapy.
- Psychological factors—any stress or emotional turmoil?
- Previous history of any gynaecological surgery.
- Family history.
- Drug history, e.g. drugs that raise prolactin levels, psychotropic drugs, progestogens, Depo-Provera®, combined pill, and other current medication.

Examination

- Check weight, height, and BMI.
- Check for signs of virilization—acne, hirsutism, clitoral enlargement.
- Thyroid examination—for goitre.
- Breast examination—for galactorrhoea.

- A full abdominal, pelvic, and vaginal examination should be undertaken. Avoid pelvic examination in girls who have never been sexually active. Look for atrophic changes in the vagina.

Investigations

It may be worth undertaking a pregnancy test in all women.

There are blood tests that can be taken in primary care that may help to make a diagnosis.

- FSH and LH, testosterone, prolactin, oestradiol, and thyroid function. Some of these may need to be repeated to obtain a diagnosis. As there is no cycle, there is no reference point for days 2–4 so they can be taken at any time. If a woman has started on hormonal medications to induce bleeding, these should be stopped for a month before blood tests are taken.
- Assess oestrogen production by progestogen withdrawal—progestogen-challenge test to initiate a withdrawal bleed.
- Pelvic ultrasound to look for polycystic ovaries and endometrial thickness. A thin endometrium, under 4mm, suggests it is under-oestrogenized.

Investigations in secondary care

These may need to be undertaken dependent on the results of primary care bloods.

- If prolactin is raised: MRI/CT may be needed to look for pituitary tumours, visual fields measurement.
- Karyotyping, if it is a POF (📖 see POF subsection p.122).
- Hysteroscopy to assess the uterine cavity.
- 24h urinary cortisol for Cushing's syndrome.
- 17-hydroxyprogesterone for congenital adrenal hyperplasia.

Secondary amenorrhoea: causes

There are multiple causes for secondary amenorrhoea. These can be broken down into the following systems, which range from the endocrine to local uterine causes. Pregnancy is still the most common cause of secondary amenorrhoea.

Physiological

- Pregnancy.
- Lactation.
- Menopause.

Uterine causes

- Cervical stenosis.
- Asherman's syndrome—intra-uterine adhesions.

Ovarian causes

- Premature ovarian failure (📖 see POF subsection).
- Resistant ovary syndrome is a functional disturbance of the gonadotrophin receptors in the ovarian follicles. It may be a cause of primary or secondary amenorrhoea and the ovary is resistant to exogenous gonadotrophin stimulation. There is elevated FSH and LH, and normal, multiple follicles are seen on ovarian biopsy.
- Chemotherapy/pelvic radiation.

Systemic diseases

- Chronic illness.
- Hypo- and hyperthyroidism.

Hypothalamic causes

- Excessive weight loss.
- Excessive exercise.
- Psychological distress.
- Chronic illness.
- Tumours.
- Idiopathic.

Pituitary causes

- Hyperprolactinaemia.
- Hypopituitarism.
- Sheehan's syndrome.

Iatrogenic

- Progestogen methods of contraception—this includes IUS, Depo-Provera®, implants, and POP (📖 see Chapter 13, p.359).
- Radiotherapy.
- Chemotherapy.
- Post-pill amenorrhoea.

Endocrine causes

- Polycystic ovarian syndrome.
- Cushing's syndrome.
- Late-onset congenital adrenal hyperplasia.
- Androgen-secreting tumours of the ovary or adrenal gland.

Secondary amenorrhoea: treatment

The treatment of secondary amenorrhoea depends on the cause, as outlined above. The following section looks at some of these. Treatment should be looking at restoring normality, replacement of hormones, aiding fertility, and prevention of long-term complications.

Generally, if there is an issue of fertility, then whatever the cause of the amenorrhoea, a referral for the woman and her partner to a specialist service, as soon as possible, is indicated. (📖 See Chapter 17, p.447.)

Physiological

- If pregnancy is found to be the cause, referral for ultrasound for dating and then appropriate management.
- Lactation—this can be discussed with the woman and an explanation that all is normal.
- Menopause (📖 see Chapter 9, p.221 and POF, p.122).

Uterine causes

Uterine causes are perhaps the easiest to deal with.

Cervical stenosis can be dilated within an outpatient setting or under a general anaesthetic.

Asherman's syndrome is when there are uterine adhesions, these again can be divided under GA in a theatre setting using a hysteroscope to lyse the adhesions, and sometimes ultrasound guidance at the same time. Once these have been divided, then, normally, a copper IUD is inserted to facilitate healing and to minimize the reformation of the adhesions. The combined pill can be given, and the IUD can be removed after 6 months.

Ovarian causes

- Premature ovarian failure. Serum FSH above 30 IU/l is suggestive of POF before age 40 (📖 see POF p.122).
- For PCOS (📖 see PCOS p.110).

Hypothalamic/pituitary causes

- Excessive weight loss—referral to dietician and, possibly, counselling. Weight should be more than 45kg and BMI >17 for menses to occur. Anorexia nervosa can be lifelong, and return of menstrual function may take months after the weight has been restored.
- Excessive exercise—advise increasing nutritional intake and decreasing energy expenditure. A 10–20% decrease in duration and intensity of exercise may restore menses.
- Psychological distress, chronic illness, and tumours—the serum FSH will be normal or low and oestrogen levels are low. Generally, if there is an issue of fertility, then a referral for the woman and her partner to a specialist service, as soon as possible, is indicated. (📖 See Chapter 17, p.447)

- Hyperprolactinaemia. If FSH is normal but prolactin is raised >800iu/l on at least two occasions, it is hyperprolactinemia. However, it is important to know the cause of high prolactin levels, which can be due to drugs, renal failure, or underactive thyroid.
  It responds well to cabergoline and bromocriptine, with monitoring of the levels. If there have been visual disturbances and an MRI shows a tumour of the pituitary gland, surgery may be indicated.

Iatrogenic

- Progestogen methods of contraception—these include LNG-IUS, Depo-Provera®, implants, and POP (see Chapter 13, p.359)—reassurance is needed that this is normal.
- Post-ill amenorrhoea—reassurance for 6 months and then referral for investigations.

Endocrine causes

Referral to an endocrinologist for:

- Late-onset congenital adrenal hyperplasia.
- Cushing's syndrome.
- Androgen-secreting tumours of the ovary or adrenal gland.
- Hypo- and hyperthyroidism—referral for treatment.

Polycystic ovarian syndrome: definition, assessment, and diagnosis

Definition

PCOS is a heterogenous, multifactorial, endocrine condition that requires at least two of the three features listed below (European Society of Human reproduction and embryology 2004):

- Oligoamenorrhoea or amenorrhoea.
- Hyper-androgenism (clinical or biochemical).
- Polycystic ovaries on ultrasound. (📖 see Fig. 16.1.)

Plus the exclusion of other conditions, such as pregnancy, congenital adrenal hyperplasia, androgen-secreting tumours, Cushing's syndrome, premature ovarian failure.

History

In addition to general gynaecological history, the following points in history are relevant:

- Age of menarche.
- Past menstrual cycles, present cycles, amenorrhoea, and/or episodes of heavy menstrual bleeding, any irregular cycles or IMB.
- Androgenic symptoms—acne, hirsutism, rapid-onset virilization, alopecia.
- Family history of coronary heart disease, obesity, diabetes, hyper-androgenism, and premature baldness in male relatives.
- Lifestyle questions.

Examination

- Height, weight, BMI, waist and hip circumference.
- Assessment of acne, facial, chest, and abdominal hair (📖 see Table 6.2, p.117).
- Blood pressure, breast examination, abdominal striae, familial balding, deepening of voice, broadening of shoulders, and a decrease in breast size.
- Pelvic bimanual examination, clitoral examination, and examination of vaginal rugae.

Symptoms

Polycystic ovaries on pelvic ultrasound without any symptoms does not constitute PCOS.

- 45% of women with PCOS are obese—android obesity with increased waist:hip ratio.
- Menstrual disturbances—manifests as amenorrhoea, oligoamenorrhoea (in 70%), abnormal menstrual cycles (in 30%).
- Hyper-androgenism—acne in 30%, male-pattern balding in 10%, and hirsutism in 70%.
- In 1–3% of adolescents—muco-cutaneous eruptions or acanthosis nigricans in the axillae, skin flexures, and nape of the neck.

Investigations

- Transabdominal scan (TAS) in women who are not sexually active.
- Transvaginal scan (TVS)—one polycystic ovary is sufficient to provide a diagnosis based on an increase in ovarian volume to more than 10ml and more than 12 (2–9mm size) ovarian follicles seen in the ovary (📖 see Fig. 6.1).
- Androgens—measure total testosterone, it should be <5nmol/l, if >5nmol/l, measure dehydro-epiandrosterone sulphate (DHEAS) and androstenedione and refer to endocrinologist to exclude adrenal causes.
- LH and FSH measurement—days 1–3 of the cycle. LH is elevated and ratio of LH to FSH is >2:1.
- Thyroid function tests and prolactin, only if amenorrhoea.
- Oestradiol is elevated but no indication to measure.
- Fasting insulin levels are elevated (not routinely measured) and there is insulin resistance.
- Glucose tolerance test after a 75g glucose load in Caucasian women with PCOS and BMI >30kg/m^2 and in Asian women with BMI >25kg/m^2.

Causes

There is evidence for polygenic inheritance. CYP21, CYP11A genes have been implicated in studies. Various aspects of the syndrome may be differentially inherited. Polycystic ovaries have a smooth, thickened, vascular capsule with hyperplasia of thickened stromal cells surrounding the arrested follicles. Microscopic examination shows thickened luteinized theca cells.

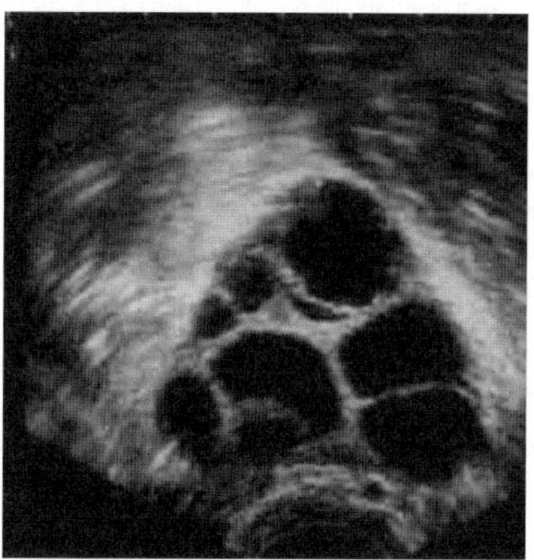

Fig. 6.1 Polycystic ovarian syndrome (stimulated ovary).

Polycystic ovarian syndrome: treatment

Of obesity

- If BMI >30, encourage patient to lose weight and discuss lifestyle issues.
- Weight loss is a desirable outcome in obese women and improves the endocrine profile and likelihood of ovulation.
- Start with decreasing the intake of carbohydrate and fat in every meal with a moderate increase in protein.
- Low glycaemic index diets may be preferable to diets with a high glycaemic index.
- Encourage moderate physical activity.
- Anti-obesity drugs—orlistat and sibutramine have been studied and are being used in primary care (see Chapter 20, p.525).
- Metformin may aid weight loss.

Of menstrual irregularity

- Consider non-androgenic or anti-androgenic combined oral contraceptive pill (COCP) for menstrual regulation, if no desire to conceive. It enables regular endometrial shedding, improves the androgen profile, and regulates the cycle. Yasmin® (30μg ethinylestradiol and 3mg drospirenone) has a more favourable effect on lipid profile and is associated with less water retention compared to other oral contraceptive pills.
- Cyclical progestogens to induce withdrawal bleeds every 3 months in amenorrhoeic women. If endometrium is thicker than 15mm, an artificial withdrawal bleed should be induced and an endometrial biopsy and/or hysteroscopy undertaken to exclude endometrial hyperplasia and cancer.
- Levonorgestrel intra-uterine system. The LNG-IUS has a significant role in providing progestogens to women with anovulatory cycles.

Of subfertility

See Chapter 17, p.447.

- Weight loss can improve ovarian function and should be the first-line treatment in obese women with PCOS.
- Induction of ovulation with:
  - Clomifene citrate 50–100mg on days 2–6 of the cycle for 6 months only. Ovulation occurs in 80% of women, pregnancy occurs in 40% of women. There is a 10% risk of multiple pregnancy. Ultrasound follicle-tracking is desirable to ensure that ovulation is taking place.[1] If endometrial thickness remains under 8mm on days 12–14 of the cycle, these are non-responders.

1. National collaborating centre for women's and children's health (2004). Fertility: assessment and treatment for people with fertility problems, Clinical guideline CGII, www.nice.org.uk (Accessed April 2009.)

- Metformin is an insulin-sensitizing agent and can improve ovulation rates. Start with 500mg daily for 1 week, increase to twice daily for 1 week, then thrice daily. Metformin decreases insulin and androgen levels and may have a direct effect on ovarian cells. Odds ratio (OR) of achieving ovulation is 3.8 compared with placebo. Metformin may be continued throughout pregnancy with a beneficial effect on miscarriage rate. The side-effects are: anorexia, nausea, flatulence, and diarrhoea.
- Metformin + clomifene citrate is an intermediate step before considering gonadotrophins. The OR of achieving pregnancy and ovulation is slightly better compared to clomifene alone.
- Gonadotrophin therapy can be used for women with metformin and clomifene citrate resistance. FSH is the choice in a low-dose regimen, which reduces the risk of ovarian hyperstimulation syndrome. Pregnancy rates are 60% and multiple pregnancy rates are 5–7%. Ovulation and pregnancy rates are significantly better in women who receive both metformin and FSH.
- Laparascopic ovarian diathermy (LOD) is reserved for clomifene-resistant PCOS. Unipolar coagulating current is used and the ovarian surface is punctured in 4–5 places to a depth of 4–10mm on each ovary. Pregnancy rate is 60%. There is no risk of OHSS and a low risk of post-operative adhesions. The effect of LOD is not long-lasting, therefore: follow by ovarian stimulation (📖 see Fig. 6.2).

Of acne and hirsutism

📖 See Hirsutism: investigations and treatment, p.118.

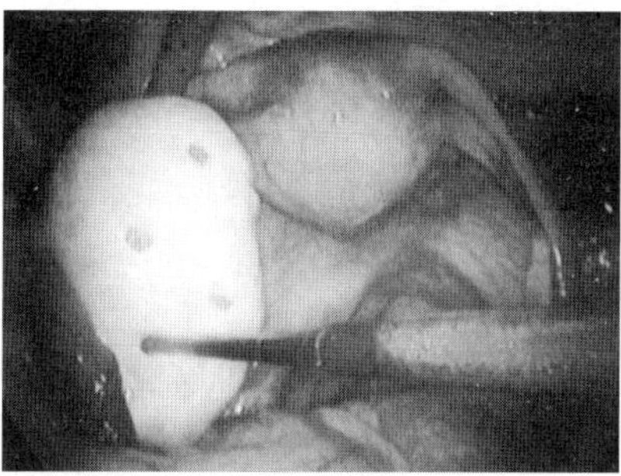

Fig. 6.2 Laparoscopic ovarian diathermy.

Polycystic ovarian syndrome: long-term complications

- Poor self-image and social life.
- 10% of obese PCOS women have Type II diabetes by age 40.
- 35% of obese women have impaired glucose tolerance test (GTT) by age 40.
- Higher risk of gestational diabetes in pregnancy.
- Insulin resistance with abdominal obesity accounts for higher prevalence of non-insulin dependent diabetes mellitus (NIDDM).
- Dyslipidemia—women have reduced high density lipoprotein (HDL) cholesterol and elevated serum triglycerides with elevated serum plasminogen activator inhibitor-1.
- Women with PCOS are more likely to develop subclinical atherosclerosis of carotid vessels and have higher risk of myocardial infarction compared to age-matched controls. Metabolic disturbances associated with insulin resistance are known to increase cardiovascular risk.
- Prevalence of treated hypertension is three times higher in women with PCOS.
- Endometrial cancer/endometrial hyperplasia. In PCOS, obesity, nulliparity, unopposed oestrogens, and subfertility are risk factors for endometrial cancer. Hyper-insulinism and hyper-androgenism may increase the potential for neoplastic change in the endometrium.
- PCOS and ovarian cancer have been poorly studied but inducing multiple ovulations in chromic anovulation may confer a slightly elevated risk.
- Breast cancer—due to obesity, hyper-androgenism and subfertility, one would expect a higher risk of breast cancer in PCOS, but there is no evidence of increase in risk of postmenopausal breast cancer.

Resources

For health professionals:

Royal College of Obstetricians and Gynaecologists. *Guideline no 33. Long term consequences of PCOS* (2007) www. rcog.org.uk (Accessed April 2009)

For women:

www.pcos-uk.org.uk

Hirsutism: overview

Definition

The excessive growth of terminal hair in a male-pattern distribution. It can result in significant social embarrassment and emotional distress.

Aetiology

70% is due to PCOS. Other causes include:

- Idiopathic hisrsutism or hyperthecosis.
- Non-classical late-onset adrenal hyperplasia.
- Cushing's syndrome.
- Thyroid dysfunction.
- Ovarian androgen secreting tumours.
- Adrenal androgen secreting tumours.
- Growth hormone secreting pituitary tumour—acromegaly.

Clinical assessment

- Racial origin—Indian subcontinent and Mediterranean countries tend to be more hirsute, compared to others.
- Elicit history of slow onset or rapid onset hair growth (rapid onset is suggestive of androgen-secreting neoplasm).
- Ask how frequently she shaves or waxes.
- Associated symptoms—obesity, acne, oligomenorrhoea, amenorrhoea, subfertility.
- Take particular note of menstrual history—if menstrual cycle is regular, the cause is likely not to be sinister.
- History of medication, e.g. danazol, glucocorticoids, testosterone.
- Symptoms of adrenal overactivity.
- Family history of hirsutism.

Physical examination

- Measure height, weight, BMI, muscle distribution.
- Look for signs of virilism—hair growth, clitoral enlargement.
- Semi-quantitative assessment of degree of hirsutism using Ferriman–Gallwey chart[1] (Ferriman and Gallwey 1961) is to assess at baseline and at follow-up to see response to treatment (📖 see Table 6.2).
- Look for signs of Cushing's syndrome—buffalo hump, central obesity, proximal weakness.
- Examine breasts.
- Examine thyroid gland.
- Examine abdomen (abdominal/pelvic mass).
- Bimanual examination.
- Acanthosis nigricans is a grey-brown velvety discoloration of the skin, usually found in the axillae, neck, and groin but may be seen in the vulval region in women with hyper-insulinemia. (📖 See Polycystic ovarian syndrome, p.110.)

Table 6.2 Ferriman–Gallwey scoring system[1]

Upper lip	1	A few hairs at outer margin
	2	Small moustache at upper margin
	3	Moustache extending halfway from upper margin
	4	Moustache extending to midline
Chin	1	A few scattered hairs
	2	Small concentration of scattered hair
	3	Light complete cover
	4	Heavy complete cover
Chest	1	Circum-areolar hair
	2	Addition midline hair
	3	Fusion of these areas with three quarters hair
	4	Complete cover
Upper back	1	A few scattered hairs
	2	Rather more still scattered
	3	Light complete cover
	4	Heavy complete cover
Lower back	1	A sacral tuft of hair
	2	With some lateral extension
	3	Three quarter cover
	4	Complete cover
Upper abdomen	1	A few midline hairs
	2	Rather more, still midline
	3	Half-cover
	4	Full cover
Lower abdomen	1	A few midline hairs
	2	A midline streak of hair
	3	A midline band of hair
	4	An inverted V shaped growth
Upper arm	1	Sparse growth affecting not more than a quarter of limb surface
	2	More than this, cover still incomplete
	3	Light complete cover
	4	Heavy complete cover
Forearm	1-4	Complete cover of dorsal surface: very light (1) to very heavy (4) growth
Thigh	1-4	As for arm
Leg	1-4	As for arm

1. Ferriman DM, Gallwey JD (1961). Clinical assessment of body hair growth in women. *J Clin Endocrinol* **21**: 1440–1447.

Hirsutism: investigations and treatment

Investigations

- Total serum testosterone measurement anytime in the cycle—elevated in only 40% of women but levels rarely correlate with severity of hirsutism or acne. In idiopathic hirsutism, levels are under 3nmol/l, in PCOS <5nmol/l and if levels are >5nmol/l, tests of adrenal function are required—refer to endocrinologists.
- Hormone tests that are not always required include follicular phase 17 hydroxyprogesterone to detect non-congenital adrenal hyperplasia, TSH, 24h urinary-free cortisol (best screening test for Cushing's syndrome).
- Measure serum prolactin, if irregular periods.
- Pelvic ultrasound—to exclude PCOS and ovarian neoplasms.
- CT scanning for assessment of adrenal glands is best done by endocrinologists.

Treatment

- Serious underlying causes are rare.
- Majority of women have benign hirsutism.
- Encourage weight loss if obesity and hirsutism co-exist.
- Direct treatment to the underlying pathology.
- Surgical removal of adrenal or ovarian neoplasm is indicated, if present.
- In primary care, cosmetic treatments, COCP, and topical eflornithine hydrochloride can be used.

Cosmetic treatment

- Waxing, shaving, and plucking.
- Electrolysis is permanent and gives better results, but is time-consuming, painful, and expensive. Can result in pit-like scars and pigment changes. It takes 3–6 months to become apparent.
- Recent developments—many different types of laser using photothermolysis techniques. It is a quick technique. Six to nine months treatment is required, some scarring, erythema, oedema, blistering may occur, not widely available.

COCP

Can be initiated in primary care. Start on a COCP with low androgenic effect. Oestrogen and progestogen suppress ovarian steroidogenesis. Oestrogen increases circulating levels of sex hormone binding globulin (SHBG), which results in decreased concentration of free testosterone in the serum (suppression can continue for 2 years after cessation of treatment). Progestins inhibit 5 alpha reductase activity and increase metabolic clearance of both testosterone and dihydrotestosterone. (📖 See Chapter 13, p.359.) Treatment is recommended for 1–2 years. The COCP can increase insulin resistance in PCOS. (📖 See Chapter 13, p.359). In the UK, Dianette® containing co-cyprindiol 2000/35 (cyproterone acetate 2mg, ethinylestradiol 35μg) is licensed for moderately severe hirsutism. However, there is evidence that it increases the risk of

VTE and is not licensed for indefinite use. Yasmin® contains drospirenone (its anti-androgenic property is similar to that of spironolactone) and ethinylestradiol. Drospirenone blocks androgen receptors and inhibits ovarian androgen production.

Anti-androgens

Cyproterone acetate reduces luteinizing hormone (LH) secretion and testosterone production, blocks androgen-receptor binding, and inhibits 5 alpha reductase activity. Cyproterone in higher doses is unlicensed for hirsutism, but can be used in secondary care. Check LFTs after 6 months and then annually due to the risk of liver toxicity with high doses only.

Topical treatments

Eflornithine hydrochloride cream inhibits an enzyme that is essential for synthesis of polyamines, which are necessary for cell division. This may be used in conjunction with COCP. There is a 58% improvement in facial hair. Use should be discontinued if no improvement in 8 weeks. Side-effects include tingling, burning, erythema, and rash.

Referral to secondary care

- Consider if sudden onset or very severe hirsutism.
- Serum testosterone >5nmol/l.
- Secondary amenorrhoea and/or infertility with hirsutism.
- Refractory hirsutism (fails to respond to standard COCP and topical treatments).

Hirsutism: medication prescribed in secondary care

Spironolactone

Used commonly if COCP contraindicated, or does not help, or as a last resort in unresponsive and severe cases.

It is an anti-androgen and aldosterone antagonist. There is a statistically significant reduction in hair growth. More effective compared to finasteride and cyproterone acetate. Less effective compared to flutamide. The dose is different in lean and obese hirsute women and lower doses should be used in elderly women. If contraception is desired, the COCP can be added. Side-effects are polydipsia, polyurea, nausea, headache, fatigue, gastritis, and ovulatory dysfunction. Treatment requires careful monitoring of renal function.

Flutamide

Another anti-androgen not widely used in the UK, and has a high cost. There is a 70% reduction in hair growth at 1 year. It is likely to interfere with normal development of a male foetus and additional contraception is required. It has minimal side-effects, though hepatoxicity can occur and can be combined with GnRH agonists.

Finasteride

Not widely used in the UK and is licensed for treatment of prostatic cancer and male-pattern baldness. At present there is conflicting evidence regarding its safety. It can be a useful alternative to spironolactone. It is no more effective than cyproterone acetate. Side-effects include dry skin, headaches, gastro-intestinal disturbances, and decreased libido. Contraception is required.

Insulin-sensitizing agents

In PCOS, they improve insulin sensitivity and corresponding improvement in hirsutism. (📖 See PCOS p.110.)

GnRH agonists

Reserved for severe cases, the agonists suppress pituitary FSH and LH secretion, resulting in ovarian suppression and improved insulin sensitivity. Residual benefits persist for 6 months after discontinuation of therapy. Side-effects are: hot flushes, vaginal dryness, decreased breast size, and mood swings. After 6 months treatment, 4% loss of bone mineral density (BMD) occurs, adding a COCP can eliminate side-effects and bone loss.

Resources

For health professionals:

Shaw RW, Soutter WP and Stanton SL (2003) *Gynaecology* 3rd edn. Hirsutism and virilisation, Churchill Livingstone, p. 387.

For women:

www.pcos-uk.org.uk

Premature ovarian failure (POF): definition, assessment, and diagnosis

Definition

POF is the cessation of menstruation before the natural age of the menopause. This is generally before the age of 40.

The clinical features are: menopausal symptoms due to oestrogen deficiency, amenorrhoea, and elevated FSH and LH with low oestradiol.

POF is caused by ovarian follicle depletion. It may occur just before or after menarche and affects 1% women under the age of 40.

It is responsible for 4–18% of women presenting with secondary amenorrhoea and 10–28% of primary amenorrhoea.

Women who are diagnosed with POF are often completely unprepared as they are diagnosed in what is usually considered the most fertile period of their reproductive life. This group of women have very special and different needs to the general menopausal population. Women of a young age have an increased risk of health problems. These include: osteoporosis and cardiovascular disease.

Assessment and diagnosis

In some women, POF may present as primary amenorrhoea (📖 see Primary amenorrhoea, p.100). However, women present more commonly with secondary amenorrhoea (📖 see Secondary amenorrhoea, p.104).

History

Careful history is needed, with particular attention to:

- Menstrual cycle—about 50% of women will have infrequent or dysfunctional bleeding leading up to POF. Ask about age of menarche and cycle length in the past. Women also may have a sudden onset of amenorrhoea after delivery or on stopping the combined contraceptive pill. Women with secondary amenorrhoea will complain of vasomotor symptoms, which may have been while menstruation was occurring.
- General gynaecological history (📖 see Chapter 3, p.21).
- Is she in a sexual relationship and planning or trying for a baby?
- History of radiotherapy or surgical removal of ovaries—as there is a known cause assessment and investigations are limited.
- Menopausal symptoms, such as hot flushes, night sweats, and vaginal dryness (📖 see Chapter 9, p.221).
- As there can be an association with other medical conditions, screening may involve looking for hypothyroidism, Addison's, and diabetes mellitus.
- Consider other causes for secondary amenorrhoea and their symptoms, such as pituitary adenomas, hypothalamic disorder, PCOS, and recent stress in her life.

- Ask about a familial component.
- Enquire specifically about psychosocial issues and explore concerns.

Examination

- Measure her BMI.
- Abdominal and pelvic examination, if her symptoms warrant it or as specified in secondary amenorrhoea, p.104.

Investigations

- Measure FSH in at least two separate cycles or months. POF is shown by raised concentrations of FSH >20IU/l. An FSH of <10IU/l is not diagnostic of ovarian failure.
- TSH.
- Autoimmune screen.
- Chromosome analysis.
- Bone density scan dual energy X-ray absorptiometry (DEXA).

Premature ovarian failure (POF): causes and treatment

Causes

There are many causes of POF and, in many cases, a cause may not be found.

Chromosomal abnormalities

There is a requirement in all women for two intact X chromosomes for normal ovarian function. In women with Turner's syndrome, one of the X chromosomes is absent, which leads to ovarian failure. Up to 30% women with POF have another female relative who is affected. The mode of inheritance here is X-linked and either dominant or recessive. Fragile X syndrome is where there are mutations. The mutations occur 10 times more commonly in women with POF.

FSH-receptor gene polymorphism and inhibin B mutation

These are mutations of the FSH-binding sites and the gene for FSH receptors and also LH receptors. The resistance to the actions of gonadotrophins can lead to the symptoms of POF.

Autoimmune disease

Autoimmune oophoritis may occur by itself or with other endocrine disorders, such as Addison's disease (3%), diabetes (2.5%), hypothyroidism (25%), lupus, Crohn's disease, myasthenia gravis, and rheumatoid arthritis. There has been some research that has shown antibodies directed to the ovary may be implicated, although this is not fully understood.

Viral infections

POF has been found after malaria and shingles. It has also occurred after mumps, but ovarian function can return when the infection has cleared.

Iatrogenic

Chemotherapy and radiotherapy can cause POF, as does bilateral oophorectomy. Hysterectomy without oophorectomy may impact on ovarian function.

Unexplained enzyme deficiencies

There are a number of these that are associated with POF. The most common is galactossaemia.

Treatment

Medical treatment

The standard treatment for POF is HRT (see Chapter 9, p.221). This is initially in higher doses (2mg estradiol valerate, 1.25mg conjugated equine estrogens with or without progestogens as needed, or 75–100μg transdermal patches) but can use lower doses, if asymptomatic. HRT is needed to maintain sexual function, to decrease the risks of cardiovascular problems and osteoporosis, and to improve symptoms of oestrogen deficiency. The bone density of patients with POF will have started to decline before the last menstrual period, with 50% of women having a decreased bone density within the first 2 years of diagnosis. HRT in this group of women can be used to the age of natural menopause. However, duration of treatment and choice of route of administration must be made on an individual basis. There is no evidence that the use of HRT in this age group increases the risk of breast cancer to over and above the peer group of menstruating women. Levels of testosterone drop by 20% after a natural menopause. Women may need to use additional testosterone, if they have low libido and/or tiredness.

📖 See general advice on the menopause, Chapter 9, p.221.

HRT is not a contraceptive and spontaneous pregnancy has been reported in women with POF. If women require contraception, then the COCP can be used as a treatment and for contraception. This can also be used in young women who wish to feel the same as their peers.

Psychological

Of major importance in this group of patients is counselling. It is essential that they have adequate information and support to aid the choices and decisions that they need to make. Information needs to be written, as well as verbal, and the use of websites, such as the Daisy Network, can form a vital support network.

Treatment for fertility

Women who are about to undergo chemotherapy and radiotherapy should be counselled in the risks to fertility. There are now fertility sparing measures that can be employed with ovum preservation (📖 see Chapter 17, p.447). Women who present with spontaneous POF should be advised that there is a spontaneous conception rate of up to 10% and that the use of drugs to induce ovulation does not help. The only successful way to achieve a pregnancy is with egg donation.

Resources

For health professionals:

Meskhi A and Seif MW (2006) Premature ovarian failure. *Current Opinion in Obstetrics & Gynaecology* **18**: 418–426.

For women:

UK site for women with premature menopause: 🖱 www.daisynetwork.org.uk
US site with multilingual support for women with premature menopause: 🖱 www.pofsupport.org
National gamete donation trust for women in need of oocyte donation: 🖱 www.ngdt.co.uk

Chapter 7

Other disorders of women's health

Fibroids: definition, assesment, and diagnosis

Fibroids are benign tumours that arise from the smooth muscle of the uterus. They are clinically apparent in 30% of women, although there are ethnic differences, and accurate estimation of prevalence is difficult, as 50% fibroids remain asymptomatic. They can vary in size from that of a pea to that of a grapefruit or a melon (📖 see Fig. 7.1). They can be:

- Intramural—develop and are maintained within the wall of the uterus.
- Submucosal—fibroids develop into, or are continued within, the wall of the uterus and are less common. Very occasionally these can prolapse through the cervix.
- Subserosal—develop in the abdomen outside the uterine wall and contribute to the characteristic irregular feel of the fibroid uterus.
- Cervical—are located in the cervix and are rare. These give rise to the greatest surgical difficulty.
- Extra-uterine—in the broad ligaments.

Assessment: symptoms

- Most fibroids are asymptomatic.
- Many women have significant symptoms requiring treatment.

Abnormal uterine bleeding

Characteristic pattern is menorrhagia (prolonged and excessively heavy), (📖 see Chapter 5, p.69). Heavy menstrual bleeding (HMB) can result in iron-deficiency anaemia, is socially embarrassing, and leads to loss of productivity in work force.

Bleeding at other times of the menstrual cycle is not characteristic of fibroids, though inter-menstrual and post-coital bleeding can be seen in women with submucosal fibroids and fibroid 'polyps'.

Pressure symptoms

- Pain in pelvic area due to increased size of the uterus, heaviness, cramps.
- Acute pain can be associated with a pedunculated subserous fibroid undergoing torsion. Red degeneration can also cause acute pain.
- Abdominal swelling.
- Pressure on bladder and/or bowel—associated with constipation and urinary symptoms.
- Pressure on the venous return can increase the risk of thrombosis.

Reproductive dysfunction

- Submucous fibroids—by blocking the tubal ostia and/or distorting the uterine cavity these are likely to cause, or be associated with, subfertility (📖 see Chapter 17, p.447).
- The role of intramural fibroids in causation of subfertility is controversial. (📖 see Chapter 17, p.447).

Pregnancy complications

Large fibroids may interfere with effective placentation and initiate abnormal uterine contractions and pregnancy loss. Other pregnancy complications include: pain, bleeding, red degeneration, mal-presentations, premature labour, postpartum haemorrhage, infection, and failure of uterine involution.

Assessment: examination, investigations

- Abdominal examination may show a pelvic or abdominal mass with an irregular contour.
- Speculum and bimanual examination.
- Full blood count, if there is HMB.
- Ultrasound TAS/TVS can identify the nature of large pelvic masses in over 80% of women in skilled hands. Difficulty may arise in the differential diagnosis of pedunculated fibroids from solid ovarian tumours. TVS is also helpful in demonstrating presence of submucosal fibroids.
- MRI is better at visualizing fibroids but, for most clinical indications, the extra cost may not be justified.
- Hysteroscopy and laparoscopy are diagnostic and often merged into treatment. Hysteroscopy or saline sonography can be helpful in assessing the protusion into the cavity and suitability for resection.
- Laparoscopy may reveal incidental pathology in the pelvis; e.g. presence of adhesions and/or endometriosis in addition to the fibroids.

Causes

- Pathophysiology of fibroids is poorly understood.
- Most fibroids develop in women in their 30s or 40s. Black women are significantly more likely to have fibroids, compared to white women.
- Being parous reduces the chance of developing fibroids.
- There may be a genetic predisposition—myomas are a common phenotype resulting from several different genetic events.
- Steroid hormone concentrations may play a role.
- Angiogenic growth factors. Abnormalities in uterine blood vessels and angiogenic growth factors may be responsible, e.g. basic fibroblast growth factor is higher in women with fibroids.

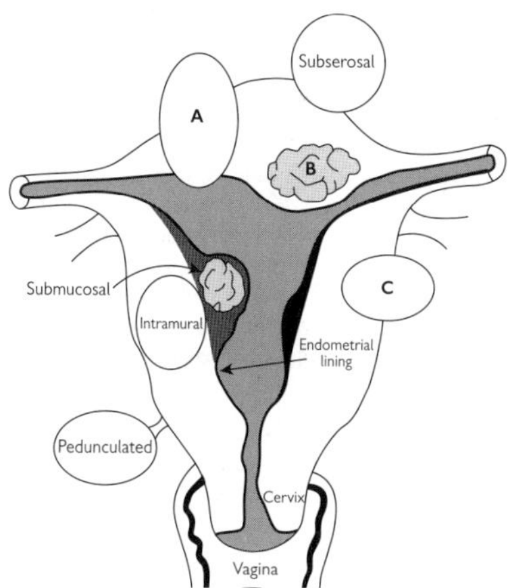

Fig. 7.1 Types of fibroids. Reprinted from Stewart E (2001) Uterine fibroids. *The Lancet* **357**: 293. Copyright 2001, with permission from Elsevier.

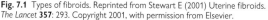

Fibroids: expectant and medical management

Size, number, location, symptoms, woman's age, reproductive plans, and whether or not the uterine cavity is distorted, are all important factors to consider in formulating a management plan.

Expectant management

Appropriate for women who have asymptomatic fibroids. This may also be used for women who request not to have interventions.

Medical treatments

Trial of medical therapy before surgery is reasonable, dependent on symptoms. It allows conservation of the uterus and avoids the complications of surgery.

COCP

COCP may decrease bleeding in some, but not all, women with HMB and a fibroid uterus (see Chapter 5, p.69). COCP is not contraindicated in women with fibroids. However, uterine volume should be monitored to ensure there is no serious enlargement in size or deterioration of symptoms.

Non-steroidal anti-inflammatory preparations

These have not been studied extensively with fibroid-related heavy menstrual bleeding. They do not appear to reduce blood loss in women with fibroids, unless they are used with tranexamic acid (see Chapter 5, p.69).

Levonorgestrel intra-uterine system

Preliminary observational studies show reduction in bleeding with fibroids. Large uterine cavities, more than 12–14 weeks size uterus on bimanual examination and presence of submucosal intracavity fibroids are some of the contraindications (see Fig. 5.1).

GnRH agonists

These initially increase release of gonadotrophins, followed by desensitization and down-regulation to a hypogonadal state resembling menopause. There is a 35–60% reduction in size of fibroid in 3 months. Discontinuation of treatment can result in regrowth of fibroids. They can be given intranasally/subcutaneously. Pre-operative administration for 3 months can facilitate surgery and increase haemoglobin prior to surgery.

With long-term therapy, severe oestrogen-deficiency can result in bone loss. Addition of low-dose oestrogen/progestin therapy or tibolone to GnRH agonists after down-regulation phase can maintain amenorrhoea and prevent osteoporosis and vasomotor symptoms.

Gestrinone

It decreases fibroid volume and induces amenorrhoea. Advantage of this drug is a carry-over effect after discontinuation.

Raloxifene

This is a selective oestrogen-receptor modulator that inhibits fibroid growth in pre-menopausal women, compared to controls, when used for 3 months in a dose of 180mg/day. There is a 30% reduction in fibroid size at 3 months. There is no hypo-oestrogenic state. Larger controlled trials are required to ascertain benefit.

Fibroid management: uterine artery embolization (UAE)

UAE aims to reduce the blood supply to the fibroids inducing shrinkage.

Eligibility for UAE

First line in women with:

- Symptomatic fibroids >3cm size.
- HMB.
- Pressure symptoms.
- Absence of submucosal, calcified, and pedunculated fibroids and adenomyosis.

- Pre-treatment fibroid mapping and MRI are desirable, with gadolinium for enhancement.
- IUD/IUS should be removed prior to UAE.
- Prophylactic broad-spectrum antibiotics are administered prior to the procedure.
- Performed by interventional radiologists, but patient selection should be in conjunction with a gynaecologist.
- Women experience pain, bleeding, and discharge post-procedure.
- Symptom improvement is seen in 62–95% of women—NICE.
- Reduction in mean fibroid volume is 40–75%—NICE.
- Embolization does not compromise fertility, pregnancies following UAE occur—the term live-birth rate is 12–20% but, they are high-risk pregnancies.

Complications of UAE

- Post-embolization syndrome, with fever, infections, and myalgia, is seen in 50% of women.
- Ovarian dysfunction occurs in 2.5–14% of women.
- Amenorrhoea rate variable—more age-related.
- Late expulsion of fibroid seen in 2.2–7.7% of women.
- There is a need for hysterectomy in 0.5–11.8% of women within 24 months.
- 12% risk of major adverse events after UAE and 20% after surgery at 1 year.
- 34% minor complication rate with UAE compared to 20% with surgery (REST study).[1]

Benefits of UAE

- More cost-effective and faster recovery, compared to surgery.
- Sexuality is significantly better after UAE, compared to surgery.
- Follow-up includes ultrasound at 3 and 6 months, and a follow-up with the gynaecologist.
- At 3 years, 20% require secondary intervention to treat persistent symptoms, which can only be myomectomy and hysterectomy—not re-embolization.

1. Edwards RG, Moss JG, Murray L (2007). The Scottish Randomized Study of Embolization and Surgical Treatment for Uterine fibroids (RESTROIDS study). *New England Journal of Medicine* **356**(4): 360–370.

Fibroid management: surgical treatment

Laparoscopic myolysis

A variation on the technique of laparoscopic myomectomy, as tissue is coagulated and not removed. Indicated for women with < 4 fibroids and who have completed child-bearing.

Myomectomy

This involves the individual removal of each leiomyoma. It is a useful option for women who wish to retain their uterus and desire future pregnancies.

Laparoscopic myomectomy

May be indicated in women with uterine size under 14 weeks or women who have a small number of <5cm size subserosal or intramural fibroids. (A deep intramural fibroid is a contraindication.) Use of an electric morcellator may be an advantage. There is controversy whether uterine wall strength will be as good after laparoscopic suturing as after conventional myomectomy.

Abdominal myomectomy

Indicated for significantly enlarged uterus and multiple myomas. The risk of unplanned hysterectomy after myomectomy is <1% for experienced surgeons. The risk of recurrence of fibroids is 50–60% at 5 years. There are disadvantages of hospitalization, blood loss, and operating time.

The risk of a second operation ranges from 10 to 25%. There is need for an elective Caesarean section with a pregnancy, to reduce the risk of uterine rupture with labour. The term live-birth rate after a myomectomy is 40%.

Hysteroscopic myomectomy

Indicated for a submucous fibroid which is <5cm size and >50% of volume of the tumour projects into the uterine cavity. The submucous fibroid may be associated with abnormal bleeding, pain, subfertility, and/or recurrent pregnancy loss. It is usually undertaken as a day case with a short recovery period. It is generally carried out by a highly skilled hysteroscopic practitioner. Fewer than 16% of women report second procedures after 9 years. There are no reports of risk of uterine rupture after a hysteroscopic myomectomy. If the fibroids are large, or there has been significant fluid absorption, then, it can be undertaken as a two-stage procedure. The subsequent fertility rates are good.

Hysteroscopic myomectomy with endometrial ablation

May be considered in submucous fibroids, when women have completed their family. The uterus should be <10 weeks size. Great care is required with choice of ablating device as the cavity may be irregular.

Hysterectomy

Fibroids are the most common indication for hysterectomy. Cumulative risk of a hysterectomy for fibroids in black women is 7–20%. There is no risk of recurrence of fibroids. Morbidity associated with hysterectomy may outweigh benefits in some women with fibroids. Laparoscopic subtotal hysterectomy can often be done as a day case, removes the mass effect, stops the bleeding, and preserves the ovaries. However, total hysterectomies may be carried out as laparoscopic-assisted or abdominal hysterectomies. (📖 See Chapter 12 for types of hysterectomy and operations.) Hysterectomy may sometimes become necessary in women with acute haemorrhage.

MRI-focused ultrasound ablation

Shows promise but is still a research tool with limited availability.

Resources

Patient information leaflets from clinical knowledge summaries:
- www.cks.library.nhs.uk
- www.nice.org.uk
- www.rcog.org.uk

Endometriosis risk factors and aetiology

Endometriosis is one of the most common benign gynaecological conditions. It is present in 10–25% of women presenting with gynaecological symptoms in the UK or USA.

Risk factors

- Primarily a disease of the reproductive years.
- Japanese women have twice the incidence of Caucasian women.
- Greater frequency in women of higher social class.
- Exposure to menstruation, e.g. early menarche, short and heavy menstrual cycles, late menopause, puts women at higher risk.
- Risk is lower among current and recent users of the COCP, compared to non-users.
- In women with a family history, the risk of developing it is seven times higher.

Aetiology

- It is the result of complex interplay between the shed endometrial tissue, the peritoneal environment, and the peritoneal lining.
- Menstrual reflux theory. Retrograde menstrual flow transports endometrial fragments through fallopian tubes into the peritoneal cavity. Some of the viable cells subsequently implant.
- Metaplasia theory. Prolonged irritation and oestrogen stimulation result in metaplasia of the original coelomic epithelium to endometrial like tissue.
- Genetic factors. Polygenic inheritance with a risk of 5–7% for first degree relatives.
- Angiogenesis—shed endometrial tissue is highly angiogenic.
- Production of antibodies against endometrial cells may have a role.
- Inadequate peritoneal defence mechanisms may determine development of the disease.
- Immune factors may be aetiological or a secondary response. In healthy women, endometrial cells misplaced into the peritoneal cavity are characterized by increased apoptosis and eliminated readily by the immune system, but, in women with endometriosis, these cells implant and proliferate in ectopic locations, to eliminate these cells a profound local immune response is set up. But the immune cells exploit this process to their own growth potential.

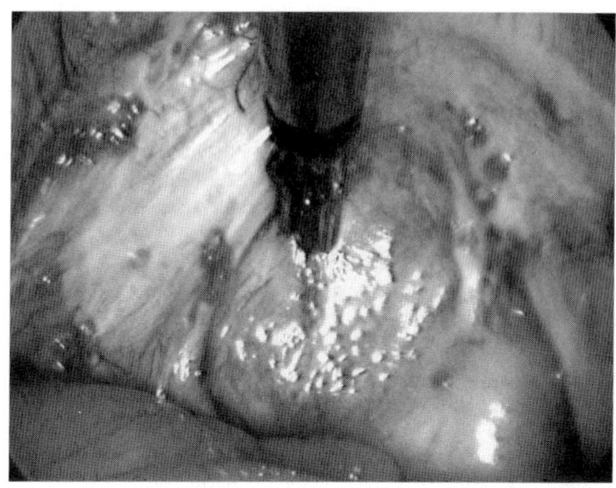

Fig. 7.2 Endometriosis—laparoscopic view.

Endometriosis assessment

History

- Gynaecological and obstetrical history.
- Some women have no symptoms and this may be found on laparoscopy for other indications such as sterilization.
- Recurrent painful periods—severe dysmenorrhoea—60–80% women—elicit cyclical nature of pain, severity and/or association with other symptoms like pelvic pain.
- Painful intercourse—deep dyspareunia—in 25–40% women.
- Chronic lower abdominal, pelvic, and lower back pain—in 30–50% women. Constant, aching, dragging pain may be exacerbated by menses, due to stretching of tissues and local production of prostaglandins within the ectopic endometrial tissue.
- Subfertility in 30–40%.
- Painful micturition in 1–2%, manifesting as cystitis or cyclical haematuria.
- Infrequent presentation is obstructive uropathy.
- Painful defecation during menses dyschezia in 1–2%, due to gastro-intestinal tract endometriosis.
- Cyclical rectal bleeding may occur, 62% of endometriotic bowel disease is multifocal, and 38% is multicentric.

Examination

- Abdominal examination is generally not rewarding but should be undertaken to exclude any masses and/or tenderness.
- Pelvic bimanual examination—the detection is improved by examination during menses—a fixed retroverted uterus with adnexal tenderness and cervical excitation is suggestive. The uterosacral ligaments are tender, but nodular posterior pelvic endometriosis is not easily palpable at vaginal examination.
- Rarely, disease may be visible in the vagina or cervix—blueberry lesions.

Assessment: investigations

- Imaging techniques like ultrasound lack resolution to visualize superficial peritoneal and ovarian implants and adhesions. However, TVS can detect ovarian endometriomata >2cm size, solid nodules within posterior vaginal wall, and/ or bladder nodules. TVS is superior to laparoscopy in detecting mild ovarian endometriosis. TVS is less expensive compared to MRI and should be first line.
- In posterior pelvic endometriosis, MRI can be combined with TVS to determine the extent of disease and MRI can pick up endometriomata >1cm size.
- Laparoscopy. Visual inspection of the pelvis at laparoscopy for endometriosis is the gold standard. It can sometimes be difficult to delineate the endometriotic lesions from fibromuscular tissue. The use of laparoscopy for diagnosis of endometriosis is important but it is an invasive procedure, has limited reproducibility, and gas ball artefacts can complicate visualization. Biopsy of at least one lesion is advisable at laparoscopy (📖 see Fig. 7.2).

- Serum marker Ca125 is elevated, though sensitivity and specificity is low. Measuring CA125 has no value as a diagnostic tool.
- IVP to exclude obstructive uropathy.
- Barium enema studies, as appropriate.
- Rectal sonography can be used to evaluate the thickness of the uterosacral ligaments and presence of rectal involvement, but seldom required.

Laparoscopic features of ovarian endometriomata

- Adherent to pelvic side-wall and posterior side of the broad ligament and/or uterus.
- There is usually a tarry thick chocolate fluid content.
- Retraction of ovarian cortex.
- Powder-burns and pink, red, blue or black spots on the ovaries.

Medical treatment of endometriosis

Symptom recurrence is common following any medical treatment of endometriosis.

NSAIDs

There is inconclusive evidence of efficacy in pain management and they have no beneficial effect on the disease. May be administered orally. Gastro-intestinal side-effects can occur.

COCP, Depo-Provera®

The COCP can be used on an extended regimen without hormone-free breaks. Can be used long term. Weight changes, menstrual disruption, and bloating can occur with injectable progestogens. eg. Depo-Provera®.

Danazol

Restricted to use for 6 months. Is rarely used due to side-effect profile of weight gain, abnormal and excessive hair growth, acne, bloating, adverse effect on lipid profile.

GnRH analogues

⚠ Restricted to 6 months use due to bone demineralization in 60% of women after 6 months. Adding oestrogen and progestogens can protect against bone mineral loss during, and for up to 6 months after treatment. Combined treatment can be continued for up to 2 years and is effective. Bone demineralization is protected by 'add back' therapy (continuous combined HRT or tibolone). Can be administered as an injection or nasal spray. Hot flushes can occur in most women due to hypo-oestrogenism.

Other medical therapy

Preliminary data show aromatase inhibitors like letrozole may be effective but associated with significant bone loss, they inhibit oestrogen production in endometriotic lesions without affecting ovarian function.

LNG-IUS

Reduces endometriosis associated pain (dysmenorrhoea, dyspareunia) with extensive pelvic and rectovaginal endometriosis. The LNG-IUS can help with adenomyosis and has similar efficacy to GnRH analogues. The benefit of LNG-IUS after surgery requires clarification. LNG-IUS inserted after laparoscopic surgery for endometriosis-associated pain, significantly reduced the risk of recurrence of moderate and severe dysmenorrhoea at 1-year follow-up.[1]

Medical treatment of endometriosis-associated subfertility (📖 see also Chapter 7, p.127)

Hormonal treatment is indicated in severe disease but is not effective in mild to moderate disease, where there may be a lost opportunity to conceive with the treatment. Treatment with GnRH agonists for 3–6 months before IVF in women with endometriosis increases the pregnancy rates.

1. Abou-Setta AM, Al-Inany HG, Farquhar CM (2006) LNG-IUS for Symptomatic Endometriosis Following Surgery, *Cochrane Database of systematic review* 4: CD0050D.

Surgical management of endometriosis-associated pain

Laparoscopic ablation/excision of endometriosis lesions

By laser or diathermy is clearly effective for a large number of women. There are limited data. More women report symptomatic improvement after initial excision surgery, compared to ablation with a 63% improvement following laparoscopic ablation and an 80% improvement following excision. The cumulative recurrence rate is 20% at 5 years.

Laparoscopic uterine nerve ablation (LUNA)

LUNA does not reduce endometriosis-associated pain and may be unnecessary. It involves division of sensory parasympathetic fibres to the cervix and the sensory sympathetic fibres to the uterus, close to their point of attachment to the cervix, using laser/electrosurgery. It may be beneficial when there is a failure to respond to conservative treatment.

Presacral neurectomy (PSN)

A complex procedure that has not been completely evaluated. Success rate is dependent on expertise. Cochrane review concludes PSN to be more effective, compared to conservative surgery alone.

Radical surgery

Total Abdominal hysterectomy bilateral sarpingo-oophorectomy (TAH BSO) removes the entire lesions in severe and deeply infiltrating endometriosis, resulting in improved pain relief[1]. In a 'frozen pelvis', a subtotal hysterectomy may be safer.

Bladder and bowel endometriosis

Management by multidisciplinary teams in tertiary centres is the preferred option. Radical extirpation of the disease confers very real benefits. Debulking of rectal lesions, disc resection, and/or large-scale bowel resection may be required. There appears to be no consensus on the range of surgical procedures required to help in advanced endometriosis.

Surgical options for endometriosis-associated subfertility

For mild to moderate disease, ablation and adhesiolysis is effective, particularly in relation to ongoing pregnancy and live-irth rates.

In severe disease, no randomized controlled trials (RCTs) are available to answer the question of whether surgery for severe disease improves pregnancy rates.

For ovarian endometriomas larger than 4cm, laparoscopic cystectomy is better, compared to drainage and coagulation of the cyst wall. Tubal flushing is associated with a significant increase in the odds of pregnancy in subfertile women. Women should be warned about the risk of poor ovarian reserve. Intra-uterine insemination improves fertility in mild endometriosis. IVF is indicated if tubal function is compromised, if there is male-factor subfertility, and if other treatments have failed (📖 see Chapter 17, p.447).

1 Royal College of Obstetricians and Gynaecologists (2006). The investigation and management of endometriosis. *Cochrane database of systematic review*, guideline **24**. www.rcog.org.uk (Accessed January 2009.)

Complementary therapy

- High-frequency TENS may help.
- Vitamin B1 and magnesium may help to relieve endometriosis related dysmenorrhoea.
- Reflexology and diet may sometimes prove helpful.
- Acupuncture may help with pain management.
- There is an enormous role of patient-support groups.

Resources

www.endometriosis.org.uk
www.clinicalevidence.org

Chronic pelvic pain (CPP): causes

Chronic pelvic pain (CPP) is defined as any pelvic pain that lasts more than 6 months. It affects approximately 1 in 6 of the adult female population of reproductive age, and is thought to be one of the most difficult problems encountered by the healthcare professional. It has the following causes.

Endometriosis

The presence of endometrium outside of the uterus.

Pelvic inflammatory disease

This may be a chronic condition of recurrent episodes of upper genital tract infection or the residual damage caused by past episodes.

Adhesions

It remains unclear whether adhesions are a cause of pelvic pain, but recent studies have suggested that destroying adhesions facilitates pain relief. It is estimated that in 40% of women with pelvic pain, adhesions are the cause.

Bowel-related pain

Irritable bowel syndrome is often diagnosed in the absence of other diagnostic features. This is a common condition that affects 20% of the population. It is a functional disease, meaning that there are usually other symptoms present, such as change in bowel habit.

Bladder-related pain

The main causes are interstitial cystitis and urethral syndrome. Both conditions have related urinary symptoms and thus are not responsible for pelvic pain alone.

Pelvic congestion

Caused by venous dilatation and engorgment of the pelvic veins.

Other causes

There are many other causes for pelvic pain, which ensure diagnosis is complex. These include:

- musculoskeletal pain;
- muscle pain;
- poor posture;
- nerve-related pain;
- referred pain;
- neuropathic pain; and
- psychologically-influenced pain.

1. Royal College of Obstetricians and Gynaecologists (2005) The initial management of chronic pelvic pain. *Guideline* **41**: 1–12. www.rcog.org.uk (Accessed January 2009.)

Chronic pelvic pain (CPP): diagnosis

History

This initial contact with the patient, if handled in an empathetic manner, will set the scene for the physical examination that will occur later and can often be emotionally stressful for the patient with pelvic pain. CPP is a complex syndrome with interplay between biological and psychosocial phenomena.[1] The clinician must remain alert at all times to subliminal indicators that may arise during consultation.

- Ask about the location of the pain, when and how it commenced, whether it is constant or intermittent, does it radiate, what makes it worse and what makes it better?
- (pqrst = palliative/provocative, quality, region, severity, timing) is a, useful acronym to describe pain.
- The use of a pain score is useful as a baseline for future consultations.
- Is it related to the menstrual cycle?
- Is it related to intercourse?
- What type of contraception is in use?
- Is there any unusual discharge or bleeding?
- Are there any symptoms affecting bowels or micturition?
- Past history of pelvic inflammatory disease (PID) and/or ectopic pregnancy.
- Sexual history.
- Menstrual history—LMP, inter-menstrual bleeding, post-coital bleeding, dyspareunia.

Examination

- Observe how the patient moves and lays on the couch.
- Check routine observations of temperature, pulse, and blood pressure.
- Abdominal examination should be undertaken to elicit site of pain, (with chronic pain the site of tenderness is more difficult to identify), if any rebound tenderness or guarding, and palpate for masses or hernia.
- Pelvic examination is undertaken to include speculum examination, observation of the mucosa, cervix, and note any discharge.
- Bimanual examination will reveal cervical excitation (pain on movement). This may indicate blood in the peritoneal cavity (ectopic pregnancy) or inflammation of the peritoneum (PID). Examination should aim to excude adnexal masses.
- Pelvic examination should be avoided if ovarian hyperstimulation syndrome or ectopic pregnancy is strongly suspected.

Investigations

- Triple swabs should be obtained to exclude sexually transmitted infections (high vaginal, urethral, and endocervical).
- Urine should be dip tested and sent for pathological examination, as appropriate.
- A pregnancy test should be performed.
- Blood samples for full blood count, and C-reactive protein should be obtained.
- Pelvic ultrasound should be undertaken to exclude pelvic pathologies.
- Laparoscopy is the gold standard investigation for chronic pelvic pain, although in 40% of cases, no cause for pelvic pain will be found. In those with abnormal findings, endometriosis and adhesions account for 85%.[2] 📖 See Fig. 7.3.

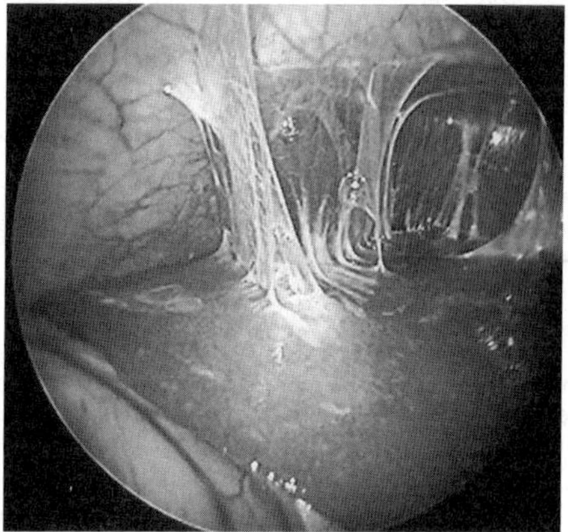

Fig. 7.3 Adhesions.

1. Tin-Chui, Li and Ledger, WL (eds) (2006) *Chronic pelvic pain*. p.11 Taylor and Francis, London.
2. Ng, C and Trew, G (2006) Common causes and protocol for investigation of chronic pelvic pain. In: Tin-Chui, Li and Ledger, WL (eds) (2006) *Chronic pelvic pain*. p.31 Taylor and Francis, London.

Chronic pelvic pain (CPP): treatment

Treatment is dependent on diagnosis. Often there is more than one treatment, as there are frequently multiple interactive problems.

Physiotherapy

Physiotherapy can be an integral facet to treatment options. The aim is to improve abnormal musculoskeletal physiology. Myofascial trigger points may be located and treated explicitly. Specific exercises may be taught. Equally, TENS (transcutaneous electrical nerve stimulation), muscle stimulators, or ultrasound may be used.

Psychological treatment

Cognitive behaviour therapies are the most widely used and provide the strongest empirical support.[1] The treatment approach provides strategies and skills for controlling pain.

Medications

Analgesics

These are used as a supportive measure. The WHO analgesic ladder[2] should be used:

- **Mild pain**—administer non-opioid medication.
- **Mild to moderate pain**—administer weak opioid plus non-opioid ± adjuvant.
- **Moderate to severe pain**—administer strong opioid plus non-opioid ± adjuvant.

Side-effects for all medications must be explained and balanced against the relief gained. Analgesics may be more effective if combined with certain anti-depressants, which have a direct effect on pain transmission (e.g. amitriptyline).

Hormonal suppression

- Oral contraceptives, such as the combined pill. Continuous use may be beneficial in suppressing the pain associated with oestrogen and progesterone withdrawal. Medroxprogesterone acetate, or the levonorgestrel intra-uterine device (Mirena®) may be used.
- Danazol, a synthetic androgen, has been found to be effective in pain control.
- Gonadotrophin-releasing hormone analogues (GnRH analogues) are used for periods of up to 6 months for symptom relief. Add-back therapy, with a low-dose hormone treatment, may be required for relief of menopausal symptoms.

CPP may originate from a specific disorder such as irritable bowel syndrome or painful bladder syndrome and treatment should be administered accordingly.

Surgery

Surgical therapy is usually aimed at removal of the suspected cause of pain. This may be endometriosis, division of adhesions, or removal of an ovarian remnant.

Laparoscopic adhesiolysis

Effectiveness is controversial, as adhesions will reform in many instances and current evidence is limited. Adhesions form in up to 90% of patients at the time of gynaecological surgery. Prevention of adhesions at the time of surgery is preferable to attempts to remove these at a later time.

Laparoscopic excision/ablation of endometriosis

Results are dependent on the skills and experience of the surgeon.

A final decision may be made to perform a total hysterectomy ± removal of the ovaries.

1 Morley, SM, Eccleston, C and Williams, A (1999) Systematic review and meta-analysis of randomized controlled trials of cognitive behavior therapy and behavior therapy for chronic pain in adults, excluding headache pain. *Pain* **80**(1–2): 1–13.

2 World Health Organization (1996) *Cancer pain relief.* WHO. Geneva.

Chronic pelvic pain (CPP): multidisciplinary chronic pain management

The Royal College of Obstetricians and Gynaecologists (RCOG) in 2005 recommended that there should be a multidisciplinary treatment approach between gynaecologists, physiotherapists, pain services, and psychologists.[1] Also, that pain clinics be established with NHS funding to support these services. Currently, only 4% of trusts have some form of multidisciplinary service for CPP.[2] Existing evidence indicates that the multidisplinary-team approach is the most effective approach for CPP.

The team should have common goals, to ensure that:

- treatable disease has been diagnosed;
- explanation and support are maximized;
- the multi-factorial cause of pain is acknowledged;
- anxiety is reduced;
- the need for cure is broken down with the woman redirected towards pain management.

Nurses are in a prime position to support and drive this type of initiative. It is recognized by Sadler that often nurses bring additional skills and expertise to the healthcare team and thus enhance its reputation.[3]
The multidisciplinary approach involves the evaluation of somatic and psychological components by all disciplines.

Where it is not possible for all disciplines to be actively involved with the patient, Pearce and Curtis describe the benefits of group meetings for patients, counselling, and information giving.[4] It is suggested that written information should be accessible on the subjects, as in 📖 Table 7.1. A patient information leaflet is available from the RCOG on *Pelvic inflammatory disease*.[1]

CPP is a common problem affecting a large proportion of women with far-reaching implications for lifestyle and social functioning. The common approach to treatment has been limited and has not focused on self-management. The aim should be to optimize treatment and to use the skills and knowledge of healthcare professionals to address and improve service provision.

Resources

www.pelvicpain.org.uk
www.endo.org.uk
www.ibsnetwork.org.uk
www.womenshealthlondon.org.uk.

Royal College of Obstetricians and Gynaecologists (2005) The initial management of chronic pelvic pain. *Guideline* **41**: 1–12.

Royal College of Obstetricians and Gynaecologists (2006) The investigation and management of endometriosis. *Guideline* **2**.

Tin-Chui, Li and Ledger, WL (eds) (2006) *Chronic pelvic pain*. Taylor and Francis, London.

Table 7.1 Information leaflets produced for the management of CPP

Acute/chronic pain	To explain the differences in the meaning of pain and the appropriate management of chronic pain.
The Medical Model	To demonstrate how the medical model does not apply to chronic pain and introduce pain physiology.
Pain Perception and the Gate Theory	To increase understanding of how pain is perceived and how pain can be altered physiologically.
Stress	To explain the effect of stress on the pain experience and introduce relaxation.
Negative thinking	To explain how the pain experience can be changed by thought processes.
Exercise	To introduce the benefits of exercise in the treatment of chronic pain including pelvic floor exercises.
Drug therapies	To explain how drug therapies may work and how to use drugs safely and appropriately.
Sleep problems	To give advice on how to improve sleep.
Healthy eating	To give advice on the benefits of diet to maintain a healthy body acknowledging irritable bowel syndrome, which may be of particular relevance.
Sexual problems	To introduce and acknowledge a subject that can be a significant problem to some women with CPP.
Alternative therapies	To introduce alternative therapies that may be helpful in the management of pelvic pain.

1 Royal College of Obstetricians and Gynaecologists (2005) The initial management of chronic pelvic pain. *Guideline* **41**: 1–12.
2 Argent, V (2003) Chronic pelvic pain. *The Pain Society Newsletter*, **Autumn**: 18–19.
3 Sadler, C (2004) At the cutting edge. *Nursing Standard* **18**(39): 16–17.
4 Pearce, C and Curtis, M (2007) A multidisciplinary approach to self care in chronic pain. *British Journal of Nursing* **16**(2): 82–85.

Benign ovarian tumours: pathology and assessment

90% of all ovarian tumours are benign and most of them are cystic. The presence of solid elements makes malignancy more likely. Fibroids, dermoids, Brenner tumours, and thecomas are benign, but may have some solid elements.

Pathology

Functional ovarian cysts

These are largely asymptomatic, are found incidentally sometimes on ultrasound, and mostly occur in reproductive age. They arise in the normal process of ovulation and are always benign. Follicular cysts are more common than luteal cysts. The smaller cysts generally resolve, some may grow up to 10cm size and become symptomatic. Multiple functional cysts can occur as a result of excessive stimulation by gonadotrophins.

Benign epithelial tumours

These are most common tumours and arise from mesothelium. They may be mucinous cystadenomata, endometrial (endometrioid), or tubal (serous) or uroepithelial (Brenner). Serous cystadenomas are most common, usually unilocular with thin fluid and bilateral in 10% cases. Mucinous cystadenomas are second most common and can grow to a large size, they are usually multiloculated. Brenner tumours are rare and generally small in size; some secrete oestrogens and can be associated with abnormal bleeding.

Benign germ cell tumours

Mostly occur in young women. Overall, 2–3% can be malignant. They arise from germ cells and may contain elements of all three germ layers. Most common is dermoid cyst: it is unilocular, <15cm and contains ectodermal (hair, teeth, sebaceous material), endodermal, and mesodermal elements. 60% of dermoid cysts are asymptomatic; torsion and rupture are rare. Mature, solid teratomas contain mature tissue and fewer cystic areas.

Benign sex cord stromal tumours

Rare—most are solid and can occur at any age from puberty to menopause. These are: granulose cell tumours (some of these produce oestrogens); theca cell tumours, many of which produce oestrogens; fibromas and sertoli leydig cell tumours, many of which produce androgens.

Assessment

Assessment: history

- Should include details of presenting symptoms, full menstrual, obstetric, family history, medication, and contraception.
- Presentation—asymptomatic, detected during pelvic examination or ultrasound or:
- Difficulties with sexual intercourse on deep penetration.
- Dyspepsia and early satiety are rare.

- Chronic lower abdominal pain and/or discomfort.
- Oestrogen/androgen effects, precocious puberty.
- Endometriomas are associated with painful heavy periods and/or dyspareunia. (📖 See Endometriosis, p.136.)
- Hirsutism, virilizm and/or acne.
- With large tumours, pressure effects on gastro-intestinal tract—bowel movements may be difficult or pressure may lead to a desire to defecate.
- Pressure effects on urinary tract are possible—frequent micturition.
- Use of POP may increase the incidence of functional ovarian cysts.
- Sudden onset of acute pain with nausea and vomiting may indicate torsion of a cyst.

*Assessment: **examination***

- Abdominal examination indicates distension by fluid or tumour and the size of the mass can be calculated by measurement.
- Bimanual examination—mass may be felt.
- Ultrasound is a primary imaging tool to demonstrate presence of the mass. TAS is better than TVS in evaluating large masses. Functional, simple, complex, haemorrhagic, dermoid, and endometriotic cysts have characteristic features. Ultrasound is not helpful in differentiating hydrosalpinx, para-ovarian, and tubal cysts from ovarian cysts.

*Assessment: **investigations***

- Examination under anaesthesia for a suspected ovarian tumour may be indicated.
- CT scanning offers no advantage over ultrasound.
- MRI is unnecessary in most cases and very seldom required.
- Chest X-ray and abdominal X-ray may be required.
- Barium enema may be indicated with bowel involvement or fixity.
- IVU, if large and suggestion of urinary tract involvement.
- A full blood count and platelet count as appropriate.
- Serum Ca125 measurement is used in various risk of malignancy indices (RMI) but may be elevated in endometriosis.
- Serum oestradiol and androgen levels may be indicated in hormone-secreting tumours.
- Alpha fetoprotein in yolk sac tumours and βhCG to exclude an ectopic pregnancy but germ cell tumours secrete this marker.
- Diagnostic laparoscopy for diagnosis and sometimes in association with the management.

Benign ovarian tumours: principles of prevention and management

Prevention

- Current use of the combined oral contraceptive pill protects against development of all ovarian cysts and tumours, except mucinous adenomas.
- Current and past use of COCP reduces the risk of epithelial ovarian carcinoma.

Management

The finding of an ovarian tumour or cyst generates considerable anxiety for women because of the fear of malignancy.

Asymptomatic woman

Simple cysts <8cm diameter, echo-free, without solid parts or papillary projections in women under 40 years, are usually benign.

- <3cm (some say up to 5cm), leave well alone—conservative treatment.
- 3–8cm, assess and evaluate every 3 months to determine symptom change and increase or decrease in size. Laparoscopy is indicated if significant increase in size of cyst or persistence.
- In women over the age of 50, such cysts are more likely to be malignant (4–18%), therefore, in this age group even if asymptomatic, only cysts under 3cm should be treated conservatively.
- >8cm size, echo-free cysts—best to remove surgically even if asymptomatic.

Asymptomatic cysts in pregnancy

- Essentially management is conservative. Most benign cysts resolve conservatively.
- It is prudent to wait until after 14 weeks gestation before removing it.
- Serum Ca125 is not a useful marker in pregnant women.
- Avoid MRI and CT in first trimester.
- At 6 weeks post-partum, surgery can be undertaken if cyst still present.

Symptomatic woman

- Emergency laparoscopy/laparotomy is indicated if severe acute pain or signs of torsion, signs of intraperitoneal bleeding.
- More chronic symptoms require rigorous evaluation and investigations.

Benign ovarian tumours: surgical treatment

Therapeutic ultrasound-guided aspiration. There is little advantage of aspiration over regular observation, as the chances of reformation of cyst are high if cyst lining is left *in situ*. There is no place for aspiration of physiological ovarian cysts, (resolve spontaneously), and for cysts in post-menopausal women.

Consider cyst aspiration only if

- Malignancy excluded.
- Simple cyst observed during ovulation induction.
- Women with symptomatic cysts where GA is a hazard.
- Risk factors for surgery, e.g. multiple laparotomies.

Surgery indicated if

- Cysts larger than 5–10cm size.
- Complex cysts that are not echo-free.
- Symptomatic cysts.
- Persistently raised CA125 in non-pregnant women, whatever the size.

Under age 35

The options are:

- Laparoscopic aspiration and fenestration of cyst.
- Laparoscopic/open ovarian cystectomy is the removal of the cyst intact without prior rupture, e.g. dermoid cysts.
- Laparoscopic/open oophorectomy, if ovary is distorted with multiple cysts or laparoscopic/open salpingo-oophorectomy.
- There is no indication to biopsy an otherwise healthy looking contralateral ovary.

Over age 35

The options are:

- Conservative surgery—oophorectomy or cyst aspiration.
- Conservative surgery, but preliminary hysteroscopy and curettage may be indicated to exclude a concomitant endometrial tumour.
- Laparotomy to remove the benign tumour, if laparoscopic approach is not feasible.

Over the age of 45/50

- Treatment should be individualized.
- Risk of malignancy index should be used to select women who require primary surgery in a cancer centre by an oncologist. (📖 See Chapter 11, p.293.)
- If laparoscopic management of ovarian cysts is undertaken in postmenopausal women, it should be oophorectomy, not cystectomy.

- If risk of malignancy index (RMI) is under 250, surgery can be undertaken in the local unit. Full staging laparotomy is undertaken with unilocular ovarian cysts over 10cm size or with any other ovarian tumours. A midline or a transverse incision allows adequate exposure.
- It should include peritoneal washings at the beginning of the surgical procedure.
- Removal of infracolic omentum, total abdominal hysterectomy, and bilateral salpingo-oophorectomy if required.
- The benefit of lymph node sampling remains unproven. (See Chapter 11, p.293.)

Resources

For health professionals:

RCOG (2003) Ovarian cysts in postmenopausal women. *Guideline* **34**: www.rcog.org.uk

Shaw, RW, Soutter, WP and Stanton, SL (eds) *Gynaecology 3rd edn*. Benign ovarian tumours p.665 Churchill Livingstone, Edinburgh.

For women:

www.2womenshealth.com

Vulval disorders

Definition

A spectrum of conditions affects the vulva, spanning the specialties of gynaecology, oncology, dermatology, and genito-urinary medicine. Multidisciplinary care of vulval disorders may involve physiotherapists and sexual therapists. Nurses in primary and secondary care take on roles in identifying conditions and referral, ongoing support, monitoring, and taking on specialist roles in multidisciplinary teams.

Cause-based classification of vulval disorders

Infectious causes

- Candida, herpes, syphilis, genital warts, Trichomonas vaginalis (TV).
- Infestation with pubic lice.

Dermatosis

- Lichen sclerosis, eczema, psoriasis.
- Chemical/irritant dermatitis.
- Contact/allergic dermatitis.
- Miscellaneous such as hydradenitis suppurativa or seborrhoeic dermatitis (look for dandruff).

Benign lumps and cysts

- Bartholin's cyst.
- Sebacious cyst.
- Congenital cysts.
- Genital warts.

Neoplastic

- Vulval cancer (📖 see Chapter 11, p.293).
- Vulval intraepithelial neoplasia (VIN).

Role of the nurse in diagnosis, assessment, and treatment

Assessment of symptoms

- Pruritis—is the itch episodic, continuous, or nocturnal? Does it affect sleep? Remember that a chronic itchy condition will lead to pain.
- Signs of atrophy that cause pain and dyspareunia—assess menopausal state.
- If pain, is there point (Q-tip) tenderness suggesting vestibulodynia?
- If ulcer—ask about duration, history of trauma, associated urinary symptoms, and test urine, systemic symptoms (suggest herpes).
- Assess impact on quality of life, psycho-sexual function.
- Inspect the vulva and perineum for:
  - Ulcers, cysts, warts.
  - Redness—universal (vestibulodynia) or localized (contact dermatitis).
  - Loss of skin texture as in lichen sclerosis and post-menopause.
  - Scratch signs and fissures indicating chronic itching.
  - Discharge; and take swabs for bacteriology and virology. Look for infective causes.
  - Pigmentation—associated with VIN.

Referral

Refer, if diagnosis uncertain, if STI suspected (unless you can manage), if biopsy necessary (VIN), if long-term monitoring or specialist counselling needed (vulvodynia, lichen sclerosis, immuno-compromised patients).

General management measures

These include the avoidance of irritants, wearing cotton underwear, using cotton gloves at bedtime to avoid effects of scratching.

Resources

Haefner, HK, Collins, ME, Davis, GD, Edwards, L, Foster, DC, Hartmann, EH *et al.* (2005) The vulvodynia guideline. *Journal of Lower Genital Tract Disease* **9**: 40–51.

Vulval cysts

Definition

Vulval skin is liable to any dermatological condition including furunculosis and sebaceous cysts. The common cyst encountered in gynaecological practice is Bartholin's cyst and abscess (see Fig. 7.4).

A Bartholin's cyst arises from obstruction to Bartholin's gland. Normally the gland opens around the hymenal membrane at positions 5 and 7 o'clock. These cysts are unsightly but tend to be painless. Infection of a cyst leads to a painful Bartholin's abscess, which presents as an emergency.

Causes

The common culprit bacterium is *Escherischia coli*, though staphylococci and streptococci can be causative. The abscess is not seen as a sexually transmitted infection, though gonococci have been reported to be rare causative bacteria.

Diagnosis/assessment

Bartholin's cyst

Presents as a painless vulval swelling, usually unilateral.

Bartholin's abscess

The diagnosis is clinical. Patients present with a painful swelling and possible fever. They may find it difficult to walk or sit. The unilateral swelling tends to be red, tense, and tender.

Treatment

Marsupialization is the treatment of choice for Bartholin's cysts and abscesses. Anaesthesia, local or general, is required. A 2.5cm incision is made on the vaginal aspect of the abscess. The pus/fluid is drained and the opening is left open to drain and close by granulation. Pain subsides quickly.

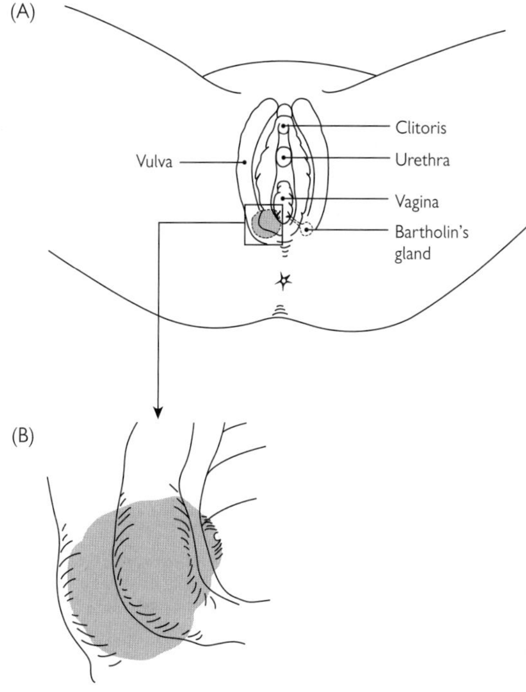

Fig. 7.4 (A) Bartholin's gland; (B) Bartholin's cyst. Reprinted with permission from Patient Pictures, Gynaecology, © 1996. Oxford: Health Press Limited.

Vulval dermatosis

Lichen sclerosis

Definition

A non-neoplastic, slowly progressive, scarring dermatosis, due to epithelial dystrophy, probably of auto-immune origin, that tends to present at the extremes of reproductive age.

Assessment

Presents with intense pruritis, with fissuring of the skin and consequent soreness and dyspareunia. Rarely, it can be asymptomatic.

The vulval skin is thin, dull white (described as cigarette-paper like), possibly excoriated and echymotic, as the skin bleeds and bruises easily. Inflammation may cause rubbery oedema. Scratching causes secondary infection. The introitus is narrowed with, at times, labial fusion. The classical description of a figure of 8/hourglass affected area extending to the peri-anal verge, is not always seen.

Diagnosis

Biopsy of the lesion is the gold standard. Two types of biopsy can be done under local anaesthesia in the outpatient department:

- Punch biopsy with Keyes 4mm punch.
- Knife excision biopsy.

Treatment

- A potent, topical steroid, such as clobetasol propionate 0.05% applied daily for 4 weeks, followed by alternate days for 4 weeks and then sparingly, as required. A 30g tube should last 3 months.
- Emollient preparations and avoidance of irritants in personal hygiene care, ensure control of symptoms.
- Regular monitoring is required, as the risk of squamous cell carcinoma is 5%.

Other dermatosis

- Psoriasis presents as well-demarcated salmon-pink lesions. The silver scales feature may not present on the vulva—it is usually associated with lesions elsewhere. The skin is thickened but not itchy. Treatment is with topical emollients +/– topical steroids and systemic treatment if widespread.
- Eczema does affect the vulva. The diagnosis may be difficult but erythema and scaling hint to eczema. Intense itching and scratching can lead to fissuring, secondary infection, and lichenification. Treatment is with emollients and moderately potent steroids.
- Chemical dermatitis is due to environmental irritants causing non-infective inflammation, excoriation, and soreness. Soaps, antiseptics, wipes, and urine in incontinent patients can cause dermatitis. Treatment is to avoid irritants, use barrier creams, and topical emollients. Prevention is through personal hygiene and keeping the area dry.
- Contact dermatitis is a true allergic reaction to local or systemic agents (drugs, latex, perfume). It is treated with short-term steroids.

Vulval intraepithelial neoplasia (VIN)

Definition

VIN is a pre-malignant intra-epithelial change with loss of epithelial maturation with atypia. VIN and vulval cancer were diseases of older women, but up to 50% of VIN is now seen in young women. VIN is classically multi-focal. The grades of VIN 1 to 3 are a continuum. The predominant type of VIN and cancer is squamous but Paget's disease leads to adenocarcinoma *in situ*.

The risk factors are similar to cervical intraepithelial neoplasia with high-risk human papilloma virus (HPV) the main oncogen. Smoking, immuno-compromised states, other genital infections, and certain dermatosis, predispose to VIN and cancer in VIN. The average risk of cancer is 8%, but higher in older women and the immuno-compromised.

Assessment

The symptom spectrum

- Pruritis.
- Lump/ulcer/warty lesion.
- Hyperkeratosis.
- Leukoplakic plaques.
- Incidental finding at colposcopy.

Diagnosis

- Vulvoscopy and biopsy.

Treatment

- Monitor low grade with vulvoscopy and biopsy; 5% acetic acid produces acetowhite changes.
- Wide, local excision for VIN 3 in unifocal lesion.
- Simple vulvectomy in selected cases.
- Medical treatment:
    - Topical cytostatic drugs, such as 5-flurouracil.
    - Immunostimulants, such as imiquimod.
    - Steroids for associated dermatosis.
- Follow-up/monitoring 6 monthly for at least 2 years after treatment.

Vulval pain

Definition

Described as soreness, vulval pain overlaps but must be differentiated from pruritis/itching (📖 see Vulval dermatosis, p.162). It may also present as dysuria or superficial dyspareunia. Vulval pain is not uncommon and accounts for at least 2% of attendances at sexual health clinics.

Causes.

Infectious causes

📖 See Vulval disorders, p.158.

Dermatosis and dermatitis

📖 See Vulval dermatosis, p.162

Bartholin's abscess

📖 See p.160.

Other conditions

- Behcet's disease.
- Vulval Crohn's disease.
- Erosive lichen planus.
- Post-radiotherapy.
- Endometriosis.

Vulvodynia

Defined as vulval pain in the absence of physical findings or neurological disorder. This is a multi-factorial condition that tends to start at a young age, causes sexual dysfunction, and by its chronicity leads to psycho-social sequalae.

Diagnosis/assessment

The pain could be episodic, cyclical, or continuous. The patient may relate it to a trigger event. Exacerbations may occur after provocation, such as sexual intercourse. Except in vestibulodynia, the pain tends to be generalized.

Vestibulodynia (previously called vestibulitis)

This is localized pelvic pain associated with erythema of the vestibular area and characterized by point tenderness. The diagnosis is based on the presence of the above three components, although erythema is not always present. Dysuria can occur if the anterior vestibule is affected.

Treatment

- Counselling, explanation, and support are essential.
- Personal hygiene advice with emphasis on avoiding irritants. Aqueous cream as soap substitute and as moisturizer. Emulsifying ointment can also be added to the regimen to use as required.
- Low oxalate diet recommended (avoid tea, coffee, spinach, peanuts).
- Lubrication during intercourse.

- If significant dyspareunia, advise the application of 5% lidocaine 20 minutes before intercourse.
- 5% topical lidocaine can be used during symptomatic flare-ups.
- Some advocate the use of the anti-histamine, hydroxyzine 25–50mg at night.
- Oral amitriptyline starting at 10mg at night and escalating the dose weekly until it works up to 100mg. Side-effects include dry mouth, constipation, and blurred vision.

Referral

Refer if diagnosis uncertain, if STI suspected (unless you can manage), if biopsy necessary (VIN), if long-term monitoring or specialist counselling needed (vulvodynia, lichen sclerosis, immuno-compromised patients).

Resources

Haefner, HK, Collins, ME, Davis, GD, Edwards, L, Foster, DC, Hartmann, EH *et al.* (2005) The vulvodynia guideline. *Journal of Lower Genital Tract Disease* **9**: 40–51.

Female genital mutilation (FGM)

FGM is defined as the partial or total removal of the external genitalia or other injury to the female genital organs for cultural or non-therapeutic reasons. Worldwide, about 100–140 million women have undergone some form of FGM, mostly practiced in Africa and in some countries in Asia and in the Middle East. It is a global problem and is now increasingly being seen in the Western world due to migration. FGM is illegal in the UK under the Prohibition of Female Circumcision Act (1985) and in 2003, it became an offence for UK residents or citizens to carry out FGM abroad.

Types of FGM—WHO classification

- Type I: excision of prepuce with or without excision of part or all of the clitoris.
- Type II: excision of the clitoris with partial or total excision of part or all of the labia minora.
- Type III: excision of part or all of the female external genitalia and stitching of the vaginal opening, i.e. infibulations.
- Type IV: unclassified.

Complications

Mortality has been reported. Type III and IV are associated with major complications which can include the following:

Immediate

- Severe pain, bleeding, and shock.
- Infections.
- Urinary retention.
- Injury to the urethra, vagina, and/or rectum with resultant urinary and/or faecal incontinence.

Long-term complications

- Sexual dysfunction—dyspareunia, anorgasmia.
- Urinary incontinence.
- Recurrent urinary tract infections.
- Paraclitoral cysts.
- PID.
- Transmission of blood-borne infections.
- Subfertility.
- Psychological disorders.

Obstetrical problems can include prolonged labour, higher Caesarean section rates, increased incidence of post-partum haemorrhage, stillbirth, and low birth-weight babies.

Women with FGM should be treated with care and empathy, preferably by female clinicians with interpreters. Defibulation can be offered before pregnancy or in pregnancy or even in labour, depending on when the woman presents to the clinician.

Eradication of the problem is the way forward, but, despite the law, FGM continues to be practiced.

Resources

Royal College of Obstetricians and Gynaecologists (2003) Female genital mutilation. *Statement* **no 3**, London, RCOG Press. ✆ www.rcog.org.uk (Accessed January 2009)

Chapter 8

Sexual health

Dyspareunia: definition, assessment, and diagnosis

Definition

There are two types of dyspareunia:

- Superficial dyspareunia is defined as pain at the onset of penetration or sexual intercourse.
- Deep dyspareunia is defined as pain during and after penetration or sexual intercourse.

It is a common but under-reported symptom, as women do not like to talk about it.

Assessment

Within women's health, asking the patient what her worries and concerns are, can often uncover the problem. It should be standard to ask women who you see, if they 'have any difficulties with sexual intercourse or desire'. This is often a useful tool to determine if there is a problem, as women are often reluctant to bring this up themselves. The patient should not feel hurried and it is important to maintain an understanding, professional atmosphere during the consultation. There are often both physical and psychological factors present. If sexual intercourse has been painful, this can lead to fear and anxiety, lack of lubrication, and then an increase of pain.

A full history (📖 see Chapter 3, p.21) and then additional flexible questions can be asked. Below is a list of some questions that may prove helpful:

- Onset and relationship of pain with women's life events.
- Relationship of pain to the menstrual cycle.
- Is there any sexual position that worsens or improves the pain?
- What sort of pain is it—burning, tearing, stabbing?
- Does the pain occur on one side more often than the other?
- Does the pain occur in relation to superficial or deep penetration?
- How long has this been a problem?
- Does the pain occur on every episode of intercourse?
- Has it shown any signs of getting better or worse?
- How often approximately do you have sex?
- Effect of the pain on the relationship with your partner?

Sexual history questioning

- Do you look forward to sex?
- When did you last change your sexual partner?
- Any relationship or work problems?
- Have you had the same pain with other partners?
- Did you have any sexual problems when growing up?
- History of recent STIs.
- Attitude to sex and sexuality.
- History of sexual abuse as a child or within current or previous relationships.

General gynaecological questions

In menstrual history, establish whether bleeding irregularities may be interfering with sexual intercourse. Details of reproductive history, including any difficulty conceiving, and elicit previous episodes of endometriosis, cysts, fibroids, and surgery.

Examination

- Tact and sensitivity to the woman's problem is important.
- The examination should be conducted in a quiet clinical room with no unnecessary staff.
- A chaperone is generally needed, regardless of the sex of the examining practitioner.
- Explain that the aim of the examination is to determine if there is any pathology causing the pain.
- If at any time she finds the pain is reproduced, advise that you will stop the examination. This will help her to feel in control.

Abdominal examination

- Inspect the abdomen for scars of major abdominal or gynaecological surgery.
- Palpate for any masses.
- Assess the mobility of the masses and tenderness.

Local examination

The examination should include full inspection of the external genitalia and, if possible, try to locate the painful area. The physical examination may be difficult and the woman's history and attitude to the examination may point to physical or psychological causes.

A particular note should be made of vaginismus when undertaking an examination and, if vaginismus is suspected, a gentle single-finger examination is first undertaken to see if the woman tolerates it. If she tolerates the digital examination, then she should be offered a speculum examination.

Bimanual examination provides useful information in relation to deep dyspareunia.

A physical examination is indicated normally with STI screening and testing. (📖 See Vaginal discharges: definition, assessment, and diagnosis, p.174.)

Investigations

- Need for diagnostic tests depends on the findings.
- Vaginal swabs, cervical swabs, and microbiological cultures may be needed (📖 see Chapter 3, p.21).
- If there is deep pain as well, then an ultrasound and possibly a laparoscopy may be indicated (📖 see Chapter 3, p.21).
- Within the history it may become apparent that there are urinary, bowel, and skeletal problems.

Dyspareunia: causes

Superficial causes

- Vulvitis—atrophic.
- Vulvitis. Caused by infections such as candidiasis, herpes, or genital warts.
- Bartholinitis. An inflammation of the glands that may present as a cyst or an abscess. There can also be pain in the area after surgery to cysts.
- Vulval dermatosis.
- Lichen sclerosis.
- Vestibulitis—this can cause pain in the vestibule.
- Vulvodynia. In vulvodynia there is a constant pain that feels like there are red-hot needles within the vulva. Generally, on examination there are no specific, obvious causes seen. It is thought that it may be brought on by a painful condition, which causes over-sensitivity of the nerve endings.
- Neoplasm.
- Vaginismus. This is the involuntary contraction of the vaginal muscles when penetration is attempted. It is generally linked to psychological dysfunction.
- Vaginitis—infective (as above).
- Imperforate hymen.
- Post-surgery. This can include any vaginal surgery like repairs, hysterectomy, TVT, and perineal stitching after childbirth.
- Post-radiotherapy (📖 see Chapter 11, p.293).
- Urethritis/caruncle.

Deep causes

📖 Many of the causes of deep pain are covered in Chronic pelvic pain, pp.144–151).

- Pelvic endometriosis.
- Ectopic pregnancy.
- Chronic pelvic inflammatory disease.
- Chronic pelvic pain syndrome.
- Ovarian cyst.
- Displaced IUD/IUS.

Dyspareunia: treatments

Treatment of both superficial and deep dyspareunia comprise medical, surgical, and psychosexual management

The treatment of dyspareunia is related to the causes.

Medical management

- For any atrophic causes, a low-dose local oestrogen cream can be used (📖 see Chapter 9, p.221). An alternative is a vaginal moisturizer or using lubricants during intercourse.
- For infective causes, treatment is aimed at treating the cause. With chronic infections this may need to be on a long-term basis.
- Bartholin's abscesses may need to be drained/marsupialized or treated with antibiotics.
- Vulval dystrophy.
- Neoplasm (📖 see Chapter 11, p.293).
- Vaginismus—this can be treated by behaviour modification and using vaginal dilatation using vaginal trainers. The teaching of how to use trainers needs to be undertaken in a private room, where there has been a therapeutic relationship between the woman and the practitioner. The smallest dilator should be used first, with gradual progression as the patient feels able. It is important to progress like this, as the patient can then overcome her fears and anxieties with the smaller sizes. Partner support and counselling directed towards reassurance and education are important adjuncts to treatment. Women may need to be referred for psychosexual counselling.
- Post-surgery and post-radiotherapy—women may benefit from lubrication, use of local oestrogen creams, and dilators, as above.
- Vulvodynia—can be managed by local hygiene and treating underlying pathology. It can also be helped by having lidocaine 5% ointment to apply prior to intercourse and, in some cases, low dosage of the tricyclic anti-depressant amitriptyline.

Surgical management

- Imperforate hymen—can be surgically incised.
- Granulomata and scar tissue after lower genital tract damage following childbirth may require corrective surgery.
- Dyspareunia associated with female genital cutting may require surgical correction.

Psychosexual management

With all causes, it is important to discuss with women the psychological impact on their relationship.

Pain can set off a cycle of problems. This can lead to fear in anticipation of sexual intercourse, which leads to decrease in sexual desire, and then decrease in lubrication. This can then move on to avoidance of intercourse and intimacy, and then relationship problems. For this, it is important that there is a sensitive and frank discussion and that the couple is offered relationship or sexual counselling, if needed.

Vaginal discharge: definition, assessment, and diagnosis

Definition

Vaginal discharge is a fluid produced by glands in the vaginal wall and cervix that drains through the vagina. Discharge can by physiological or pathological.

Physiological discharge

Normal vaginal flora (lactobacilli) colonize the vaginal epithelium and may have a role in defence against infection. They maintain the normal vaginal pH between 3.8 and 4.4. The quality and quantity of vaginal discharge will vary during the menstrual cycle; each woman will have her own sense of normality and what is acceptable or excessive for her. Women who have used hormonal contraception may find this differs when they change methods.

Pathological discharge

An increase in the amount of vaginal discharge, an abnormal odour, or consistency of the fluid can be pointers of an infection or other pathological causes listed in 📖 Fig. 8.1.

Assessment and diagnosis

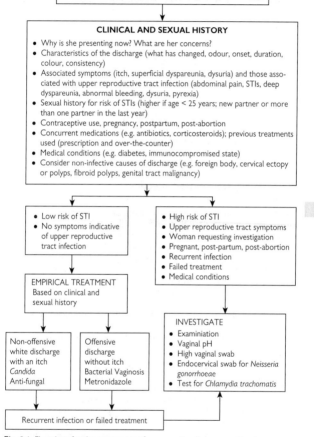

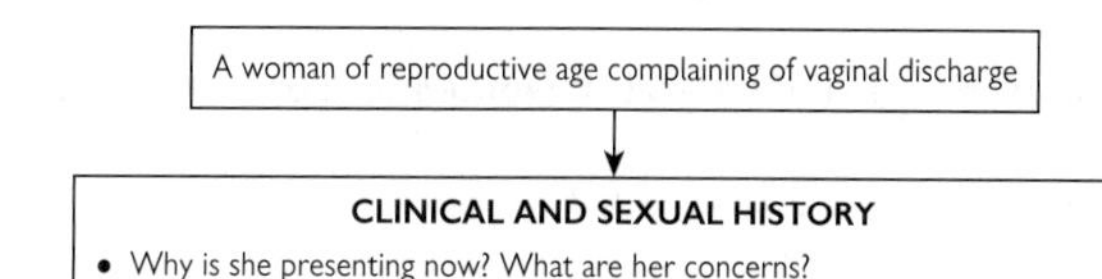

CLINICAL AND SEXUAL HISTORY

- Why is she presenting now? What are her concerns?
- Characteristics of the discharge (what has changed, odour, onset, duration, colour, consistency)
- Associated symptoms (itch, superficial dyspareunia, dysuria) and those associated with upper reproductive tract infection (abdominal pain, STIs, deep dyspareunia, abnormal bleeding, dysuria, pyrexia)
- Sexual history for risk of STIs (higher if age < 25 years; new partner or more than one partner in the last year)
- Contraceptive use, pregnancy, postpartum, post-abortion
- Concurrent medications (e.g. antibiotics, corticosteroids); previous treatments used (prescription and over-the-counter)
- Medical conditions (e.g. diabetes, immunocompromised state)
- Consider non-infective causes of discharge (e.g. foreign body, cervical ectopy or polyps, fibroid polyps, genital tract malignancy)

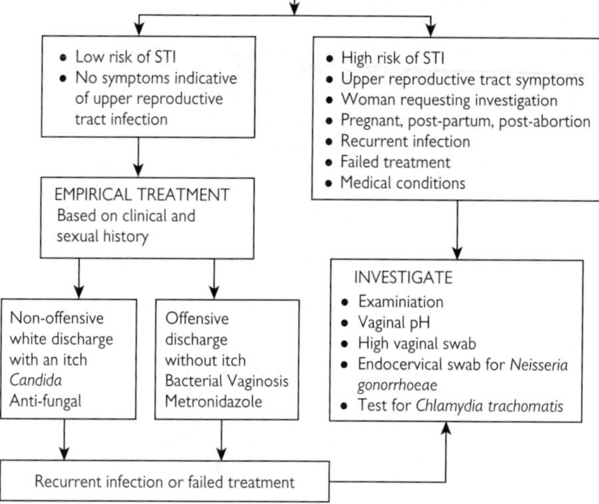

Fig. 8.1 Flowchart for the assessment of women attending non-genitourinary medicine settings complaining of vaginal discharge. Adapted from FFPRHC and BASHH Guidance—The management of women of reproductive age attending non-genitourinary medicine settings complaining of vaginal discharge (January 2006).

Vaginal discharge: causes

Causes of vaginal discharge in women of reproductive age[1]

- Physiological.
- Infective non-sexually transmitted.
  - Bacterial vaginosis.
  - Candida.
- Infective (sexually transmitted).
  - *Trichomonas vaginalis.*
  - *Chlamydia trachomatis.*
  - *Neisseria gonorrhoeae.*
- Non-infective.
  - Foreign bodies (e.g. tampons, condoms).
  - Cervical polyps and ectopy.
  - Genital tract malignancy.
  - Fistulae.
  - Allergic reactions.

Non-sexually transmitted infections

Bacterial vaginosis

Bacterial vaginosis (BV) is the commonest cause of infective vaginal discharge. BV is characterized by an overgrowth of anaerobic organisms that replace normal lactobacilli, leading to an increase in (pH ≥4.5). *Gardnerella vaginalis* is commonly found in women with BV, but the presence of *Gardnerella* alone is insufficient to make a diagnosis of BV. Signs and symptoms are outlined in Table 8.1. BV is associated with a new sexual partner and frequent changes of partner, although can be seen in virgins. Increased rates of BV can occur in certain groups of women, such as black African women, smokers, and lesbians. BV is also associated with pelvic infection after induced abortion and in pregnancy with pre-term delivery and low birth-weight babies.

► Recurrent BV is seen in women who experience prolonged bleeding.

Candida

Candida albicans is a vaginal commensal found in 10–20% of asymptomatic women. Acute vulvovaginal candidiasis (VVC) is caused by an overgrowth within the vagina of yeasts—usually *C. albicans* (80–95% of cases) or *C. glabrata* (5%). VVC affects about 75% of women at some time during their reproductive life, with 40–50% having two or more episodes. Candidiasis occurs most commonly when the vagina is exposed to oestrogen, especially in women aged 20–30 years and in pregnancy. Antibiotic use and diabetes may precipitate VVC. There is no good evidence that hormonal contraception increases VVC, nor is there evidence that tampons, sanitary towels, or douching cause candidiasis. 🕮 Signs and symptoms are outlined in Table 8.1.

Sexually transmitted infections

Trichomonas vaginalis

Trichomonas vaginalis is a flagellated protozoan that can cause vaginitis. Women with TV commonly complain of vaginal discharge and dysuria (due to urethral infection). Typical signs and symptoms are given in 📖 Table 8.1. Trichomoniasis is less common in affluent countries but reaches high levels (often 10–20%) among poor women in developing countries, as well as among disadvantaged women in affluent countries. Trichomoniasis has been ranked by the WHO as the most prevalent non-viral STI in the world, with an estimated 172 million new cases a year.

Table 8.1 Summary of symptoms and signs (including point of care test for vaginal pH) associated with common infective causes of vaginal discharge in women of reproductive age[1]

Bacterial vaginosis	**Candida**	**Trichomoniasis**
SYMPTOMS		
Thin discharge	Thick white discharge	Scanty to profuse or frothy yellow discharge
Offensive or fishy odour	Non-offensive	Offensive
Associated symptoms	Associated symptoms	Associated symptoms
No itch	Vulval itch or soreness	Vulval itch
	Superficial dyspareunia	Dysuria
	Dysuria	Low abdominal pain
SIGNS		
Discharge covering vagina and vestibule. No vulval inflammation	Normal findings or vulval erythema, oedema, fissuring, satellite lesions	Vulvitis and vaginitis. So-called strawberry cervix (uncommon 2%)
POINT OF CARE TEST—VAGINAL pH		
≥4.5	<4.5	≥4.5

1. Adapted from FFPRHC and BASHH Guidance: the management of women of reproductive age attending non-genitourinary medicine settings complaining of vaginal discharge (January 2006).

Vaginal discharge: investigations and treatment

Investigations

- Take cervical and urethral sampling for microscopy and culture for gonorrhoea (rectal and oropharyngeal culture is only appropriate if indicated by sexual history).
- Cervical nucleic acid amplification test (NAAT) for chlamydia. If cervical swab not possible, then urine NAAT.
- Microscopy and culture of vaginal discharge for *Candida* is not always necessary.
- Microscopy of vaginal discharge provides an immediate diagnosis of trichomonas, but, culture is more sensitive.

Non-sexually transmitted infections: treatment

Bacterial vaginosis

Oral regimen (cure rate: 70–80%):
Metronidazole 2g stat, single dose, or 400–500mg twice a day for 5–7 days.

⚠ Avoid alcohol and advise if metallic taste in the mouth.

Avoid stat dose when breast feeding.
Clindamycin 300mg twice a day for 7 days is an alternative.

► Advise condom use if on combined oral contraceptive pill (COCP)—apply the 7-day rule (📖 see Chapter 13, p.359).

Vaginal regimen (cure rate: 70–80%):
Metronidazole gel 0.75% 5g for 5 nights, or clindamycin cream 2% 5g for 7 nights.

► Advise latex barrier methods may be damaged.

All regimens are safe in pregnancy.

Suppressive regimens:
Metronidazole 400mg twice a day before and after menstruation, or metronidazole gel 0.75% twice a week for 4–6 months.

Lifestyle/hygiene advice:
Avoid local irritants, no soap, alcohol, and/or perfume products, (shower preferred to (bubble) bath), avoid vaginal douching, and avoid antiseptics. Aqueous cream can be used externally as soap substitute.

Counselling/patient education:
Nature of infection (non STI, but possible transmission between lesbians, imbalance in normal vaginal flora), possible trigger factors (e.g. personal hygiene, period, unprotected sex), possible complications in pregnancy: miscarriage, premature rupture of membranes.

Candida

Vaginal regimens (cure rate 80–95%):
Clotrimazole pessaries 500mg single dose, or 200mg for 3 nights, or econazole pessaries 150mg single dose (Ecostatin-1®), or 150mg for 3 nights, or miconazole cream 2% 5g for 10–14 nights. Creams can be applied to vulval and peri-anal areas.

⚠ Advise latex barrier methods may be damaged.

Oral regimens:
Fluconazole capsule 150mg single dose.

⚠ Avoid oral regimens in pregnancy, may be teratogenic. Topical treatment may require a longer duration.

Suppressive therapy:
Fluconazole 100mg once a week for 6 months, or clotrimazole pessary 500mg once a week for 6 months.

Lifestyle/hygiene:
As above for BV, additionally avoid tight fitting clothing, nylon underwear, allow skin to breathe.

Counselling/patient education:
Nature of infection (non-STI, but possibly transmittable to uncircumcized male partners, fungal overgrowth), ascertain presence of underlying condition (immunosuppression, diabetes, pregnancy), or use of antibiotics.

Sexually transmitted infections: treatment

Trichomonas

Oral regime (cure rate 95%):
Metronidazole 2g single stat dose, or 400–500mg twice a day for 5–7 days. Metronidazole is not known to present a problem in pregnancy, but avoid stat dose.

Counselling/patient education:
Nature of infection (STI), possible complications if not treated (e.g. vestibulitis, cervicitis), partner notification, screening and treatment, recommend screening for other STIs considering window periods, advise no sexual intercourse for 1 week after self and sexual partner(s) have been treated, additional condom use if on COCP.

Gonorrhoea

🕮 See Gonorrhoea: overview, p.184.

Chlamydia

🕮 See Chlamydia: overview, p.188.

Resources

For women: www.ckslibrary.nhs.uk

Sexual health in context

Close links exist between the fields of sexual health and reproductive health as illness/disease/psychological well-being/interventions in one area can impact on others. According to World Health Organization (2005), sexual health encompasses:
- HIV and reproductive tract infections;
- unintended pregnancy and abortion;
- sexual well-being (sexual dysfunction, pleasure)
- violence related to sexuality and gender;
- certain aspects of mental health;
- genital mutilation;
- the effect of physical disabilities and chronic illnesses on sexual health;
- infertility.

Vulnerability to sexual ill health, therefore, goes beyond medical conditions. In the UK, sexual health has a public health function and one of the aims of services is to reduce the increasing burden of STIs and unintended pregnancies by providing a wide range of accessible and high-quality services in a variety of settings, which include general practice, community and voluntary sector sexual and reproductive health clinics, and specialist GUM services

Sexual history

- Taking a good sexual history is a prerequisite to good care.
- An assessment that involves asking relevant questions to acquire the right information to effectively guide examination, testing, and/or referral.
- Find out the most important causes for concern.
- Creates opportunities to appropriately inform and advise patients on risk reduction of STIs and sexual health.
- May identify association with current health problems.
- Some screening services have patient self-management with minimal clinician involvement.

Factors facilitating an effective SH consultation—clinicians should:
- Allow adequate time for the consultation.
- Ensure a confidential environment and emphasize confidentiality.
- Be non-judgmental.
- Avoid embarrassment.
- Be knowledgeable on STIs, at-risk behaviours, tests available, and targeted interventions.
- Have well-developed communication skills: asking sensitive questions, giving information, listening, recognizing verbal and non-verbal cues in patient.
- Be aware of, and use, guidelines on consent (e.g. Fraser guidelines and <16 Department of Health Guidance) Mental Capacity Act and child protection, where appropriate, or acts applicable in your country.

Main elements of a sexual history

Approach to taking a sexual history

- In a comprehensive sexual history, both the clinician and the patient need to avoid embarrassment.

- Framing of questions is important.
- Choice of terminology is crucial.
- Some patients prefer to use common language, others may prefer to discuss the issue in medical terms.
- Social and medical history should always be explored.

Risk assessment

- Presenting complaint/reason for testing/presentation at clinic.
- Age—to establish competency/meet service criteria.
- Past STIs—to establish if any symptoms due to recurrent/untreated infection.
- Current/recent antibiotic use/medication—to check for drug interactions/contraindications.
- Sexual partners, gender, last sexual intercourse, condom use, type of sex in last 3–6 months or most recent partners—establishes risk factors for some STIs, sites for sampling, timing of when to test to cover incubation/window period of some infections.
- LMP and contraception—some medications contraindicated/unlicenced for use in pregnancy or interact with hormonal contraception.
- If symptomatic, check if:
  - abnormal vaginal discharge;
  - genital sores/pain/lumps;
  - urinary symptoms;
  - lower abdominal pain;
  - vulval skin problems.

The 5 Ps

Incorporates all aspects of a good sexual history:

- Partners.
- Prevention of pregnancy.
- Protection from STI.
- Practices.
- Past history of STI.

Planning: specimen collection, diagnosing

- Based on assessment, decide which tests to offer and where to sample, i.e. if includes examination/screening only/referral—important to ensure patients understand what they will be tested for, why, and give consent.
- Discuss any findings with patient and how results will be given.

Health promotion

- Based on risk assessment, raise/discuss safe sex, condom use, as appropriate.
- Partner notification if also being treated for an infection at the time.

The level of detail, depth of information, and relevance of some elements of the sexual history will vary, depending on if patient is having screening only, has symptoms, complexity of any problem, the services offered in that setting and referral pathways.

Partner notification

This is defined as the process of contacting and notifying sexual partners of an individual diagnosed with an STI, that they may be exposed to an infection and need treatment and tests. The aim is to break the chain of infection, i.e. prevent re-infection to the treated individual from an untreated partner, and/or to stop an infection being passed on to new partners.

Main types of partner notification (PN)

Patient referral

This takes place when the patient (referred to as the index patient), with the diagnosis of an infection, is encouraged and helped to inform their sexual partner(s) of the need for treatment and testing. The patient may then decide to do this verbally, send a message, or give a contact slip. The aim is that the patient takes the initiative to inform their sexual partner of the infection and the partner attends in good time for treatment and tests.

Provider referral

Where a patient is unable or unwilling to tell their sexual partner(s), the clinician undertakes to do this (this may be after an agreed period) with the details given by the index patient. The health advisor or clinician is obliged to maintain the confidentiality of the index patient, including the diagnosis, if they do not wish to be identifiable.

The contact slip

Patients with an STI have an option to give or send a contact slip to their partner(s). The purpose is that, hopefully, a contact will respond quickly and attend a recommended clinic. This slip of paper is recognized across sexual health services in the UK and gives key basic information, some of which the clinician completes:

- The clinic where the index patient was treated.
- A national code for the infection.
- The date the index patient was treated.
- The unique number of the patient (not a name).

By using a code for the infection and a number for the patient, the patient's identity and diagnosis is protected.

In some cases, if the index patient agrees, the name of the infection may be written on the slip.

⚠ Contact slips are never given for HIV, more support is needed here compared to other STIs.

Key points when undertaking PN with a patient who has an STI

- Establish understanding of infection, inform and advise.
- Inform of the need to treat, importance of partner treatment.
- Highlight the risks of re-infection if partner untreated and any possible health complications for self and partner or future partners.
- Develop strategies with patient to overcome embarrassment, anger, fear, or other barriers that may prevent them telling partners.

- Establish how they would inform their partner—would they use a contact slip or tell them in person?
- Be objective—listen, explain, challenge any misconceptions, give facts.
- Health promotion—safer sex to prevent/reduce future risks.

Consultation with the contact or partner who presents for treatment

- Check they know what infection they have been in contact with.
- If they bring a slip with a code and are unaware what infection they may have been exposed to, be careful not to break the confidentiality of the index patient by divulging what this means. This is often difficult, as patients would like to know what they are being treated for. You can only offer the treatment and tests unless their own STI tests are subsequently positive for a specific infection.
- Give epidemiological treatment, where needed, and offer/refer for STI screening.

Most STIs are notifiable for advice, screening, and treatment. There are specific issues with HIV partner notification, where the aim is to get as many partners in for counselling and testing rather than break the chain of disease.

Resources

www.ssha.info
For advice, contact health advisers at your local GUM clinic.

Gonorrhoea: overview

Also known as 'the clap' or GC, this infection is caused by a Gram-negative bacterium called *Neisseria gonorrhoea* and affects mucosal sites, such as the endo-cervix, urethra, pharynx, rectum, and conjunctiva.

Epidemiology

It is the second most commonly transmitted bacterial STI in the UK.

At-risk groups in the UK

- Those under the age of 25 years.
- Men who have sex with men.
- Black ethnic groups.

Transmission

Occurs when infectious fluids come into contact with mucosal surfaces. Risk of transmission from a single episode of sexual intercourse from an infected male to female is 40%. About 30% of babies born to infected mothers develop ophthalmia neonatorum.

Incubation

Generally a short incubation period ranging from as little as 2–10 days.

Table 8.2 Gonorrhoea: signs and symptoms

Female	Men
Mucopurulent cervical discharge	Green/yellow urethral discharge and dysuria
+/– contact bleeding of the cervix (up to 50%)	
Up to 50% have no signs	
Women with pharyngeal and rectal infection are often asymptomatic	
Increased or abnormal vaginal discharge (up to 50%)	
About 12% of women with urethral infection experience dysuria	
Lower abdominal pain (~5%)	

Differential diagnosis in women

Difficult to achieve if based on signs and symptoms only. as these mirror other infections as well (📖 see Table 8.2).

Investigations

- Culture—gold standard test and recommended as the first choice where women are symptomatic or where GC is highly suspected. Sensitivities to antibiotics are also given in lab report.
- Rapid test—microscopy (30–57% sensitive).
- NAAT test—a DNA test for screening, often offered as a combined test with chlamydia screening. A positive result should always be confirmed by taking a sample for culture at the time of treating, as false-positive results have occurred. Also NAAT tests do not give sensitivities to antibiotics.

Specimen collection

Sample can be taken from mucosal sites. Use the specified manufacturer's swab kits for NAAT tests and culture. Some names of NAAT testing kits include Aptima Combo and Probetec.

NAAT tests from women who are asymptomatic can be self-taken, low vaginal swabs.

Storage and transport

Outside GUM, samples for culture should be taken with the specified swab for insertion into an Amies Charcoal or Stuart's medium. The sample, once taken, should get to the lab within 24h. If samples are kept overnight in the clinic/ward, they should be stored in a fridge ideally at 4°C, but aim to get to the lab as soon as possible next day.

Complications

These occur in 3% of women.

Complications

- Salphingitis and endometritis.
- Bartholinitis and skenitis (paraurethral gland infection).
- Perihepatitis.
- Less common disseminated infection—arthritis, endocarditis.
- HIV transmission can be facilitated.
- Neonatal conjunctivitis if untreated infection in pregnancy.

Gonorrhoea: treatment and notification

Treatment

Depends on site of infection, local antibiotic sensitivities, and national recommendations.

Cephalosporins are currently the first-line treatment, although this differs for pharyngeal infection. Gonococcal antibiotic resistance is becoming an increasing problem, particularly with gonorrhoea that has been acquired abroad, and some quinoline-resistant gonorrhoea has emerged, which responds better to third-generation cephalosporins.

Pregnant women

First line is, amoxicillin or ceftriaxone 250mg IM single dose, if allergic to penicillin. Cefixime 400mg orally can be used. Pregnant women should not be treated with tetracyclines or quinolones.

Partner notification

All partners for the last 10 days to 3 months should be notified to have tests and treatment. Points to cover include:

- Nature of the infection, transmission, importance of treatment for herself, and partner treatment.
- Once she is treated, no sex until partner treated and for 1 week after he is treated.
- Check the patient understands the risk to herself and/or partner or future partners if she has an untreated infection and continues to have sex or if re-infection occurs from an untreated partner.
- Risks to herself include PID or tubal damage, which may lead to subfertility problems or ectopic pregnancy risk (see Chapters 15 and 17, p.415 and p.447).
- Discuss how she intends to inform any partners.
- Agree on how to follow up to check treatment-compliance, if relevant, partner treatment, and any risk of re-infection.
- Offer condoms.

What the patient needs to know

- GC is highly infectious and the longer it is left untreated, the more likely it will get passed on to a partner, especially new partners.
- GC can cause complications for women such as PID, which is often quite painful and may affect fertility in the future.
- She must tell her partner or partners to get treated or last known partner, if contactable.
- If she is unable to tell a partner, health advisers in a GUM clinic can help with this.

Resources

Sherard J *Gonorrhoea*: www.themedicine publishing.com (Accessed January 2009)
UK management guidelines: www.bashh.org (Accessed January 2009)

Chlamydia: overview

Caused by the bacterium *Chlamydia trachomatis*. Sero-variants D-K primarily affect the genital tract.

Transmission

- Primarily sexually acquired via unprotected vaginal, oral, anal intercourse or genital contact with an infected person.
- Has also been found on nasopharynx and eyes without genital tract infection.

Epidemiology

The most common bacterial STI in the UK. In 2006, the highest rates in women were in ages 16–19.

Risk factors

- Change of sexual partner or more than one partner at the same time.
- Under the age of 25.
- Not using barrier method of contraception.

Table 8.3 Chlamydia: signs and symptoms

Women	Men
Asymptomatic (70%)	Urethral discharge
Contact bleeding on cervical cytology or swab	Dysuria
Post-coital/inter-menstrual bleeding	
Unusual vaginal discharge	
Dysuria	
Deep dyspareunia	
Mucopurulent cervical discharge	

Tests

Asymptomatic women

The recommended test is Nucleic Acid Amplification Test (NAAT), a DNA test that is highly sensitive and specific, and can be used on non-invasive specimen samples, such as urine and self-taken low vaginal swabs (currently only the Aptima NAAT is licensed for vulvo-vaginal swabs). The recommended manufacturer's testing kits should be used and local lab advice sought on sites for specimen collection. Although NAATs are more than 99% specific, false-positive results can occur, particularly in low-prevalence populations.

Symptomatic women

Here the endocervical swab remains the recommended optimal specimen for detecting *Chlamydia trachomatis* by NAAT.

Specimen collection

As a guide:

- If female and asymptomatic—patient can take a low vaginal swab. Urine samples not usually recommended for women, as sensitivity of the NAAT test is reduced compared to swabs
- If female and symptomatic—an endocervical swab should be taken. Men—first-catch urine samples are the recommended specimen.

Chlamydia: treatment and partner notification

Treatment

First-line treatment is a stat dose of azithromycin (1g) or doxycycline 100mg twice a day for 7 days. Choice of drug is dependent on cost (the latter being cheaper) versus compliance. Both have equal effectiveness in clearing uncomplicated infection and a test of cure is not necessary but, if wanted, should be done 5 weeks after treatment.

Pregnant women

Untreated infection can be passed to the baby via the birth canal resulting in pneumonitis and/or eye infection.

Erythromycin is the recommended treatment for pregnant women but is associated with poor tolerance, resulting in patients not completing the course. Test of cure is recommended at 3 weeks for women receiving this treatment. Many sexual health clinics now treat pregnant women with azithromycin, although this is out of licence use (BASSH guidance).

Complications

- Risk of PID, if untreated infection.
- Chlamydial perihepatitis.
- Sequalae of chronic PID—ectopic pregnancy.
- Chronic persistent pelvic pain.
- Chlamydial pneumonitis in baby with maternal untreated infection.

Partner notification

- Check understanding of the nature of the infection, treatment, transmission.
- Partner(s) from the last 6 months or last known partner. If last sexual intercourse >6 months, should be contacted for epidemiological treatment and screening.
- Offer a contact slip/establish how partner will be informed.
- Discuss the risk to self, partner, or future partners, if untreated, or risk of re-infection if a partner remains untreated, e.g. PID.
- Advise no sex from treatment to completion, until current sexual partner is treated and for 1 week after.
- Offer condoms and advise on usage.

What to discuss with the patient

- What is chlamydia and how it is transmitted?
- Chlamydia is often asymptomatic, particularly in women, and, although tests are accurate, no test is absolutely so.
- What are the complications of untreated chlamydia?
- The side-effects of treatment and the importance of compliance.
- Interactions between antibiotics and the COCP.

Resources

Further reading on *Chlamydia trachomatis* can be found on:
www.hpa.org.uk
www.bashh.org.uk/guidelines

Pelvic inflammatory disease (PID): definition, causes, and diagnosis

Definition

The result of an infection in women, ascending from the endocervix or other pelvic organs, causing one or more of the following:

- Salpingitis.
- Endometritis.
- Parametritis.
- Tubo-ovarian abscess.
- Pelvic peritonitis.

PID may be acute or chronic, and a patient may present with or without symptoms (📖 see Table 8.4).

Causes

- *Chlamydia trachomatis* (60%).
- *N.Gonorrhoea* (implicated in 14% of PID cases in a British study).
- Non-sexually transmitted micro-rganisms from the vaginal tract, such as *Mycoplasma hominis*, anaerobes, *E. coli*, and staphylococci.
- Descending infections from appendicitis.
- Ascending infections post-procedural, such as insertion of IUD, hysteroscopy.

Associated factors

- Women under age of 25.
- Multiple partners.
- Past history of STIs.
- Termination of pregnancy.
- Insertion of an IUD within the last 3 weeks.

Table 8.4 Clinical features suggestive of PID

Symptoms	Signs
Lower abdominal pain	Fever >38 degrees
Deep dyspareunia	Guarding/rebound on bimanual examination
Post-coital or inter-menstrual bleeding	Cervical excitation and adnexal tenderness, adnexal mass on bimanual examination
Abnormal vaginal discharge	Mucopurulent discharge on cervix
Irregular vaginal bleeding	
Rectal discomfort	

Examination and investigations

- Bimanual examination. Clinical symptoms and signs lack specificity and sensitivity, the positive predictive value of a clinical diagnosis ranges from 65 to 90% compared to laparoscopy.

- Endocervical swabs for chlamydia and GC culture. If either of these tests are positive, this supports the diagnosis of PID; if negative, does not exclude these infections as possible causes, as tests can be negative after infection has ascended. A positive NAAT for gonorrhoea should be confirmed by culture prior to treatment because of high false-positive rates. A high vaginal swab for *Trichomonas vaginalis* is also recommended but its value in the management of PID is questionable. Bacterial vaginosis has been associated with PID. The presence of clue cells, and leukocytes on microscopy is associated with a 5-fold risk of PID.
- ESR or C reactive protein tests may help in supporting a diagnosis, if either are raised.
- Pregnancy test, if required to rule out ectopic pregnancy.
- Check patient's temperature.
- Laparoscopy—allows samples to be taken from the fallopian tubes, but there is not enough evidence to support routine use due to:
  - High cost.
  - Inter-observer variability.
  - Intra-observer variability.
  - Potential difficulty in diagnosing mild intra-tubal inflammation or endometritis.
- Transvaginal ultrasound scan may help where diagnosis is difficult, but, evidence does not support routine use. Is useful if suspected adnexal or pouch of douglas mass to look for pyosalpinges or tubo-ovarian abscess.

Differential diagnosis

To consider in women presenting with lower abdominal pain:

- Ectopic pregnancy.
- Acute appendicitis.
- Urinary tract infection.
- Endometriosis.
- Torsion of an ovarian cyst.
- Constipation/bowel problems such as irritable bowel syndrome (IBS).

Careful discussion should be based on current evidence and individual patient history.

Complications

- Fitz–Hughes–Curtis syndrome.
- Chronic pelvic pain or adhesions.
- Ectopic pregnancy.
- Infertility—8% after a single episode, 20% after two episodes, and 40% or more after three episodes.

Pelvic inflammatory disease (PID): treatment

The Royal College of Obstetricians and Gynaecologists (RCOG) recommends a low threshold for empirical treatment. Generally, if cervical motion tenderness +/– adnexal tenderness on bimanual examination, empirical treatment should be given. Do not await the outcome of STI tests.

In mild to moderate PID

Broad-spectrum antibiotic treatment to cover the main likely causes i.e. *N.Gonorrhoea*, *Chlamydia trachomatis* +/– anaerobes (treatment for anaerobes is of greater importance in severe PID).

In severe acute PID

Or severe pain and diagnostic doubt on surgical emergency, refer for hospitalization and management.

Treatment in pregnancy

In all cases of suspected PID, a pregnancy test should be undertaken to rule out ectopic pregnancy; erythromycin is the preferred antibiotic.

In an intra-uterine pregnancy, PID is rare, but cervicitis can occur, which is associated with increased maternal and foetal morbidity.

Recommended outpatient treatment regimens for PID

- IM ceftriaxone 250mg single dose + doxycycline 100mg bd for 14 days + metronidazole 400mg bd for 14 days;

OR

- Oral ofloxacin 400mg bd for 14 days + metronidazole 400mg bd for 14 days.

Partner notification

- Partners should be screened, then given empirical treatment for chlamydia, gonorrhoea, and/or other STIs.
- Patient should not have sex until she has completed her treatment and her sexual partners have been treated.
- Where screening for CT and GC is not possible, empirical treatment to cover both infections should be offered to the partner.

Follow-up

Review in 72h to check resolution of symptoms and a bimanual examination and, if improving, thereafter in 2 weeks to check compliance with treatment, response to treatment, abstinence from SI, and to check on partner notification and treatment.

Women with PID and IUD

Current advice from the RCOG and the FSRH is leaving the device *in situ* in women with mild PID and ensuring review at 72h and in 2 weeks. This sounds sensible and is workable. This also enables a full discussion with the woman regarding her susceptibility to infections within her current sexual relationship.

The British Association for Sexual health and HIV (BASHH) suggest considering removal. It is important to follow local guidelines.

Women with HIV and PID

Antibiotic therapy is the same as for women who are HIV negative, as response tends to be good. If severe symptoms, parenteral therapy may be considered.

Resources

Health professionals:

www.rcog.org.uk/resources/Pelvic_Inflammatory_Disease_No.32.pdf

www.bashh.org/guidelines/2005/pid_v4_0205.pdf

Women:

www.rcog.org.uk/resources/public/pdf/acute_PID_2004.pdf

Hepatitis B (HBV)

Hepatitis B is a blood-borne virus that causes inflammation of the liver. About 10% of those infected may not clear the virus and remain infectious.

Risk factors

- Injecting drug use with contaminated equipment
- Receiving infected blood or blood products vertical transmission from an infected mother
- Sexual transmission higher in some groups e.g. sex workers, men who have sex with men
- Needle stick/sharps injury
- Practices e.g. tattooing piercing, using infected equipment
- Living in endemic countries

Transmission

The main route of transmission in UK is via unprotected sex and injecting drug use. Other routes of transmission include: needlestick injuries in health professionals, transfusion of infected blood products, piercing and tattooing with unsterile equipment, living in institutions, and coming from endemic countries.

Incubation period

2–6 weeks.

Symptoms and signs

- Asymptomatic or flu-like symptoms, nausea, fever, unwell, lethargy,+/– pale stools.
- About 30% develop jaundice.

Tests

Recommended to check for acute/previous/chronic infection or previous vaccination if hepatitis B suspected or if patient is from a high-risk group and considering vaccination.

- Core antibody (tests for previous infection or natural antibodies).
- Surface antibody (tests for previous vaccination and indicates if a vaccination course or booster is required).
- Surface antigen (if positive suggests current or infection that has not cleared).
- Ig M antibody to Hep B core antigen (to determine if acute or chronic infection).
- Hepatitis B antigen/antibody and Hep B DNA (to determine if high or low infectivity).

Prevention

- Avoiding and/or minimizing exposure to the risks, e.g. condom use, sterile disposable needles for tattoos.
- Routine screening of transfused blood and blood products.
- Using universal precautions in healthcare settings.

- Vaccination (a course of three injections) for high-risk individuals and all newborn infants:
  - persons from endemic areas;
  - sex workers;
  - alleged sexual assault;
  - men who have sex with men and their partners;
  - partners and household contacts of hepatitis B carriers;
  - injecting drug users and their partners/household contacts;
  - those living in institutions, e.g. prisons;
  - HIV positive individuals.
- Prevention of vertical transmission from HBsAg and HbeAg positive mothers to newborns—vaccinate newborn.
- Post-exposure prophylaxis—hepatitis B immunoglobulin.
- Preventing transmission in women with liver transplants.

Chronic HBV

Chronic carriers are those who have not cleared an acute infection naturally after 6 months (the Hep B surface antigen test remains positive). Such persons have no symptoms for many years but are at risk of developing liver cirrhosis and liver cancer. This risk increases in persons who are also HIV positive, on immuno-suppressant drugs, or with chronic renal problems. 90% of babies born to infectious mothers (hep B eAntigen positive) will become chronic carriers unless vaccinated at birth.

Contact tracing testing +/– vaccination

Consider partners or household contacts from the time when the patient remembers having symptoms (2 weeks before the onset of jaundice). This may be difficult for persons coming from endemic countries, where infection may have been acquired vertically or in early childhood.

Treatment

Lamivudine, adefovir dipivoxil, possibly pegylated interferons in the long term, reduce liver damage and lower risk of liver cancer in patients who respond to treatment.[1] Patients are usually managed by a specialist (hepatologist or physician experienced in liver disease).

Advice

Patients should be informed of the long-term implications of the condition, advised on alcohol, risk of transmission to partners and household contacts, and prevention measures, such as condom use, getting partners/household contacts tested and vaccinated. No unprotected sexual intercourse should take place until the partner is tested and vaccinated.

Resources

www.bashh.org

1 Aggarwal, R and Ranjan, P (2004) Preventing and treating hepatitis B infection. *BMJ* **329**: 1080–1086.

Hepatitis C (HCV)

Hepatitis C is a common disease but is often under-diagnosed. Hepatitis C is caused by a blood-borne RNA virus, which, like HBV, can cause inflammation of the liver, but the effects of the infection vary from one individual to the other. There are 11 genotypes of HCV. Genotype 1 is the most common in the UK

Prevalence

The estimated prevalence is between 0.4 and 1% of the UK population.

Transmission

- From infected blood transfusions or products prior to 1987.
- Use of, or exposure to, contaminated needles is the major route of transmission in the UK.
- Vertical transmission.
- Sexual.

Only 20–40% of women infected will clear the virus naturally. Infection lasting more than 6 months is considered chronic.

⚠There is no vaccine at present to prevent this infection.

Incubation

Takes up to 6 months.

Common risks

- Injecting drugs sharing contaminated needles/equipment.
- Received infected blood transfusions or blood products.
- Dental care or medical care in countries where infection control is poor.

Other risks

- Regular sexual partner of someone with HCV.
- Tattoos, piercing, other practices involving needles where infection control poor e.g. FGM.
- Accidental exposure to blood where there is a risk of exposure to HCV.

Symptoms

- May take years or decades to develop.
- Most people at the time of transmission are unaware and have no symptoms.
- Some may feel unwell.
- Jaundice is uncommon.

Complications

One in five with chronic HCV may eventually develop severe liver damage, which could lead to primary liver cancer or liver failure.

Tests

- Antibody test (anti-HCV)—takes up to 3 months for antibodies to become detectable in blood.
- RNA test (HCV RNA):
  - If +, suggests unresolved infection.
  - If after 6 months it is negative and the anti HCV +, this suggests the infection has cleared but the person may not be immune to further infection.

Prevention in primary care

- Provide hepatitis A and B vaccinations to all those using IV drugs and MSM (men who have sex with men).
- Information on safe sex including condoms.
- Easy convenient access to local needle exchanges or run a needle exchange in the surgery.
- Advice to stop smoking.
- Monitor weight and provide help with weight reduction.
- Discuss alcohol and advise to stop drinking alcohol.

Treatments

Combined pegylated interferon and ribavirin help to reduce the viral load in about 55% of patients with chronic HCV.

HIV and HCV co-infection

HIV positive patients who also have HCV co-infection and are on HAART, have a 2- to 3-fold increased risk of developing hepatotoxicy. However, the majority of co-infected patients are able to use HAART with careful monitoring (such as ultrasound scans, fibroscan, liver biopsy, blood tests) and are often jointly managed by the HIV physician and local hepatology team.

Nurses have a role in supporting co-infected patients by:

- Discussing safe sex and prevention of transmission to new or long-term partners.
- Advising and referring patients who are planning a pregnancy for specialist advice.
- Advising on avoidance of alcohol and reducing/stopping smoking.
- Helping to cope with side-effects of pegylated interferon drugs, such as weight loss, anorexia, depression, and hair loss by referring appropriately.
- Supporting adherence to HIV medication and treatments.

Resources

www.bashh.org
www.bhiva.org
www.dh.gov.uk/immunisations
www.hpa.org.uk
www.nhshepcfaceit.preppario.net

Anogenital warts (benign epithelial skin tumours)

Cause

The double-stranded DNA human papilloma virus—there are several strains associated with genital warts, most common ones are types 6 and 11.

Transmission

- Mostly sexually through genital to genital skin contact.
- Can occur even if there are no visible warts.
- Increased risk of transmission to a partner if warts are present.
- Poor evidence of transmission from fomites.
- Mother to baby transmission during vaginal delivery possible.

Prevalence

- Most commonly diagnosed viral STI in UK.
- In 2006, there were 47% new diagnoses in GUM clinics in women with highest rates in the 16–19 age group.

Incubation

Weeks to months.

Features

- Can appear anywhere in the genital area.
- Perianal lesions common.
- Rarely cause physical discomfort.
- May be itchy, sore, and cause irritation especially around the anus.
- Psychological distress as a result of the disfigurement.
- Occasionally warts can grow so large as to affect urination, defecation, and childbirth.
- Children born to women with cervical and vaginal warts may develop laryngeal and/or genital warts.

Presentation

- Single or multiple.
- May be flat, fleshy, soft, or keratinized, pigmented, or pedunculated lumps. Size varies, but may increase over time if untreated or if immuno-compromised.

Diagnosis

- Usually based on appearance and naked eye examination.
- External genital and speculum examination.
- Biopsy should be considered in secondary care if the lesion is atypical or pigmented.
- Good lighting and clinical diagnostic skills are essential.

Treatment

Treatment depends on the site, number, size, appearance of warts, and patient preference. The most common treatments for external genital warts are:

- Cryotherapy—clinician applied freezing of individual external warts using liquid nitrogen spray. Often a weekly or twice weekly treatment.
- Podophylotoxin 0.15% cream—patient applied treatment to external warts (except if lesion area is >4cm square). Avoid in pregnancy.
- Imiquimod—an immune response modifier. Suitable for home use. Not licensed in pregnancy.
- Other treatments include clinician applied trichloracetic acid, excision under anaesthetic, electro surgery, and laser treatment. All have limited impact in clearing the virus.
- No treatment is an option.

Cervical warts—may not require colposcopy, unless there is clinical concern or diagnosis is uncertain.

Recurrence

- Most likely in the first 3 months after treatment but varies.
- Warts generally clear within 2 years but may be longer especially if immuno-compromised.

Partners

Should check themselves for warts. If in long-term relationship, very likely already exposed to genital HPV. Transmission is more likely when warts are visible. Condoms may not provide complete protection.

Pregnant women

Warts can increase in size and proliferate in pregnancy but often disappear once pregnancy is over.

Caesarean section is generally not indicated unless vaginal introitus studded with warts or there are large cervical warts

Prevention

- Condom use may be beneficial in new relationships.
- Vaccines for preventing high-risk HPV types 16 and 18 now available and a quadrivalent vaccine, which includes protection against low-risk types 6 and 11, is an effective option.

Resources

www.bashh.org/guidelines/2007Natguidemgxagw2007.pdf (Accessed Nov 2008.)

Genital herpes

Caused by the double-stranded DNA herpes simplex virus (HSV), which is a member of the herpes family. Disease episodes may be primary or recurrent.

Types

- Type 1—causes cold sores on lips and mouth, and usually transfers to the genitalia via oral sex.
- Type 2—confined to genitals only and transmission is via direct genital skin contact, especially mucosal contact. Transmission is even possible if there are no visible sores or ulcers (asymptomatic shedding).

Incidence and prevalence

Incidence rates are highest in the 20–24 age group and prevalence of type 2 infections is 10–30% in developed countries

Symptoms

- Severity of symptoms is determined by primary immunity to HSV.
- Tingling sensation preceding the formation of a blister or vesicle.
- +/– fever, neuralgia.
- Vaginal discharge may reflect vaginal ulcers or cervicitis.
- +/– more severe symptoms such as difficulty passing urine.

Signs

- Painful ulcer at the site of the blister or vesicle when it is broken.
- Enlarged and tender inguinal nodes.
- +/– increased vaginal discharge.
- Ulceration usually occurs as multiple small ulcers.

Common differentials

- Behcet's disease.
- Chancroid (often a single painless ulcer with indurated edges found in primary syphilis).
- Fissure—superficial linear tear in the vulval skin particularly in the folds of the labia and often caused by *Candida*.

Diagnosis/signs and symptoms

- Clinical appearance based on naked eye examination.
- DNA test with PCR or virus culture of lesion. Swab sample of the fluid from the vesicle or from base of vesicle/ulcer. The sample is inserted in the specific viral medium. The sample has to be kept refrigerated and cold-chain maintained until it reaches the lab.
- Antibody testing is not helpful as it lacks specificity.

Treatment

- Topical anaesthetic gel helps with localized pain, but, sensitivity can occur.
- Saline bathing.

- Oral antivirals (aciclovir, famciclovir, or valaciclovir) for 5 days can reduce severity and duration of symptoms. These antivirals are most effective if taken within the first 5 days of an outbreak or while new lesions are forming. 5–7 day treatment is best. Longer treatment is required for up to a year if recurrences occur.

Complications

- Urinary retention requiring catheterization is rare.
- Aseptic meningism.

Partners

- If in a long-term relationship, it is likely the partner has already had exposure to the virus.
- Partners should check themselves for any sores or ulcers.

Pregnant women

Management, including type of delivery, depends on gestational age and whether primary/recurrent episode of herpes. Women should be asked at their first antenatal visit if they or their partners had genital herpes in the past. Caesarean section is recommended for all women presenting with primary genital herpes at the time of delivery and/or if infection occurs within 6 weeks of delivery.

Recurrences

The first episode or primary episode is often the most painful and subsequent episodes are more tolerable. Patients learn to recognize prodromal symptoms, such as tingling or itching, in the same area of previous herpetic ulcers and can use antivirals to prevent or reduce an outbreak. Recurrences are more likely in the first year of a primary diagnosis and are more likely with HSV Type 2.

Episodic treatment

- Patient-initiated antiviral treatment considered for persons who experience <6 outbreaks in a year and can use with onset of symptoms to prevent or reduce an outbreak.
- Prophylactic or suppressive treatment—offered where patient has >6 episodes in a year and antiviral treatment is taken every day with regular follow-up. Long-term treatment with aciclovir can prevent recurrences and is thought to be safe.

Genital lumps and ulcers

Genital lumps

Common causes

Normal

- Vaginal papillae.

Sexually acquired

- Genital warts (HPV) (See Anogenital warts, p.200).
- Syphilis-related (lumps that resemble genital warts called condylamata lata and present in the secondary stage of syphilis).
- Bartholin's abscess: a lump may appear on the left or right Bartholin's gland area, occasionally due to a gonococcal infection, feels warm to touch and may be tender on touch. STI testing is recommended.
- Molluscum contagiosum: caused by the pox virus, not a true STI as commonly found in children but usually sexually acquired in adults. Presents as small round, raised pearly lumps with a dent or core in the middle. Incubation period 3–12 weeks and can be present for up to about 9 months.

Physical

- Skin tag.
- Haemorrhoids.

Trauma

- Folliculitis—due to waxing/shaving.

Dermatological

- Cysts—usually form under the skin in the area of the Bartholin's glands; often painless, not raised and may increase or decrease in size. Antibiotics usually not required.
- Other—any lumps that are discoloured, atypical, should be reviewed carefully and consider referral to an appropriate specialist.

Diagnosis

Good history taking and clinical examination skills are the key to an accurate diagnosis. History of any previous diagnosis of lumps, of the possible causes, as mentioned below, how long the lump(s) present and any self-treatment help in reaching a correct diagnosis or indicates the need for referral elsewhere.

Treatment

- Treatment is dependent on the cause.
- Treatment for primary syphilitic sore and genital warts.
- Cryotherapy is indicated for molluscum contagiosum and can be administered in the GUM clinic.
- Urgent marsupialization and antibiotics for Bartholin's abscess.

Genital ulcers

Patients often describe any breaks in the genital skin as a sore.

Most common types of genital ulcers and the causes

HSV ulcer or lesion

(📖 See Genital herpes, p.202.)

Chancre

A sore that presents in primary syphilis infection, usually as a single, painless ulcer with raised, indurated edges. It appears at the site of entry (could be mouth as well) and, depending on the location, may not be noticed by a patient and eventually heals on its own within a week or so. Clinicians should ask about recent travel to or from endemic areas, or sexual activity in high-risk groups, e.g. sex workers. A syphilis blood test that tests for Ig G may be negative in early infections.

Anyone with a suspicious sore should be sent urgently to a GUM clinic, where a sample of fluid from the sore is taken and examined under dark ground microscopy for evidence of treponemes (the parasites that cause syphilis).

Fissures

Often small, linear, superficial tears in the folds of the labia minora and majora, or posterior fourchette, usually caused by *Candida* (thrush). Women may complain of burning and soreness. They are often present with other typical signs suggestive of *Candida,* such as thick vaginal discharge, and vulval itching.

Other less common causes of genital ulceration

- Trauma.
- Behcet's disease—multi-organ disease, where symptoms include painful ulceration in mouth and/or genital area.
- Crohn's disease.
- Vulval dysplasia and severe dermatitis.

Diagnosis

- Good history taking, including a thorough sexual history, is important.
- Note should be made of worsening symptoms and/or systemic symptoms.
- Visual examination with good lighting is an essential aid to diagnosis or may sometimes indicate the need for referral.

Treatment

Treatment depends on the cause and has been discussed elsewhere for herpes and candidal infections. For primary syphilitic chancre—consider parenteral procaine penicillin, but, treatment is best carried out in GUM clinics.

Resources

www.bashh.org

Human immuno-deficiency virus (HIV)

Definition

A RNA virus that infects protective cells of the immune system, CD4 cells. Over time, these CD4 cells die from continued viral replication and attack. As numbers decline, the person's immune system becomes compromised. This process often takes place over a number of years.

⚠ There is currently no vaccine or cure.

Risk factors

In the UK, HIV is higher in:

- men who have sex with men;
- heterosexuals from migrant black communities, mainly from sub-Saharan Africa;
- injecting drug users sharing needles.

Signs and symptoms

- Primary infection or sero-conversion may involve flu-like symptoms, but not always.
- Such symptoms may occur in the first few weeks after contracting the infection.
- Patient is often asymptomatic afterwards and for many years.

HIV testing

Consent must always be sought.

❗ Where a patient is unable to consent, seek advice from specialists in GUM (genito-urinary medicine), if necessary.

Pre-test discussion

Highly anxious or high-risk patients may need more in-depth counselling—consider referring such patients to GUM specialists or counsellors. General points to cover with someone testing for HIV:

- Reason for testing/benefit of knowing a result.
- Confidentiality of test and what happens with results.
- Window period, if relevant.
- What result are they expecting?
- Limitations of testing and the window period.
- What support would they have if a test was to be positive?
- How will they obtain the result?
- Other concerns—symptoms or high-risk sexual activity, which would require specialist advice, e.g. need for PEP.
- Need full STI screening.

Preventon and risk reduction strategies

- Promoting condom use. There is compelling evidence that in sero-discordant couples, consistent condom use protects the sero-negative partner against infection.
- Post-exposure prophylaxis (📖 see PEP, p.208).
- Partner notification is desirable but not mandatory, and an environment favourable to disclosure must be encouraged.

- Male circumcision may reduce the risk of infection in men but whether it reduces the sexual transmission of HIV from men to women is not known.

Screening tests for HIV

Antibody test

Checks only for antibodies to the HIV virus. The window period (length of time for antibodies to the virus to appear in the blood) is 3 months. A rapid Point of Care screening Test will only test for HIV antibodies but the result can become available within half an hour.

Combined antibody and P24 antigen test

As well as antibodies, this picks up the antigen circulating in the blood and detects early infection, making the window period shorter (on average 6 weeks). Most UK hospital labs now offer a combined antibody and antigen test (check with your local lab).

For both tests a venous blood sample is required.

A person testing positive for HIV should always have a confirmatory test.

Pregnant women

Vertical transmission has dramatically reduced in the UK due to the antenatal programme of screening for HIV. An HIV +ve pregnant woman could still take antiretroviral drugs to prevent vertical transmission.

Highly active anti-retroviral drugs (HAART)

These medicines do not cure HIV but help to control viral replication and sustain the immune system. There has been a two-thirds reduction in AIDS-related deaths in the UK as more HIV +ve patients have a better life-expectancy on HAART. The choice of drugs is dependent on viral load, CD4 count, and other illnesses, which may be present at the time. There are side-effects associated with these drugs, which can affect patient compliance. Adherence is important, as viral resistance to drugs can occur if patients do not comply with treatment plans.

Progressive illnesses

(Formerly called AIDS-defining illnesses.) Occur if HIV is poorly controlled and include:

- Malignancies, e.g. lymphoma.
- Opportunistic infections, e.g. tuberculosis.

Post-exposure prophylaxis (PEP)

A combination of anti-retroviral drugs, which are given to women who are at high risk of exposure to HIV in order to prevent sero-conversion. These are often administered over a period of 4 weeks, with regular follow-up blood tests and reviews usually in a GUM clinic.

PEP for sexual exposure

The detailed risk assessment is based on the type of sexual activity, if the source or contact was from a high-risk group or prevalent area, and if the person was known to be HIV +ve. Such information helps clinicians weigh up the benefits to the patient of taking PEP vs the potentially severe side-effects and whether to recommend PEP or not.

PEP for a sharp injury

The risk of transmission from a single percutaneous exposure is estimated to be 0.3%. This risk increases if a deep injury occurred, or if a visibly blood-stained sharp or hollow-bore needle had just been in an artery or vein, or high-source HIV viral load.

In occupational-related exposure, if the source is known, e.g. a patient, they could be asked to consider an HIV test. The outcome could greatly affect whether someone should take PEP or not.

Timing of PEP

PEP works best if started within 72h (ideally within 24h) from exposure, although may be considered or recommended up to 2 weeks after exposure in someone at very high risk of acquiring HIV. Regular follow-up during the therapy is important to ensure adherence.

Resources

www.bashh.org/guidelines/2006/hiv_testing
www.bashh.org/guidelines/2006/pepse
General advice on HIV or PEP: www.tht.org.uk

Sexual dysfunction: history taking and useful prompts

Introduction

Disorders of sexual function may be the result of organic disease processes but more commonly they are due to psychological and emotional factors. Sexual problems are brought to medical settings because people do not know where else to go. The medical setting may sometimes not be the correct one, and the nurse's task may be to assess the problem and refer on appropriately. Without adequate information, the next step will not be clear, so good history taking is crucial.

Taking a comprehensive history of a sexual problem is dependent on both the ease and comfort of the nurse in dealing with this topic, and the willingness of the patient to open up such a sensitive area to that individual. A number of factors need to be taken into account to facilitate this.

General points

- Confidentiality needs to be clarified. The patient may well want to know how confidential her answers will be, how they will be recorded, and what will happen to them.
- Permission giving may be required from the nurse. The patient may be worried about the appropriateness of using explicit sexual language. The nurse should also seek permission before pursuing any line of investigation that the patient may feel uncomfortable with.
- Comfort with the topic is an essential ingredient of effective history taking. Discomfort with the need to be explicit is very common among our patients, as we do not discuss sex frankly in our culture, even when it is going well. It is, therefore, much more difficult when it is going badly. If we as clinicians are embarrassed or uncomfortable, then the difficulty in speaking out is doubled.
- Attitude needs to be open and non-judgemental, as any hint of criticism will close the patient down, and make further history taking very difficult.
- Language may need to be negotiated. Some words can be offensive or unacceptable to some people, or they may not have a word to describe or name something that needs to be explored.
- Taking time is crucial to good history taking in this sensitive subject. Rushing will mean people give inaccurate information, as they are often trying to express something they have never previously put into words.

Guidelines for areas to explore

- History of presenting symptom and its precise features: How long has it been going on? How was it first noticed? How is the patient's life and her relationship affected by it? What remedies have been tried so far? Has anything made it better/worse?
- What is happening in the patient's sexual life/relationship/family now?

- Medical history to include medical conditions, e.g. hypertension, depresssion, for which treatments like beta-adrenoceptor blocking drugs and selective serotonin re-uptake inhibitors may have been prescribed.
- Specific factors of relevance are: treatment for subfertility/or control of fertility, lost pregnancies, menstrual history, contraception.
- Sexual history to include: early sexual learning, sex education, childhood development, any interruptions, e.g. illness, loss of close relative, parental divorce, abusive events, trauma.
- Relationship history—first experience with a partner, same sex experiences, development of sexual relating, why relationships came to an end, the place of sex in relationships.

The woman's views on the reasons why her symptoms are occurring are important, as she will often be right. As sex is a multi-faceted, socio-psychological matter, it is impacted by many factors. These can include cultural and religious influences, life events, family and relationship problems, financial and social pressures, and so on. The successful resolution of a sexual problem needs to take account of whatever other factors may have a bearing on the well-being of the patient.

Referring on

Many women expect to be referred on for specialist help with a sexual problem, so it is useful to have knowledge of available facilities in your area.

Women very often have a good idea, both of what the problem is and what would be a good way forward. It is wise to ensure they know what the next step may involve before implementing it, however. Many women referred for therapy with a sexual problem have a fear that they will be asked to 'perform' for the therapist. In those circumstances they are unlikely to attend!

Female sexual arousal disorder

Definition

Sexual arousal in women brings about both physiological and psychological change. When a woman complains of a reduction in these changes, despite appropriate stimulation and a conducive emotional atmosphere, she may be experiencing arousal problems.

However, since a woman can undergo the physiological changes of sexual arousal without being consciously aware of them, she might believe she is experiencing arousal problems, when in fact, she is simply not psychologically/emotionally connecting to her bodily sensations of arousal. In other words, she is blocking her awareness of arousal.

Physiological changes of arousal

- Increase in respiratory rate, pulse, and blood pressure.
- Pelvic engorgement and swelling of the vulva.
- Ballooning and deepening of the interior third of the vaginal barrel.
- Vaginal lubrication.

Psychological changes of arousal

- Sense of excitement, well-being, elation.
- Wish for closeness with the partner.
- Feelings of emotional warmth, pleasure, openness.

Emotional atmosphere

For women, the ability to become sexually aroused is bound up with emotional atmosphere and the quality of the relationship with their partner. If the emotional environment is not conducive to the release of those neurotransmitters necessary for arousal to occur, arousal will be inhibited.

Underlying illness

Presentation of a sexual arousal problem can be the first symptom of an underlying illness that can be treated. Therefore, accurate diagnosis is crucial. Differential diagnosis must involve careful consideration of both physiological and emotional factors, in order to devise the most appropriate treatment strategy.

Psychological support

Treatment

The treatment of choice will depend on the cause(s) of the arousal problem, but it is worth bearing in mind that the commonest causes are emotional, in which case personal or relationship counselling is very often the advisable next step.

Where a physiological cause is found, it is likely that there will be a degree of psychological distress to the woman, and possibly to her partner also, and it would be important not to overlook any needs for support in this area. (📖 See Sexual dysfunction: treatment options, p.216.)

Physiological causes of sexual arousal disorder

- Inappropriate or insufficient stimulation.
- Neurological disease including multiple sclerosis.
- Vascular disease, such as hypertension, arteriosclerosis.
- Endocrine disorders.
- Any chronic pain condition.
- Drug side-effects.
- Mental illness.

Psychological causes of sexual arousal disorder

- Emotional stress or discomfort for any reason.
- Relationship stresses, inequality, lack of closeness.
- Cultural or religious influences and conditioning.
- Problems with intimacy or commitment.
- Fear of sex, sexual abuse, trauma.

Resources

Crowe, M (2005) *Overcoming relationship problems.* Constable Robinson, London.
Self help guide for couples in trouble, with useful homework exercises and good examples. Since relationship stress is so frequently a factor in arousal problems, this seems a good place to recommend it.

Hypoactive sexual desire disorder

Definition and classification of female sexual dysfunction (FSD)

Implicit to any discussion about a dysfunction is a consideration of normal functioning. There is much debate about this as satisfaction and fulfillment are more important to women than physiological events.

A classification that has been widely accepted is the American Psychiatric Association's *Diagnostic and Statistical Manual of Mental Disorders* (4th edn) (DSM IV-TR) which covers the physiological events of desire, arousal, and orgasm. Pain is also included.

DSM IV classification of sexual dysfunction

- Hypoactive sexual desire disorder (HSDD).
- Female sexual arousal disorder.
- Female orgasmic disorder.
- Sexual pain disorders—vaginismus and dyspareunia.

Definition of HSDD

HSDD or loss of libido is an absence of, or marked reduction in, a woman's desire for sex. It can be noticed by changes in frequency of dreams, fantasies, masturbation, and wish for contact with a partner.

Incidence

- Up to 46% of women in relationships never feel the need for sex.
- 23% of women not in relationship would say they do not experience sexual desire or libido.
- The incidence of loss of libido is, therefore, hard to quantify, but up to 34% of women are dissatisfied with their sexual lives.

Not necessarily a problem

Changes in libido are part of the hormonal and reproductive life of a woman, and could, therefore, be considered normal. If there has been a change that is causing distress to the woman or her partner, then it might become a problem.

Causes of loss of libido

Hormonal

- Hysterectomy and oophorectomy, menopause, pregnancy and childbirth, thyroid imbalance, conditions and drugs that cause hyperprolactinaemia.

Psychological distress

- Depression or anxiety, sexual phobia, sexual trauma, sexual abuse, grief and loss, family demands, work stress, insufficient knowledge about sex.

Relationship stresses

- Unexpressed resentment or anger, violence, infidelity, loss of intimacy, gender issues/inequality.
- Partner's sexual problem.

- Erection or ejaculation problems in the partner, changes in partner's sexuality, e.g. addiction, orientation confusion.
- Other sexual problems.
- Fear of sex, fear of pregnancy, avoidance, dyspareunia, vaginismus.

Assessment of HSDD

There are numerous diagnostic tools and validated inventories for sexual dysfunction, which assess various components of the disorder and scales that assess female sexual distress. All have self-reported versions available and take less than half an hour to administer. A full discussion of these inventories is out of the scope of this handbook.

Treatments

Pharmacological

Where there is imbalance, HRT may have a positive effect. Medical treatment of depression or other psychiatric conditions can also be helpful.

Couple therapy

This would be indicated where relationship issues are detected, and can be successful using a wide variety of approaches, including psychodynamic cognitive behaviour therapy, systematic therapy, and others.

Help for partner

Where there is a need to resolve or ameliorate a problem in the partner, that can be discussed and advice for further action given.

Management of the underlying sexual problem

If there is pain, phobia, fear, sexual trauma, or sexual abuse underlying the loss of libido, the appropriate help can be offered.

Adjustment

If the situation underlying the loss of libido is unlikely to be resolved, and if the woman can respond and enjoy sexual contact with her partner, then it need not be an obstacle to a fulfilling and happy sexual relationship.

Resources

American Psychiatric Association (1994) *Diagnostic and statistical manual of mental disorders* (4th edn). Washington DC American Psychiatric Association.

Kashak, E and Tiefer, L (2001) *A new view of women's sexual problems.* Haworth Binghampton.

Sexual dysfunction: treatment options

Introduction

The selection of treatment for sexual problems is dictated by what is revealed in the patient's history, identification of the sexual health problem, and her choice in discussion with the health professional.

Physical

- Surgical removal of hymeneal tag or a rigid hymen, if present. It should be emphasized that this is exceedingly rarely encountered, although sometimes the physical reaction to attempted genital examination can make full evaluation difficult.
- Vaginismus training using vaginal dilators, usually combined with psychological help to reduce fear, and may include biofeedback and anti-anxiety medication, along with counselling.
- Pelvic floor exercises can improve muscle tone and vaginal awareness.

Pharmacological

- Modification of reversible causes can be achieved by HRT and/or testosterone after a hysterectomy where indicated by abnormal blood levels. Topical oestrogen may also be beneficial after the menopause.
- Lubricants such as Sylk® and Replens MD® to aid vaginal dryness. Care should be exercised if latex contraceptive products are used, as natural oils can harm the latex.
- Creams and gels recommended for use in vestibulodynia and other vulval pain syndromes, possibly combined with oral medication, such as tricyclic anti-depressants.

Psychological

- Cognitive restructuring of unrealistic expectations and incorrect beliefs.
- Education of the woman and her partner, since lack of accurate information can give rise to performance pressure and fear of failure.
- Relationship evaluation and couple therapy, by professionals trained in understanding the impact of relationship patterns on sexual expression and function and the methods to resolve these.
- Individual counselling and psychotherapy, where indicated by history of trauma, sexual abuse, childhood influences, co-dependency, addictions.

Combined approaches

- Genital examination, if acceptable, can reveal hidden beliefs and emotional blocks in relation to the woman's self perception, body image, and relationship to her sexuality.
- Sensate focus and self-sensate focus, where the schedule outlined on p.217 is adapted for a single person.
- Psychosexual therapy/sexual and relationship therapy, which might include both of the above, and attend to couple relationship dynamics, systemic aspects of the couple, and all facets of sexual functioning.

Sensate focus

Ground rules

- Agree a ban on intercourse and genital touch until the programme includes these.
- Set up twice-weekly session times to spend on this, increasing from 20 to 60 minutes over 4 weeks.
- Speak during these times only if the touch of the partner is unpleasant or painful, as concentration is important.
- Emphasis is on the personal experience/learning of each partner, not on giving pleasure or aiming for any particular outcome.

Stage 1

Taking plenty of time, each person explores the other's body, avoiding breasts and genitals, avoiding trying to arouse the other, and concentrating on the physical and emotional feelings experienced in both 'active' and 'passive' roles. After 2 weeks, 4 sessions, there should be enough familiarity and trust to include breasts, asking for what is preferred, and experimenting with a range of touches, to include oils if liked.

Stage 2

Maintaining the ban on intercourse, genital touching can be included, to explore what types of touch feel pleasurable, to familiarize the couple with each other's genital responses, and to aid communication about each other's sexuality. If liked, proceeding to mutual masturbation to orgasm could be included after a few sessions.

Stage 3

Initially maintaining the ban on full intercourse, as before, the couple would experiment with including vaginal penetration and containment without thrusting for a few moments at each session, increasing the movements gradually session by session until full intercourse becomes easy and comfortable.

Resources

Consensus view of European experts: www.ipm.co.uk

d'Ardenne, P and Morod, D (2003) *The counselling of couples in healthcare settings: a handbook for clinicians*. Whurr London.

Contains practical information for dealing with a range of problems.

Female orgasmic disorder

Definition

It is the persistent or recurrent delay in, or absence of, orgasm following a normal sexual excitement phase, despite appropriate stimulation and a conducive emotional atmosphere (although some authorities prefer the term pre-orgasmia, if the condition is primary). It may be primary, if the woman has never experienced orgasm in any circumstances, or secondary, in which case, for some reason, she has ceased to have an orgasm. Also, female orgasmic disorder may be situational, where the woman is orgasmic in some situations and not others, e.g. being able to orgasm on her own but not with a partner.

Causes of anorgasmia

These may be physiological, psychological, or anatomical, and whatever the cause, there is likely to be a degree of emotional distress, usually a feeling of not being fully a woman, not measuring up to others, and a sense of shame and inadequacy. The main causes are physiological, psychological and anatomical (📖 see p. 219 for causes of anorgasmia).

Treatment

Education

Where there is a lack of accurate and useful information about the normal anatomy and physiology of orgasm, basic sex education is an important part of treatment.

Normalization

Many women with this problem believe they are the only sufferers, so reassurance that as many as 34% of women have sexual problems and about 10% of women have anorgasmia can be helpful.

Bodywork

This would include learning to masturbate to orgasm, possibly using aids (see below), practising Kegel's pelvic floor exercises to strengthen the pubbococcygeal muscles, sensate focus programme either for the woman alone or with a partner, experimenting with lubricants.

Sex aids

Sex toys and vibrators can be very helpful in this condition. Main's operated devices are more effective for women who have never achieved orgasm

Vielle orgasm enhancers are latex finger cots with protuberances to increase stimulation to the clitoris.

Couple therapy and counselling

These are useful where there may be underlying issues between the couple, or where the woman may benefit from deeper exploration of any emotional blocks to orgasm.

Causes of anorgasmia

Physiological causes

- Any disease that affects the nervous system or the blood supply to the genital area.
- Hormonal imbalance, particularly hyperprolacitinaemia, menopause, thyroid imbalance.
- Any drug treatment that affects the nervous system, particularly SSRIs.
- Genital surgery where the nerve supply may have been implicated.

Psychological causes

- Fear of intimacy/commitment/need to control.
- Relationship stresses.
- Fear of sex.
- Past sexual trauma.

Anatomical causes

- Insufficient or inappropriate stimulation.
- Poor pelvic fit between partners can cause orgasm difficulty with intercourse, simply because the male pelvis does not press the woman's vulva at the correct angle for her.
- Weakening of pelvic floor causing reduced intravaginal sensitivity.

Resources

Heiman, J, LoPiccolo, J (1988) *Becoming orgasmic: a sexual growth programme for women.* Piatkus Books, London.

Useful self-help guide for women, a bit old-fashioned but it does not sensationalize and is very sound.

Komisaruk, B, Beyer-Flores, C and Whipple, B (2007) *The science of orgasm.* Johns Hopkins University Press Baltimore.

Interesting for clinicians as it gives overview covering many aspects and approaches to this wide subject.

Chapter 9

Menopause

Menopause: overview

Definition

The permanent cessation of menstruation that is caused by ovarian failure. This can only be diagnosed a year after the last menstrual period, and is, therefore, a retrospective event.

The period that leads to this change is called the peri-menopause. This is characterized by biological and endocrine changes, which lead to symptoms and irregular bleeding.

It is estimated that at least 80% of women have at least one menopausal symptom but 45% find them troublesome and may seek help.

The menopause occurs in all women who live long enough. As life-expectancy extends, the menopause is now seen as a mid-life event, with the mean age at menopause being 52 years old; however, the range is 45–58.

It is estimated that 80% of women have menopausal symptoms but only 10–20 % receive hormone replacement therapy (HRT). With all of the controversy about HRT, it is essential that women receive accurate information in order for them to make an informed choice about whether to take HRT or not. Women with menopausal symptoms can generally be managed by their GP, practice nurse, or in well-woman clinics. However, specialist menopause clinics have a role to play in the management of women.

Physiology of the menopause

As the ovaries become unresponsive to FSH, the cycles become anovulatory. Follicular development fails and there is no production of oestrogen. The low oestrogen leads to a raised FSH, followed by a rise in LH.

History and examination

A general history (see Chapter 3, p.21) with the addition of:

- Assessment of the menopausal status—LMP and any menopausal symptoms.
- Full past gynaecological, medical, and surgical history, including history of hormone-dependent malignancies, osteoporosis, and thromboses/emboli (DVT/PE).
- Special attention to bleeding patterns, identifying any abnormalities, and investigating this prior to commencement on HRT.
- Indications for HRT—menopausal symptoms, premature ovarian failure, and risk factors for osteoporosis.
- Past use of hormones, i.e. COCP, HRT and whether any side-effects.
- Her need for contraception and a discussion around conception in the peri-menopause (see Chapter 13, p.359).
- Family history of cardiovascular disease (CVD), osteoporosis, DVT, breast cancer, bowel cancer, or ovarian cancer.
- Smoking and alcohol.
- Height, weight, BMI, waist circumference, and blood pressure.
- Pelvic, abdominal, and breast examination, if clinically indicated in relation to past/current disease, any symptoms or family history.
- Teaching breast awareness.

Symptoms of the menopause

Short-term symptoms

These are the most common reasons for women presenting to health professionals for help and advice, and are helped by HRT.

- Vasomotor symptoms.
- Psychological symptoms.
- Urinary and vaginal symptoms.
- Irregular bleeding/change in bleeding patterns: 3–7% cycles are anovulatory between the ages of 26–40 years and this rises to 12–15% between 41 and 51 years (see Abnormal bleeding at the menopause, p.240).
- The peri-menopause may be associated with reduced fertility.

Vasomotor symptoms: hot flushes

These are described as periods of inappropriate heat loss; they occur in about 75% of women. Frequency is variable from 1–2/week up to 20/day. They start prior to the final LMP and increase in incidence in the first year after the last period. Some women can suffer for more than 5 years. Each episode lasts for between 2.5 and 3.3 min. Women complain of intense heat, sweating, shivering, and tachycardia. At the time of the flushes, women can also suffer from faintness, weakness, vertigo, nausea, vomiting, insomnia, and palpitations. When they occur at night, there is a decrease in rapid eye movement. Sleep is disturbed, with more frequent waking. This leads to tiredness. Night sweats affect 75% women and can lead to irritability, anxiety, depression, fatigue, and inability to concentrate.

The pathophysiology varies from individual to individual. The onset of hot flushes is due to a decrease in the concentration in oestradiol and not the absolute oestradiol levels. There are changes in plasma levels of serotonin, adrenaline, and noradrenaline—the latter two can cause supraventricular tachycardias, peripheral vasodilatation, and anxiety. Untreated hot flushes will cause no long-term harm.

Psychological symptoms

These occur in about 25–50% of women. There is debate as to whether these symptoms are related to a lack of oestrogen or secondary to other symptoms, e.g. persistent night sweats lead to poor sleep that contributes to a reduced concentration span that affects memory and ultimately mood. Psychological symptoms may also be multi-faceted, taking into account past experiences, culture, and perceptions of the menopause.

Psychological symptoms

- Deterioration in memory and neurological function.
- Depression.
- Anxiety.
- Irritability.
- Mood swings.
- Lethargy.
- Lack of energy.
- Nervousness.
- Confusion.
- Loss of libido.
- Forgetfulness.
- Difficulty in concentration.
- Loss of confidence.
- Low self-esteem.

Urinary and vaginal symptoms

- Vaginal dryness.
- Painful sex.
- Recurrent vaginal infections.
- Recurrent urinary tract infections.
- Urinary incontinence.

Urethral and vaginal tissues are oestrogen-sensitive. The lack of oestrogen can lead to a lack of lubrication and a short and narrow vagina, which can lead to painful sex, lack of libido, and sexual dysfunction. Sexual dysfunction is a combination of both psychological and urogential symptoms.

Investigations

- FSH measurement is of limited value in diagnosis, unless there is doubt with symptoms. It has more value in POF (📖 see Chapter 6, p.99). The rise in FSH is gradual and there is a wide fluctuation in the climacteric period.
- Similarly LH, oestradiol, progesterone, and testosterone are of no value in assessing ovarian function.
- Measurement of oestradiol is of benefit only in monitoring levels when symptoms persist despite use of non-oral HRT.
- Thyroid function tests (TFT) (free T4 and thyroid stimulating hormone) can be measured if the presenting symptoms are lethargy, weight gain, hair loss, and flushes, or if the diagnosis of menopause is in doubt, particularly if non-response to HRT.
- Measurement of 24h urine for catecholamines, 5-hydroxyindolacetic acid, and methylhistamines to exclude the rarer causes of hot flushes, such as phaeochromocytoma, carcinoid syndrome, and mastocytosis, is generally carried out by specialists.
- Investigations required due to a positive personal medical or family history—thyroid, clotting screen, lipid profile, cervical smears, and mammogram.
- Bone density scan if risk factors for osteoporosis, POF, corticosteroids >5mg prednisolone/day, positive family history, especially first-degree relative, eating disorders, and height loss. Bone density may also be useful in helping women to decide whether or not to take HRT.
- Vaginal or abdominal ultrasound may be indicated to investigate abnormal bleeding or abnormal findings on examination.

Prevention of long-term health problems

Although in the short term, problems of the menopause can impact on quality of life, in the long term they do no harm. As discussed in the section on POF, the long-term consequences may be osteoporosis and an increased risk of cardiovascular disease. Osteoporosis is covered in a subsequent section and the role of HRT in primary prevention of cardiovascular disease remains unclear. Some studies do suggest that HRT started in the peri- and early menopause may be of benefit. Genito-urinary atrophy may cause dyspareunia and apareunia and can significantly affect quality of life.

Treatments: HRT and alternatives

The treatment will depend on the symptoms and their severity. Women with an early menopause should be managed as in the section on POF. If symptoms are mild, then they may respond to lifestyle changes, education, and reassurance.

Lifestyle advice

- Counselling.
- Reassurance.
- Diet—including weight management.
- Increased exercise.
- Relaxation.
- Maintain sexual activity to improve vaginal health.
- Avoid trigger foods for hot flushes—spicy food, caffeine, alcohol.
- Stop smoking—as part of a healthy lifestyle it can help reduce flushes.
- Maintaining mental activity.
- Vaginal dryness may be helped with lubricants and moisturizers.

HRT was the standard treatment for the menopause until the publication of the Million Women and the Women's Health Initiative studies. These cast doubt on the safety of long-term HRT and have led to the current guidance from the Committee on Safety of Medicines (CSM) that HRT should be used at the lowest dose for the shortest duration, primarily for the relief of menopausal symptoms.

With all treatments it is important to stress that they may take at least 3 months to see any benefit. If symptoms are severe and impact on quality of life, then hormone replacement therapy may be indicated. If women complain of vaginal symptoms, local HRT is likely to help.

HRT

HRT is medication that contains one or more female hormones, normally oestrogen and progestogen. It is used to treat the short-term symptoms of the menopause, such as flushes, by aiming to reproduce the effect that the hormones would have produced if they had been produced by the ovaries.

It is available as systemic and local treatments, and in different types, dose, and delivery systems to enable therapy to be tailored to each woman.

HRT is available as:

- Sequential (continuous oestrogen and cyclical progestogen) for women who are peri-menopausal.
- Continuous combined therapy (continuous oestrogen and progestogen), which is for post-menopausal women (bleed-free therapy). It is a 'misnomer' as some women will get irregular bleeding in first 6 months.
- Long-cycle HRT has 3 months of continuous oestrogen and tri-monthly cyclical progestogen.
- Oestrogen-only for women who have had a hysterectomy.
- Local treatments with topical oestrogen vaginally for women with vaginal symptoms only.

HRT delivery systems:
- Tablets.
- Transdermal patches and gel.
- Implants (subcutaneous).
- Vaginal (cream, ring, pessary, tablet).
- LNG-IUS.

► The most common HRT is oral.

If symptoms are minor, then women may benefit from lifestyle changes only as outlined before. The current thinking is that women should take the lowest dose of HRT for the shortest duration to relieve symptoms, with review of risks at regular intervals. In starting HRT, women should be advised to persevere for at least 3 months before changing a therapy if needed, and that sometimes they may need to try several therapies before finding one that is suitable for them.

⚠ Caution—HRT is different to the COCP and there are no breaks for bleeding and women should be encouraged to continue with no breaks in the treatment.

Duration of treatment

Treatment should be for the shortest time possible to stop symptoms. This is generally suggested up to 3–5 years for vasomotor symptoms. In POF, it is suggested to use HRT up to the age of 52 and then to re-assess risk factors and individualize as appropriate.

Stopping HRT

There is no evidence of a difference between immediate cessation or tapering the dose down first before discontinuation. But with the publication of studies that have led to large numbers of women stopping HRT suddenly, there are reports of return of severe symptoms.

Women can be put onto the lowest dose possible or they may like to try alternate tablets as a way of weaning themselves off. This is not possible in practical terms with sequential therapy.

Types of therapy

Sequential therapy

This can be via any delivery system but tablets and patches are the most common sequential therapies.

It mimics the natural cycle with continuous repeat cycles. Women have oestrogen for 28 days and then progestogen for 10–14 days, following this there is a withdrawal bleed. It is used in the peri-menopausal period and can help to regulate menstrual irregularities and relieve menopausal symptoms. This gives a monthly bleed. Long-cycle HRT therapies are designed for a 3-monthly bleed, as apposed to a monthly bleed, when women are unable to tolerate progestogens.

Continuous combined therapy

This is HRT with oestrogen and progestogen tablets or patches that are taken for 28-day cycles. This makes the endometrium atrophic and leads to no bleeding but a reduction of the symptoms. It is only suitable for women who have not had a period for a year. It gives better protection of the endometrium from hyperplasia and is not associated with PMS-like symptoms, which are not uncommon with sequential therapy.

If women are peri-menopausal and are sensitive to oral progestogens or require a near non-bleed therapy, then an IUS may be used. With systemic oestrogen, the Mirena® IUS is licensed for 4 years only for this indication.

Oestrogen-only therapy

This is used for women who have had a hysterectomy; it can be given as tablets, patches, and implants. More recent studies have shown a lower risk of breast cancer but using this in women with an intact uterus increases the risk of ovarian and endometrial cancer.

⚠ Women who have had a TAH and BSO for endometriosis may need to use combined therapy due to the risk of reactivation of the disease in the pelvis and then a re-occurrence of pain.

It can be difficult to decide when to switch women from sequential to continuous therapy. In general terms it is estimated that 80% of women will be post-menopausal by the age of 54, so this can be a good time to try. Women who had periods of over 6 months of amenorrhoea in their 40s and raised FSH will be menopausal a few years after taking HRT. Therapy can be changed and women warned that they may have some irregular bleeding for 6 months. If the bleeding continues after this, then it is prudent to investigate and, if all is normal, switch back to sequential.

Treatment: modes of delivery

Oral

Oral medication is absorbed by the gut and passed into the hepatic portal system, where it is metabolized into the active ingredient in the liver. This means that larger doses are needed for a therapeutic effect and the levels of circulating hormones vary and may not be enough to control symptoms.

Table 9.1 Oral delivery

Advantages	Disadvantages
Cheap	Disrupt the ratio of oestradiol to oestrone
Convenient	Needs compliance
Familiar	Nausea, affected by GI conditions May not be suitable where there is liver pathology Hypertension – through effect on angiotensinogen High lipids Past history of DVT/PE

Transdermal

Oestrogen can be given in the form of patches or gel. Transdermal progestogens can currently only be given as a combined patch. It is absorbed via the skin and associated with stable hormone levels and symptom control. The patches are applied on the abdomen, thighs, back, deltoid, or buttocks once or twice a week.

Table 9.2 Transdermal delivery

Advantages	Disadvantages
Normal ratio of oestradiol to oestrone	Problems with adhesion
Avoids the liver	Skin irritation
Can be perceived as natural	Visual reminder
May be preferred in women with diabetes, liver problems, and GI problems	Compliance

Implants

Implants of oestrogen and/or testosterone are given into the subcutaneous fat of the abdomen or buttocks on a 6-monthly basis. The levels of oestrogen achieved are generally higher compared to tablets or patches.

Table 9.3 Implants

Advantages	Disadvantages
Good control of symptoms	Needs to be inserted by a healthcare professional
Minimum compliance, administered twice a year	Prolonged use may be associated with tachyphylaxis—levels of oestrogen normal but symptoms of oestrogen withdrawal noted, i.e. the body clock is reset to higher levels of oestrogen
Can give testosterone for libido	
Avoids the liver	
Cheap and convenient, particularly after a hysterectomy	

In the event of tachyphylaxis with implants, the effects of the oestrogen can last up to 2 years, so in women who have a uterus, they may need to continue progestogens for 2 years after the last implant.

Vaginal

Local therapy can be administered to women who have atrophic vaginitis and/or urethritis without the systemic effects from HRT. It can be given in the form of creams, pessaries, rings, or vaginal tablets. The frequency of use is normally reduced after 2–3 weeks with discontinuation and assessment of need for further treatment after 3 months, dependent on the product.

Table 9.4 Vaginal delivery

Advantages	Disadvantages
No bleeding	Regulation can be difficult
Effective for urogenital symptoms	Messy
Can be used with systemic HRT for persistent local symptoms	Can be difficult to use in the elderly
Convenient	

Practical prescribing

In general, there are few absolute contraindications to HRT. These are: pregnancy, undiagnosed vaginal bleeding, active hormone-dependent tumours, and recent VTE event. In practice, women may need to be managed within a specialist clinic, with or without HRT.

When to refer to specialists

- Women with co-existing medical conditions requiring HRT.
- Multiple treatment failure.
- Previous or high risk of hormone-dependent cancer.
- Implant therapy.
- Abnormal bleeding in HRT users.
- Premature ovarian failure.

Other conditions can often cause some anxiety. Some of these are listed in 🕮 Table 9.5.

Table 9.5 Contraindications to HRT

Condition	Comments
Abnormal smears, cancer of the cervix	No contraindication
Angina	No contraindication
Asthma	HRT OK if stable—oestrogen may improve problem but progestogens may make it worse
Benign breast disease	No contraindication
Breast and ovarian cancer	Treated patients should be seen by specialist clinic. Women with family history need counselling and genetic referral
Coeliac disease	Increased risk of osteoporosis. Transdermal better
Crohn's disease	Increased risk of osteoporosis. Transdermal therapy
Depression	No contraindication, progestogens may exacerbate problem
Diabetes	No contraindication—if seen in specialist service, consider transdermal therapy
DVT/PEt	Individualize and decision to treat with HRT made in conjunction with haematologist
Endometrial cancer	Complete surgical resection—the merits of HRT and non-hormonal alternatives to be discussed on an individual basis

Table 9.5 Contraindications to HRT (*continued*)

Condition	Comments
	Incomplete—individual options need to be explored, high-dose progestogens may be considered, if appropriate
Endometrial hyperplasia	HRT can be administered if indicated
Endometriosis	No contraindication—can cause re-activation of disease, consider continuous combined therapy or tibolone even after hysterectomy to suppress deposits
Epilepsy	No contraindication—consider transdermal
Fibroids	No contraindication—may enlarge and will require monitoring of size and amount of bleeding
Gall bladder disease	Advise transdermal therapy/non-oral
Hypertension	No contraindication. Blood pressure may rise on conjugated equine oestrogen
Lactose intolerance	Consider non-oral therapy
Liver disease	Check LFTs prior to treatment—advise non-oral
Migraines/headaches	No contraindication—discontinue if problems worsen. If cyclical try continuous combined
Ovarian cancer	Do not consider if endometrioid ovarian cancer
Renal failure	No contraindication—may cause fluid retention
Rheumatoid arthritis	Due to steriods and immobility increased risk of osteoporosis—HRT can be used and does not increase risk of flare ups
Sickle cell disease	No contraindication
SLE	May deteriorate on HRT
Smoking	No contraindication, but cessation reduces symptoms
Stroke	May be considered, no contra-indication, but reassess risk factors and no HRT for three months after the episode
Thyroid disease	No contraindication—thyroxine will need to be monitored and may need to be increased

HRT: side-effects

As with all medication there can be side-effects with HRT. It is, therefore, of paramount importance when starting women on HRT to counsel about these and to warn women to be realistic. HRT is not a quick fix.
Side-effects are common in the first few weeks and normally resolve after 3 months.

If side-effects persist it is important to establish if they are related to the oestrogen or the progestogen, or to other incidental pathology.

Oestrogen-related side-effects

- Breast tenderness/engorgement.
- Nausea.
- Leg cramps.
- Bloating.
- Nipple sensitivity.
- Headaches.
- Dyspepsia.

These usually resolve, but if they do not, consider changing to a different oestrogen.

They can be worse if the patient is more than 5 years past the menopause. This can be minimized by starting with a very low dose.

Otherwise observe the patient and wait, reduce the dose or change the mode of delivery.

Progestogen-related side-effects

These are often worse in cyclical regimes and can appear as pre-menstrual like symptoms:

- Fluid retention, bloating.
- Breast tenderness.
- Abdominal cramps.
- Anxiety.
- Mood changes, depression.
- Headaches.
- Acne.
- Dysmenorrhoea.
- Clumsiness.
- Bleeding problems.

These can be reduced or alleviated by changing or adjusting the type of progestogen (testosterone to progesterone derivatives or vice versa) or by changing the route (transdermal) or the frequency of administration (long-cycle HRT).

Consider the use of the progestogen-only IUS, if neither oral or transdermal progestogen is tolerated.

Weight gain is often a reason that women will not start or decide to stop HRT. RCTs show no evidence of a link with HRT.

HRT: risks

Thrombosis

There is a risk of thrombosis in taking HRT. This is higher in the first years and with oral therapy. The risk is theoretically low ranging from 1/1000 to 3/10,000, if there are no other risk factors. In terms of absolute risk, there are 2 extra cases per 1000 women for 5 years use of oestrogen HRT at ages 50–69 and 8 extra cases per 1000 women for 5 years use of combined HRT at ages 60–69.

Risk factors include:

- Cardiovascular disease—pulmonary hypertension, atrial fibrillation.
- Massive obesity.
- Personal history of thrombosis.
- History of thrombosis on the combined oral contraceptive pill or in pregnancy.
- Strong family history of thrombosis.

Breast cancer

A woman in the UK has a lifetime risk of breast cancer of 10%. Women who have never used HRT aged 50–70 years old have a risk of 45/1000. The risk of breast cancer is increased on HRT in addition to the background risk that a woman may have in relation to family history and other medical factors. HRT use confers a similar risk year on year, similar to that of a late menopause. This increased risk does not apply to women with POF or those <50, suggesting that it is the lifetime exposure to oestrogen that confers the risk. If a woman has a specific family history, she should be referred for genetic counselling prior to the commencement on HRT to establish her individual risk. The risk is higher with combined HRT and lower in the Women's Health Initiative (WHI) in study with oestrogen only HRT. There is variation in risk with different studies. Updates can be found on the British Menopause Society website.

Aged 50–59

- For every 1000 women between the ages of 50 and 59 taking oestrogen-only HRT for 5 years, 2 will develop breast cancer.
- For every 1000 women between the ages of 50 and 59 taking oestrogen-only HRT for 10 years, 6 will develop breast cancer.
- For every 1000 women between the ages of 50 and 59 taking combined HRT for 5 years, 6 will develop breast cancer.
- For every 1000 women between the ages of 50 and 59 taking combined HRT for 10 years, 24 will develop breast cancer.

But mortality rates are lower in women who develop breast cancer while on HRT.

Endometrial cancer

In women who have a uterus there is a slightly increased risk of endometrial cancer and hyperplasia, especially if oestrogen-only HRT is used. This is significantly reduced with the addition of progestogen.

Non-hormonal and alternative menopause therapies

Non-hormonal options

With the decrease in the use of HRT, non-hormonal alternative treatments can include:

- Clonidine—originally developed as an anti-hypertensive. Is the only licensed non-hormonal preparation for menopausal flushing. It can help in some women (50µg twice daily), however, the evidence is conflicting and effects wear off after a few months.
- Anti-depressants, such as selective serotonin re-uptake inhibitors and noradrenaline re-uptake inhibitors like fluoxetine. Venlafaxine is the most convincing in studies, side-effects can sometimes preclude use. ⚠ This is an unlicensed use.
- Gabapentin shows limited evidence in relief of hot flushes (about 50% improvement).
- Progestogens may help in vasomotor symptoms; however, doses that are effective may increase the risk of vascular disease and safety of these doses with regard to breast is uncertain.

Alternative therapies

Many women will use these, as there is a perception that they are natural. However, there may be concerns on safety and it is important to ascertain whether women are using any other over-the-counter or herbal or other preparations. Also, women should be encouraged to try one preparation at a time to assess efficacy and to limit cost. There is currently a lack of long-term evidence in relation to alternatives. Patients should be encouraged to check a practitioner's qualifications, how long they have been practicing, and how much it will cost.

Herbal remedies need to be used with caution in women who have a contraindication to oestrogens. Interactions with medication can lead to a decrease in efficacy of the prescribed medication and/or irregular bleeding. The following are alternative therapies:

- Phyto-oestrogens are plant substances that have a similar effect to oestrogen. They can be added to foods to enrich them or are found commonly in soya products. The two main groups are isoflavones and ligans. There is a growing body of evidence that redclover isoflavones are well-tolerated in healthy women and reduction in hot flushes ranges from 20 to 50%. However, further research is warranted on safety.
- Progesterone transdermal cream has been advocated for the treatment of hot flushes. Insufficient published data show positive effect on hot flushes. Some women use a combination of oestrogens with progesterone cream with no guarantee of endometrial safety.
- Black cohosh—a plant from North America that may help with flushes; caution is needed, as there have been some reports of liver toxicity.
- Others include: St John's Wort, ginseng, evening primrose oil, dong quai, kava kava, gingko, wild yam cream, liquorice root, valerian root, and Angus castus.

- Homeopathic therapies are based on concept of 'minimal doses' and 'similars'.
- Acupuncture, reflexology, acupressure, massage, Reiki, Alexander technique, Ayurveda, and magnetism show little effect on menopausal symptoms but have been tried.
- Dehydroepiandrosterone (DHEA) is a steroid secreted by the adrenals and is thought to help with memory, libido, and well-being. There is no evidence to show that DHEA has any effect on hot flushes.

Abnormal bleeding at the menopause

This can manifest as abnormal bleeding in the peri-menopause, or post-menopause and irregular bleeding on sequential or continuous combined HRT. It is important to investigate, as it can signify cancer of the endometrium or cervix—though uncommon. It is much more likely that no cause will be found or that the bleeding is from benign pathology. If women are on HRT, bleeding can be one of the reasons for discontinuation, as they find the side-effect annoying.

Abnormal bleeding that may require investigation includes:

- Change in menstrual pattern.
- Inter-menstrual bleeding.
- Post-coital bleeding.
- Post-menopausal bleeding that occurs a year after the LMP.
- Breakthrough bleeding on sequential HRT and/or change in pattern of withdrawal bleeds.
- Bleeding that occurs on continuous combined HRT after the first 6 months of initiating therapy and bleeding after a phase of amenorrhoea.

In assessing risk factors for bleeding, the relevant risk factors for endometrial cancer need consideration.

Risk factors for endometrial cancer

- Nulliparity.
- Late menopause.
- Diabetes.
- Obesity.
- PCOS.
- Unopposed oestrogen.
- Family history of endometrial cancer.

Assessment

All women should have:

- Abdominal examination.
- Pelvic and speculum examination.
- Smear, pregnancy test, and swabs, if indicated.
- Ultrasound scan. This is to assess the endometrial thickness and any pathology, such as fibroids and polyps. Some have a 4mm cut-off value for endometrial thickness in women who are post-menopausal or on continuous HRT. In women on sequential HRT in the peri-menopause, there is no standard measure of endometrial thickness. If possible women should have an ultrasound performed just after a bleed.
- Hysteroscopy and/or biopsy may be indicated.
- Reassurance, as about 40% of women will be found to have pathology such as polyps, fibroids, hyperplasia, with a minority having a cancer.

After assessment, women may be reassured and monitored or referred for further investigations, such as hysteroscopy and biopsy.

Dependent on the findings, women may be managed as for menorrhagia, IMB, or PCB (📖 see Chapter 5, p.69).

Abnormal bleeding on HRT

Up to 60% of HRT users have abnormal bleeding. In some women, it may be due to the wrong HRT, e.g. if they are too young for continuous combined HRT.

Women on sequential HRT should have regular withdrawal bleeds that are not too heavy or painful. Some women have amenorrheoa and this may not need investigation. Abnormal bleeding on HRT is relatively rare and includes post-coital bleeding and inter-menstrual bleeding.

Causes of bleeding include:

- Cervical and endometrial polyps.
- Submucosal fibroids.
- Uterine malignancy.
- Bleeding on continuous combined therapy—check if post-menopausal and on correct therapy. If within first 6 months observe, if persists investigate.
- Idiosyncratic—this can be reduced by changing the type of oestrogen, progestogen, or the route of administration.
- Spontaneous ovarian activity.
- Endometrial hyperplasia.
- Unscheduled bleeding may be due to the woman's underlying cycle. Initiating the progestogen 12 days prior to the expected start of menstruation can prove helpful.

Women should be investigated if they have abnormal bleeding. This could be performed in a one-stop clinic environment where there is access to ultrasound, endometrial biopsy, and hysteroscopy, if needed.

► For women who are on HRT, check compliance. Check if there has been a change in medication.

A thickened endometrial in a woman on HRT or any irregularity of the endometrium should be considered abnormal and a hysteroscopy and endometrial biopsy performed.

If investigations have been performed and are normal then the following can be tried:

- If the bleeding is heavy, painful, starts too early, or prolonged, the type and/or dose of progestogen can be changed, or an LNG-IUS considered.
- Spotting early in the cycle—increasing the oestrogen may help.
- If breakthrough bleeding is a persistent problem, then it needs to be investigated. This can be due to poor compliance, drug interactions, GI upset, or stress.
- Consider a wash-out period and stopping HRT for 6 weeks.
- Synchronize with cycle so progestogen intake occurs in luteal phase.
- Absorption/compliance problems—change route.
- If suitable, consider changing to bleed-free preparations.
- Consider the use of the LNG-IUS, vaginal progestogen gels, e.g. Crinone®.

Sexual dysfunction at the menopause

Around the time of the menopause there can be many changes in a woman's life; these can include changes in sexual activity. Sexual function decreases in both sexes with aging. This seems to be more pronounced in women and has led to speculation that this could be linked to changes within the menopause. There is evidence that oophorectomy decreases circulating testosterone, which has a negative impact on sexuality and libido.

There is now a recognized term 'female sexual dysfunction', which is further divided into four disorders.

Female sexual dysfunction

- Class one: sexual desire disorders; a lack of thoughts, desires, and receptivity, which causes distress or sexual aversion disorder.
- Class two: sexual arousal disorders; inability to maintain sexual excitement.
- Class three: orgasmic disorder; inability to have an orgasm.
- Class four: sexual pain disorders; includes painful sex, vaginismus, and genital pain.

In practice, manifestations may overlap with pain maybe being the underlying cause of the problem. Many of these problems can be related to the lack of oestrogen and the associated vaginal problems. In addition, there may be life factors that come into play.

Treatment

The treatment of sexual dysfunction falls within the remit of numerous members of the multidisciplinary team, e.g. women may need local oestrogen cream, testosterone patches, and counselling. The addition of oestrogen helps, but addition of testosterone supplements can help further.

- Testosterone can be administered in the form of implants and, more recently, patches. However, gel that is licensed for males can sometimes be used.
- Tibolone is useful in women who require continuous HRT and have a low libido, as this is also licensed for the improvement of libido.
- There are two in the relationship and male-partner issues need to be taken into account (📖 see Chapter 8, p.167).

Osteoporosis

Definition

Osteoporosis is a disease process in its own right but can also result from a longer-term deficiency of oestrogen. It is characterized by low bone mass and destruction of bone structure, which may lead to increased fracture risks. In the menopause, the lack of oestrogen causes an increase in bone turnover and an imbalance between resorption and formation of bone. Once bone mass has been lost it is hard to replace. Bone mass is at its peak when women are in their 30s and declines from then on. However, in the presence of risk factors, peak bone mass may not have been reached or bone mass diminishes, so there is a higher risk of osteoporosis.

Prevalence

It affects 1 in 3 women and 1 in 12 men. Women who have an early menopause are more at risk but there are other factors that impact on risk (see Box).

The risk of developing osteoporosis is not related entirely to the menopause, as bone mass can be affected by the following factors:

- Race.
- Sex.
- Hereditary factors, including a past family history.
- Hormonal factors.
- Exercise.
- Low dietary calcium.
- Early menopause <45 years old.
- High intake of alcohol.
- Smoking.
- Low body weight.
- Nulliparity.
- Episodes of amenorrhoea.
- Sedentary lifestyle.
- The long-term use of steroids either oral or inhalers.
- Hyperparathyroidism.
- Cushing's syndrome.
- Other chronic diseases, e.g. rheumatoid arthritis.

Diagnosis

Osteoporosis and osteopenia can be diagnosed with DEXA (duel energy X-ray absorptimetry) scan of the hip and spine. The individual density is plotted against the normal range for a young adult to give the T-score. Osteopenia and osteoporosis are defined by the number of standard deviations below the mean. A T-score of –2.5 indicates osteoporosis and –1 to –2.5 SD equates to osteopenia.

Treatment

Women who are worried about bone density, and who have no risk factors, can be advised on a diet high in calcium and vitamin D, and weight-bearing exercises.

Before the publication of the WHI study, HRT was considered first-line treatment in the prevention of osteoporosis. The current advice is not to use HRT as a first-line treatment in the absence of any other symptoms in women of a normal menopausal age. However, HRT is effective at maintaining bone density.

Most of the options work by inhibiting bone resorption.

- Calcium and vitamin D—recommendations for the daily requirement of calcium can vary from 700mg–1500mg.
- Bisphosphonates—are used in the prevention and treatment. They need to be given on an empty stomach and can cause GI disturbances. This can be reduced by giving weekly or monthly preparations and asking the patient to stay upright for ½h after taking the tablets.
- Raloxifene—this is a SERM (selective estrogen receptor modulator) that is licensed for vertebral fractures, but limited evidence in relation to hip fractures. It has an increased risk of VTE and fatal stroke and does not reduce the risk of coronary heart disease. It can cause hot flushes, making it not ideal for menopausal women. However, it reduces the risk of breast cancer.
- Teriparatide—parathyroid hormone used in severe osteoporosis.
- Strontium ranelate—needs to be taken on an empty stomach and can cause stomach upset.
- Hip protectors—used to decrease the impact of falling on the hip.

Cardiovascular disease (CVD)

Coronary heart disease (CHD) is the leading cause of death in women, but it is generally thought to be a man's disease. The presentation in women tends to be different. Women are generally older and present with different symptoms.

- The risk of cardiovascular diseases such as myocardial infarction (MI) and stroke increases with age and after the menopause. Studies have shown that there is an increase in events in women who have had their ovaries removed, which would suggest a protective effect of oestrogen.
- Within a menopause consultation, assessment, and discussion around risk factors for heart disease and stroke, as well as other risk factors that can be found within the medical history, such as hypercholesterolemia, smoking, obesity, and stress, should be undertaken. This should include measurement of blood pressure, BMI, and waist circumference. Advice on lifestyle changes that can help to reduce risk is important.
- In the 1990s, observational studies showed a 40% reduction in incidence of coronary heart disease in HRT users.
- RCTs for primary prevention—WHI and secondary prevention RCTs do not confirm the results of observational studies. These studies have shown a higher risk of stroke and MI in women. This is generally thought to be as women in the trials were older and had other risk factors for development of such problems and started on HRT more than 10 years after the menopause.
- Re-analysis of WHI and nurses' health study—show timing of initiating HRT is crucial and that oestrogens may have a protective role in CHD in age 50–59. It is suggested that starting at the time of the menopause may be beneficial. Further studies are needed in this area.
- Higher doses of oestrogen have the potential to cause vascular harm.
- Background incidence of stroke is 4/10,000 at age 50–59 and 9/10,000 at age 60–69, there are one and three additional cases respectively with both oestrogen only and combined HRT for 5 years use.

Resources

For health professionals:
- www.medscape.com
- www.bms.org.uk

For women:
- www.bms.org.uk
- www.menopausematters.co.uk
- www.patient.co.uk
- www.womens-health-concern.org

Chapter 10

Bladder and urogenital prolapse

Assessment of urinary incontinence

Types of urinary incontinence

Stress urinary incontinence (SUI)

The involuntary leakage of urine on effort or exertion, e.g. on sneezing or coughing. It is the commonest presenting symptom for which women seek advice.

Urge urinary incontinence

Involuntary leakage accompanied by, or immediately preceded by, a strong desire to void. Overactive bladder (OAB) is a symptomatic diagnosis when the patient experiences urgency, frequency, urge incontinence, and/or nocturia.

Mixed urinary incontinence

When the woman complains of SUI and urge incontinence at the same time.

Voiding difficulties

Generally the bladder will empty almost completely. When the bladder is unable to empty completely, this may be due to an under-active detrusor muscle, stricture, constipation, urinary tract infection, or surgery.

There are many factors affecting bladder function and a person's ability to cope with continence 🕮 see Table 10.1.

Table 10.1

Factors affecting bladder function	Factors affecting ability to cope with incontinence
Urinary tract infection (UTI)	Immobility
Faecal impaction	Environment
Drug therapy	Mental function
Endocrine disorders, e.g. diabetes insipidus	Emotions
Bladder pathology—stones, cancer	Poor patient care

Assessment

General gynaecology assessment needs to be undertaken (🕮 see Chapter 3, p.21). However, further symptoms need to be explored, dependent on the patient's presenting urinary symptoms.

- Urinary symptoms—since when (e.g. since hysterectomy)? was the onset sudden? linked to any specific time (e.g. when the weather is cold/after drinking lots of alcohol)?
- Nocturia—when the bladder wakes you at night; defined as more than two episodes.
- Urgency—desperate need to get to the toilet; a sudden, compelling desire to pass urine that is difficult to defer.
- Urge incontinence—leakage of urine on the way to the toilet.
- Frequency—frequent trips to the toilet (normal is 6–8 times a day).
- Stress urinary incontinence—leakage with coughing, sneezing, or increasing intra-abdominal pressure.

- Urinary tract infections (UTIs), which have been treated by the GP. If the patient has had more than four infections in one year, she needs to be investigated.
- Frank haematuria—visible blood in the urine.
- Voiding difficulties—does the patient feel like she is emptying her bladder fully, poor stream, hesitancy?
- Previous treatment, pelvic, and abdominal surgery.
- Drug therapy.
- History of pelvic organ prolapse.
- Fluids—type of fluids drunk, how much, when?
- Bowels—how often she opens her bowels, whether she uses laxatives, whether she digitates vaginally or anally. The assessor may find it useful to use the Bristol stool scale to determine how the stool looks to aid treatment.[1] Is there concomitant faecal incontinence?
- Obstetric history—parity, duration of labour, tears, sutures, instrumental deliveries, recency of childbirth.
- Quality of life questionnaires—these can be a useful adjunct in assessing the impact of urinary incontinence and bladder dysfunction. Questionnaires commonly used are Kings Health Questionnaire (KHQ), the Incontinence Impact Questionnaire (IIQ), or the incontinence short questionnaire (ICI) form. The international consultation on incontinence short questionnaire is a validated combined symptom and quality of life questionnaire. It is comprised of four questions that measure symptoms of urinary incontinence and their impact on the quality of life.

Physical assessment and local assessment

Look for focal neurological signs, e.g. altered sensation in the distribution of the sacral nerves (S2–S4) or loss of local reflexes, such as clitoral–anal reflex.

Abdominal examination followed by vaginal examination—the assessor should be looking for the following during a vaginal assessment:

- Pelvic organ prolapse—type and severity.
- Any pelvic masses.
- Assessing pelvic floor strength and tone—by inspection (drawing up of the anus, lifting of the posterior wall of the vagina, and narrowing of the vaginal introitus) or by digital palpation (e.g. Oxford Score).
- Looking for evidence of a sore vagina/atrophic vagina.
- Evidence of lichen sclerosis, *Candida*, or sexually transmitted infections (STI).
- The assessor should also ask the woman to cough to see if there is any leakage of urine (cough test).

Resources

www.NICE.org.uk

1. Lewis, S and Heaton, KW (1997) Stool form scale as a useful guide to intestinal transit time. *Scand J Gastroenterol* **32**(9): 920–924.

Investigations of urinary incontinence

Urinanalysis

Mandatory as a screening tool for haematuria, glycosuria, pyuria, and bacteruria. Microscopic haematuria in the absence of infection should be investigated only if persistent.

Mid stream urine (MSU)

Dipstick for nitrites and leucocyte, and send off for microscopy culture and sensitivity (MC&S) if positive.

Frequency volume chart

This will provide useful information about bladder function and the degree of incontinence. The patient records her intake and type of fluid, the volumes taken and voided, as well as the time of each micturition, day and night. This should be completed for at least 3 days.[1]

Post-void residual urine volume (PVR)

Perform a PVR, using a bladder scanner or an in and out catheter, if no scanner is available. Any PVR of 150ml or over (this amount may vary from unit to unit) should be considered significant. If the PVR remains high, she may need to learn how to perform intermittent self-catheterization.

Pyridium (phenazopyridine)

A urinary dye, 200mg three times a day can be used to detect incontinence if there is doubt, e.g. in women where a fistula is suspected.

Flow rate

📖 See Urodynamics, p.252.

Urodynamic studies

Not required as part of the initial management of incontinence, except when:

- there is voiding dysfunction;
- high PVR urine volumes;
- severe stress incontinence such that surgery is indicated as first line treatment;
- failure of conservative measures.

1. National Institute for Health and Clinical Excellence. *The Management of Urinary Incontinence in Women.* www.nice.org.uk. (Accessed January 2009)

Urodynamics 1

Types of urodynamics

Urodynamics is a term used to describe a combination of tests that look at the ability of the bladder to store and expel urine. They study the pressure, volume, and flow relationships in the lower urinary tract. Urodynamic investigations are not 100% sensitive or specific, therefore a detailed history and examination are still vital components of patient assessment.

When to perform urodynamics

Urodynamics are often performed prior to bladder neck surgery or prolapse surgery if the woman is also complaining of urinary symptoms. A prolapse can often mask symptoms of urinary incontinence, so performing urodynamics with a ring pessary *in situ* (which will simulate the anatomy following a prolapse repair) may reveal occult stress incontinence that could then be rectified with a continence procedure at the same time as the pelvic floor repair.

Some hospital units perform urodynamic investigations on all women not responding to conservative treatments. The indications may vary from unit to unit.

Indications for urodynamics

- Failure of conservative therapy for incontinence.
- Past history of prolapse/continence surgery.
- Women with concomitant pelvic organ prolapse and incontinence.
- Mixed urinary symptoms.
- Voiding difficulties.
- Painful bladder syndromes and recurrent cystitis.

Uroflowmetry

This plots the flow rate of urine over time and represents it graphically (see Fig. 10.1). It can be used to screen for voiding difficulties. Women should be encouraged to attend the clinic with a comfortably full bladder so they can void 'normally' on the toilet.

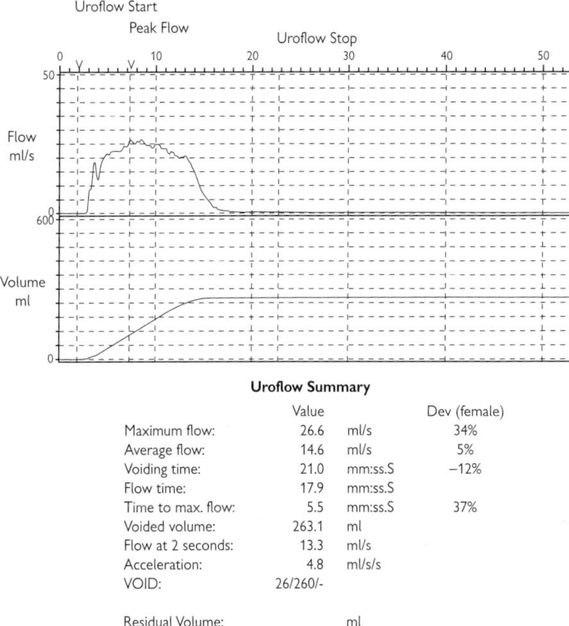

Uroflow Summary

	Value		Dev (female)
Maximum flow:	26.6	ml/s	34%
Average flow:	14.6	ml/s	5%
Voiding time:	21.0	mm:ss.S	–12%
Flow time:	17.9	mm:ss.S	
Time to max. flow:	5.5	mm:ss.S	37%
Voided volume:	263.1	ml	
Flow at 2 seconds:	13.3	ml/s	
Acceleration:	4.8	ml/s/s	
VOID:	26/260/-		
Residual Volume:	________	ml	

Fig. 10.1 Uroflow chart.

Resources

www.NICE.org.uk

Urodynamics 2

Cystometry

The recent NICE guidelines[1] for the treatment of stress urinary incontinence in women do not recommend performing cystometry prior to any bladder neck surgery, unless there is clinical suspicion of detrusor overactivity, there has been previous surgery for stress incontinence, or there are symptoms suggestive of voiding difficulties. This has caused much debate amongst urogynaecologists and urologists performing bladder neck surgery, and many units still perform urodynamics prior to this type of surgery.

The patient is catheterized following the flow-rate test. A fine pressure catheter (which measures the pressure in the bladder or intra-vesical pressure) is passed into the bladder along with a filling catheter and a pressure catheter is inserted into the vagina or anus; this catheter measures the pressure in the abdomen as the bladder is filled.

The bladder is then filled rapidly at 50–100ml/min with normal saline. A slower fill may be used for those with neurological disorders. The patient is asked to state when she can feel her bladder filling, when she gets the first sensation to void, and when her bladder feels full. During the test, the patient is asked to cough at regular intervals to ensure correct placement of the pressure lines. The filling catheter is then removed and she is asked to perform a series of provocation tests, which may include coughing, star jumps, heel bouncing, listening to running water, and hand-washing. Any urinary leakage is noted, along with any rise in intra-vesical pressure that may indicate an over-active detrusor muscle.

Video-urodynamics—videocystourethrography (VCU)

This is used for complex cases in tertiary units only. It combines X-ray imaging of the bladder neck with cystometry by filling the bladder with urograffin instead of saline. Video-urodynamics is especially useful to detect detrusor-sphincter dyssenergia in those with spinal cord injury, where voiding difficulties are caused by the failure of the urethral sphincter to relax at the same time the bladder contracts.

Urethral pressure profilometry

Can provide useful information about urethral function, but there are limitations related to artefacts and reproducibility.

1. National Institute for Health and Clinical Excellence. *The Management of Urinary Incontinence in Women.* www.nice.org.uk (Accessed January 2009.)

Ambulatory urodynamics

Ambulatory urodynamics can be used for the diagnosis of detrusor over-activity and the aim is to perform measurements under more physiological conditions, but this test is not routinely available in units offering urodynamic testing in the UK. An intra-vesical and intra-abdominal line is inserted, but no filling catheter is used. The bladder fills naturally with urine from the kidneys. A small recording device is worn and the information can be downloaded for review at a later date. This test is indicated when simple urodynamics fail to pick up stress incontinence or detrusor over-activity (DO) but the woman's symptoms are highly suggestive of the disorder.

Although overactive bladder (OAB) is a symptomatic diagnosis, the diagnosis of detrusor over-activity (DO) can only be made following urodynamic investigations.

Overactive bladder (OAB): overview

Symptoms and terminology

Overactive bladder syndrome (OAB) is a term used to describe a symptom complex in those suffering with urinary urgency, frequency, and nocturia, with or without urge incontinence.

Detrusor over-activity (DO) has been defined by the International Continence Society as the 'occurrence of uninitiated, spontaneous, or provoked detrusor contractions during bladder filling' while the woman is attempting to inhibit micturition.

A patient may have symptoms of OAB, but may not have DO. Urodynamic investigations need to be performed to make a diagnosis of DO.

⚠ Some medication used in the treatment of other unrelated medical conditions can cause side-effects that can lead to symptoms of OAB, e.g. diuretics, alpha blockers.

Prevalence

The prevalence varies with age, 1 in 6 women are affected by bladder problems; in the elderly it could be seen in as many as 80% of women.

Aetiology

- Most cases of OAB are idiopathic.
- Diabetes mellitus.
- Neurological disorders such as multiple sclerosis, spinal injury, Parkinson's disease, cerebrovascular accident, tropical spastic paraparesis can result in DO.
- Drugs such as diuretics.

Clinical presentation

- Frequency.
- Urge.
- Noctura is present in up to 70% of women.
- Urgency in 80% of women.
- DO may be associated with a history of childhood enuresis.

Examination

- Check that the bladder is not palpable to exclude retention.
- Single digit transvaginal bladder palpation is useful as it may exhibit urgency on bladder palpation.
- Examine for neurological lesions—cranial nerves, sacral dermatomes, muscle wasting, weakness of reflexes in the lower limb, and decrease in tone of the anal sphincter.

Investigations

MSU

Urinalysis must be performed on all patients presenting with symptoms of OAB to rule out a UTI, as symptoms are very similar.

Frequency volume chart/bladder diary

These are an essential tool in discovering the extent of a patient's bladder problems. The sensitivity and specificity in diagnosis of DO is 90%.

NICE suggest that a bladder diary (see Fig. 10.2) should be completed for at least 3 days whilst covering normal activities. Women are asked to record when they pass urine and write down the voided volumes, if possible. They are also asked to record how much they drink, when, and what they are drinking. It is then possible for the nurse to run through and reiterate fluid advice according to the chart.

Urodynamics

Urodynamics should not be performed before conservative treatment has been tried for at least 6 weeks (NICE 2006). Urodynamics can help to assess:

- bladder sensation;
- bladder compliance; and
- detrusor activity.

There are problems regarding their reproducibility, validity, and accuracy. Two patterns seen on urodynamics are.

- Phasic DO: where contraction of the detrusor occurs spontaneously or as a result of provocation during cystometry.
- Terminal DO: there is no activity during filling, but at the end of filling, there is involuntary DO that results in incontinence.

Time	IN	OUT	WET	How urgently I needed to get to a toilet
07.00				
08.00				
09.00				
10.00				
11.00				
12.00				
13.00				
14.00				
15.00				
16.00				
17.00				
18.00				
19.00				
20.00				
21.00				
22.00				
23.00				
00.00				

Fig. 10.2 Bladder diary/frequency volume chart. Reproduced with kind permission of Guy's and St Thomas' Foundation Trust.

1. National Institute for Health and Clinical Excellence. The management of urinary incontinence in women www.nice.org.uk (Accessed January 2009.)

Treatments for overactive bladder

Treatments for a woman presenting with OAB are simple.

- Caffeine reduction and fluid advice.
- Bladder retraining and frequency volume chart completion.
- Pelvic floor exercises.
- Medication.

Pelvic floor exercises (PFE), fluid advice, and bladder retraining have been explained in the conservative management section of this chapter.

Drug therapy

Drug therapy is prescribed in order to reduce symptoms of urgency, frequency, and urge incontinence associated with OAB. NICE[1] recommend that drug therapy should be considered if conservative therapy (PFE, bladder retraining, and caffeine reduction) fails to improve symptoms after a period of 6 weeks. Patients with symptoms of voiding difficulties should have a bladder scan performed prior to starting any anticholinergic medication, to ensure they are emptying their bladder properly. If patients have a significant PVR volume, starting antimuscarinic medication may make this worse and cause recurrent urinary tract infections.

Anticholinergic drugs

There are a number of anticholinergics available that help to reduce symptoms of OAB (e.g. oxybutinin hydrochloride, tolterodine tartrate, trospium chloride, solifenacin succinate, fesoterodine, darifenacin) They act on muscarinic receptors by blocking acetylcholine.

Oxybutinin has antihistamine properties in addition to being antimuscarinic. Oxybutinin is available in two oral forms (immediate and extended release form) and a transdermal preparation. Recent guidance suggests that immediate release should be tried first, but if side-effects are anticipated or occur, other drugs should be used.

Side-effects

They all have the potential to cause side-effects of constipation, dry mouth, and dry eyes, as muscarinic receptors are found in other parts of the body and these too are blocked, so women must be counselled about this prior to commencing them on the medication. They should be advised on measures to reduce these side-effects, should they occur.

Oestrogens

Post-menopausal women with symptoms of OAB, who have vaginal atrophy, may benefit from a course of topical oestrogen. However, oestrogens have no proven benefit on detrusor over-activity.

Tricyclic anti-depressants

Imipramine has antihistaminic, anticholinergic, and local anaesthetic properties. Side-effects include tremor, anticholinergic side-effects, and fatigue.

Vasopressin analogues

Desmopressin has been used to treat nocturia and nocturnal enuresis, since it decreases urine production by 50%. Hyponatraemia is a major side-effect, so monitoring is required.

1. National Institute for Health and Clinical Excellence. The management of urinary incontinence in women www.nice.org.uk (Accessed January 2009.)

Specialized treatments

More invasive and specialized treatments include:

- Botulinum toxin type A—seven types of botulinum are known. Type A is beneficial in idiopathic DO for up to 1 year, while type B has shown some short-term benefit in the treatment of refractory DO. ⚠ This use is unlicensed.
- Neuromodulation uses electrical stimulation of the sacral nerves to treat DO. This is only undertaken in specialist units.
- Denervation—the idea is to denervate the micturition reflex.
- Urinary diversion can be into the abdominal cavity, by construction of an ileal conduit, or outside the abdomen, by inserting a suprapubic catheter for continuous drainage.
- Continent diversion, such as mitrofanoff pouch, and clam cystoplasty to increase the bladder capacity.

These last two surgical procedures are only considered if every other treatment avenue has been explored and with in-depth counselling, as they may be associated with significant potential complications. There is a 5% risk of adenocarcinoma with clam cystoplasty and cystitis and calculus formation can occur.

Stress urinary incontinence: overview

Definition

Stress incontinence has been defined as the involuntary loss of urine on effort or exertion, or sneezing or coughing or any rise in intra-abdominal pressure. It is not associated with urgency and is generally associated with smaller volume loss than urge incontinence. Stress urinary incontinence is the most common cause of incontinence in the UK. It represents around 50% of all incontinent women.

Risk factors

There are many possible causes, some of which are listed below.

- Pregnancy/childbirth—the number of deliveries, the length of the second-stage of labour, i.e. quick or protracted with many hours pushing, whether instruments were used, i.e. forceps, ventouse, whether there was a tear and/or stitches. High parity and instrumental delivery are associated with a high prevalence of post-natal incontinence.
- Caucasian race is associated with higher prevalence, as opposed to Black and Asian.
- Menopause—reduction in oestrogen production may have an indirect effect on symptomatology.
- Obesity.
- Constipation—straining weakens the pelvic floor muscles.
- Chronic cough—weakens pelvic floor muscles.
- Heavy lifting—increase in intra-abdominal pressure puts pressure on pelvic floor muscles.
- Previous gynaecological surgery.
- High impact sports, i.e. running, trampolining.
- Smoking.

Assessment

Symptoms

Leakage of urine when the woman coughs, sneezes, gets up, walks, runs for a bus, and so on.

Physical assessment

- A vaginal assessment to assess for prolapse, possible excoriation of vulval skin, atrophy, and general tissue status, as well as pelvic floor strength and tone.
- It is ideal to assess the patient's pelvic floor (using the modified Oxford Grading System) to ensure she has the correct technique—as bearing down not tightening the muscle, for example, will weaken the pelvic floor muscle not strengthen it. The patient will then be able to practice a routine set specifically for her and her current pelvic floor strength.
- A cough test should also be performed to check for the presence of urinary leakage. This can be done whilst the patient is in a supine position, whilst observing the urethral orifice.

The basic continence assessment, with frequency volume chart and urinalysis, should be undertaken.

Investigations

Pad tests

Office or home-based pad tests can detect urine loss after the patient is asked to cough, climb the stairs, or bend down. The pad is weighed before and after use.

Urodynamic investigations

Previously performed prior to continence surgery. However, since the introduction of the NICE guidelines, the suggestion is that urodynamics are not required for symptoms purely suggestive of stress incontinence. There has been considerable debate as to whether urodynamics are indicated in such circumstances. In most units that provide surgery for stress incontinence, urodynamics are still used to confirm the presence of stress urinary incontinence before any surgery is undertaken (📖 see Urodynamics, p.252).

Perineal ultrasound

This can be a helpful aid to urodynamics by demonstrating bladder neck opening and hypermobility in stress urinary incontinence but is rarely used.

1. National Institute for Health and Clinical Excellence. The management of urinary incontinence in women ☞ www.nice.org.uk (Accessed January 2009.)

Stress urinary incontinence: treatment

Conservative treatments should always be tried before considering any form of surgery.

- Pelvic floor exercises (PFMT)—with vaginal assessment of pelvic floor muscle strength and correct routine set (📖 see Conservative treatments of urinany incontinence, p.266).
  A Cochrane review has suggested a 56–75% short-term success rate in stress incontinence with PFMT.
- Vaginal cones/devices These devices support the urethra and can be worn during physical activity, e.g. Contrelle or Contiguard (📖 see Conservative treatments, p.266).
- Vaginal ring pessaries, where there is significant prolapse (📖 see Pelvic organ prolapse: overview, p.286).
- Prevention of constipation.
- Smoking cessation.
- Weight loss of 5–10% of body weight has been shown to be useful for primary and secondary prevention and treatment.

Advantages of conservative therapies are that many women's symptoms are cured or improved to the point that they don't require surgery, with its potential problems.

Specialist treatment

These treatments tend to be used in hospitals by specialist physiotherapists, continence advisors, or urogynaecology specialist nurses.

- Electrical stimulation.
- Biofeedback.
- Pelvic floor educator.

📖 See section on electrical stimulation and biofeedback for more details.

Duloxetine

Duloxetine is a combined serotonin and noradrenaline re-uptake inhibitor. In >50% women there is a significant improvement in symptoms.

Side-effects

Not uncommon and include nausea that is self-limiting in more than 80% women by 1 month.

Other drugs used include imipramine, topical oestrogen, and alpha adrenergics.

Surgery

Mid-urethral tapes

Tension-free vaginal tape (TVT) or transobturator (TOT) are now the most common surgical procedures performed for women with stress urinary incontinence. The aim is to support the mid-urethra at the level of the rhabdosphincter with a polypropylene tape.

With TVT, an 80% cure rate has been seen at 7-year follow-up.

At 7 years, tape erosion/extrusion is seen in under 1% of women. Complications include bladder injury and voiding difficulties.

Surgical treatment of SUI

- Mid-urethral tapes
- Retropubic suspension:
  - Colposuspension
  - TVT (transvaginal tapes)
  - TOT (transobturator tapes)
- Urethral injectables or Bulking agents:
  - GAX collagen
  - Silicone
  - Polyacrylamide hydrogel

Colposuspension

This has now largely been replaced by mid-urethral tapes. It is a retropubic elevation of the bladder neck. Cure rate is 80% and about 50% of women are satisfied with the procedure. Problems include: angulation of the vagina with the risk of developing enterocele, vault prolapse, and rectocele. New symptoms of voiding difficulty and overactive bladder are not uncommon.

Urethral injectables

Peri-urethral bulking agents are placed around the mid-urethra and bladder neck in order to support and enhance urethral competence. Treatment may have to be repeated and is not long-lasting. Results show 50% improvement in 2 years. High costs limit use. Indications are:
- frail elderly women unsuitable for GA or other surgery;
- intrinsic sphincter deficiency.

Resources

Pantazis, K and Freeman, RM (2006) Investigation and treatment of urinary incontinence. *Current Obstetrics and Gynaecology* **16**(6): 344–352.

Specialist treatment of stress urinary incontinence

Electrical stimulation

Neuro-muscular electrical stimulation (NMES) is a technique whereby small electrical impulses applied to the body may affect nerve or muscle tissue within the field of stimulation.

NMES has been shown to produce contraction of the pelvic floor muscles. It can be used:

- to assist in the production of muscle contractions in those women who either have an extremely weak contraction or are unable to contract their muscles at all;
- to inhibit detrusor over-activity by the sensory feedback it produces.

Inclusion criteria

The NICE guidelines[1] suggest that electrical stimulation is considered in women who are unable to actively contract their pelvic floor muscles.

Electrical stimulation should be used when a woman has no (or minimal) voluntary movement of the pelvic floor muscle. Specialists with expert knowledge are able to decide after thorough vaginal assessment if this treatment is suitable.

Contraindications for electrical stimulation

- DVT.
- Pacemaker.
- History of genital tract neoplasia.
- Pregnancy.
- Copper IUD—not Mirena® IUS.
- Active bleeding.
- Reduced sensation.

Use of the machines

Machines can be bought on the internet or directly from the manufacturers. Physiotherapists and continence services often have machines that are loaned out to suitable women for use at home. The machines are pre-programmed to enable easy use; however, programmes can be adapted and used to suit individual needs (see Fig. 10.3).

Biofeedback

Biofeedback relies on the principle of relaying information about a normally subconscious physiological process to the conscious awareness of the individual. This information is relayed in a visual signal, which often helps the patient to improve their muscle contraction and consequently pelvic floor strength. It can help to motivate those:

- women who are finding it difficult to do pelvic floor exercises at home;
- women who are unsure of whether they are doing the exercises correctly; and
- women who believe that pelvic floor exercises are a waste of time.

1. National Institute for Health and Clinical Excellence. The Management of Urinary Incontinence in Women. www.nice.org.uk (Accessed January 2009.)

Vaginal cones

📖 See p.268.

Pelvic floor educators

This was developed from the periform vaginal probe, which is often used with the electrical stimulation machine.

The body of the educator is retained in the vagina whilst the wand remains external. When the pelvic floor muscles are contracted correctly, the wand moves away from the body. The wand will move upwards if a valsalva manoeuvre (the patient bears down) is performed. This educator can be given to the patient and used at home to ensure the correct muscles are being utilized.

Intra-urethral and intra-vaginal devices

Intra-urethral devices are silicone cylinders that are self-inserted or removed at the woman's discretion, i.e. during physical exercise. They act by occluding the urethra or urethral meatus. The only one currently marketed is Femsoft (Rochester Medical).

Intra-vaginal devices support the bladder neck to help correct stress urinary incontinence. They work with varying degrees of success and can be used if the practitioner and woman feel it appropriate. They are not frequently used as they are often associated with UTI and women find them uncomfortable.

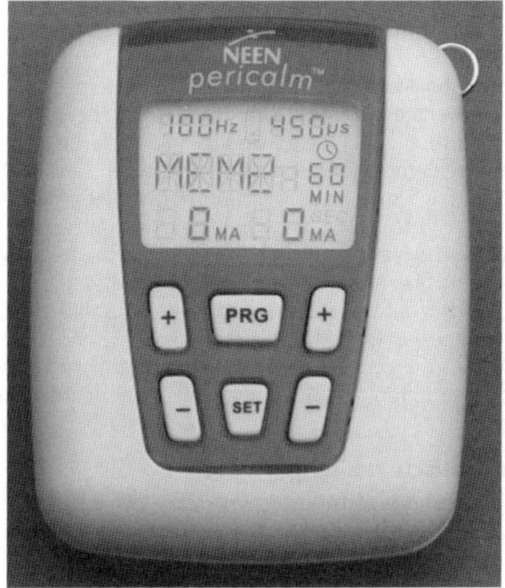

Fig. 10.3 Electrical stimulator. Reproduced with permission from Mobilis Healthcare.

Conservative treatments of urinary incontinence

Many simple treatments can be given to women presenting with urinary symptoms/urinary incontinence. Often a very simple lifestyle change can improve a woman's quality of life. However, patients need motivation, and a thorough understanding of their symptoms and problems for conservative treatments to be a success. The nurse needs to show empathy and understanding, as well as provide plenty of support.

The NICE guidelines suggest that conservative therapy should be offered as first-line treatment to women with urinary incontinence.

Bladder retraining

The aim of bladder retraining is to restore the woman suffering with urgency, frequency, and urge incontinence to a more normal and convenient pattern of micturition. The patient should aim to void every 2–3h or even longer, without any urgency or urge incontinence. Drug therapy is often used to compliment bladder retraining (📖 see Treatments for overactive bladder, p.258). NICE suggests that a minimum of 6 weeks bladder retraining should be offered to women with urge or mixed urinary incontinence.

The patient needs to understand why bladder retraining is important and how it will help to improve her symptoms. She also needs to have an understanding of how the 'normal bladder' functions and why her bladder isn't behaving in a normal way. This should help her to be more compliant with treatment.

The patient should complete a frequency volume chart (📖 see Treatments for overactive bladder, p.258) for 3 days so her pattern of voiding can be seen. She should then be advised to hold on for as long as possible when she gets the urge to go to the toilet to pass urine—even if she is only able to hold on for 5 minutes longer than normal. Her bladder will soon stretch and get used to having larger volumes in it and, as a consequence, she will decrease the number of visits she makes to the toilet. She must be warned, however, that her symptoms may become worse initially as she starts the treatment, but that she should persevere, as things will get better.

Repeat frequency volume charts are an excellent way of showing any progress made in the reduction of frequency and urgency, as reduction in frequency can often be slow and cause the patient to become de-motivated.

Pelvic floor muscle training (PFMT)

PFMT is a programme of repeated voluntary pelvic floor muscle contractions that is taught by a physiotherapist or a specialist nurse. Pelvic floor exercises increase the strength and tone of the pelvic floor muscles. Training improves muscle strength. The 3rd International Consultation on Incontinence (ICI)[1] and NICE recommend that a trial of supervised pelvic floor exercises of at least 3 months (8 contractions 3 times a day) should

1 Hanno P (2005) International consultation on incontinence—Rome, September 2004. Forging an international consensus: progressing painful bladder syndrome/interstitial cystitis. *International Urogynaecology Journal* **16**: S2–S34.

be offered to women with stress or mixed urinary incontinence. It is essential that women are doing the exercises correctly because if the incorrect technique is adopted (if the patient bears down) then more damage can be done to the muscle. A vaginal assessment should be performed and the pelvic floor correctly assessed before a suitable programme devised to suit the individual's needs.

Indications for PFMT

- Stress incontinence.
- Mixed incontinence.
- OAB syndrome.

The Oxford Grading System

This is often used when assessing pelvic floor strength and length of contraction.

0 nil concentration.
1 flicker.
2 weak.
3 moderate.
4 good.
5 strong.

To perform the slow twitch exercises

1. Close and draw up the muscles around back passage, as if you are trying to stop passing wind. Make sure that you do not contract your buttock muscles while you do this.
2. Now close and draw up the muscles around your vagina and urethra, as though you are trying to stop the flow of urine.
3. Hold for five seconds. Try not to hold your breath and breathe normally. Try to increase this hold to 10 seconds, if possible.
4. Then slowly relax and let go.
5. Repeat 5–10 times in total.

To perform fast twitch

1. Pull up muscles as before.
2. Hold for 1 second and relax.
3. Repeat 5–10 times or until your muscles feel tired.

Fluid advice

It is essential, in order to maintain bladder health, that 1.5–2l of fluid are consumed each day. Many women with bladder problems and incontinence restrict what they drink to prevent urinary leakage or frequency. Dehydration can cause the urine to become more concentrated and, as a result, can cause urinary frequency and urgency. Frequency/urgency can also be caused by excessive fluid intake of 3l+/day. It may be useful to look at the colour of the urine to assist women in ascertaining that they are drinking an optimum amount of fluid (📖 see Table 10.2).

Table 10.2 Bladder irritants

Drinks which irritate the bladder	Drinks which don't irritate the bladder
Caffeine—tea, coffee, hot chocolate, green tea	Milk
Citrus drinks such as orange juice, tomato juice	Decaffeinated tea and coffee
Carbonated drinks	Water, squash
Alcohol	Bovril
	Herbal teas such as chamomile

Constipation management

Straining to open bowels can cause weakening of the pelvic floor muscles and can cause prolapse. It is essential, therefore, that patients are given advice on preventing constipation. The Bristol Stool Scale is a tool commonly used to ascertain the severity of the problem (📖 see Fig. 10.5).

Patients should be advised to drink the required amount of fluid a day, take regular exercise, and ensure they are eating sufficient dietary fibre. Other measures include drug management with stool softeners, bulking agents and suppositories. They should also be advised on the correct position to adopt whilst sitting on the toilet.

Vaginal cones and pelvic floor educators

In SUI, vaginal cones may be a helpful addition to pelvic floor exercises (PFE). They are graded weights that are inserted into the vagina inside a plastic cone. One cone with weight in is inserted into the vagina and is held there for up to 30 minutes twice a day. The cone is held in by the contraction of the pelvic floor muscle. By gradually increasing the weight of the cone, the strength of the pelvic floor may be increased. They are particularly useful in women with pudendal nerve damage, who may not have good sensory feedback when doing PFMT (📖 see Fig. 10.4). Cones should not be used by women with utero-vaginal prolapse.

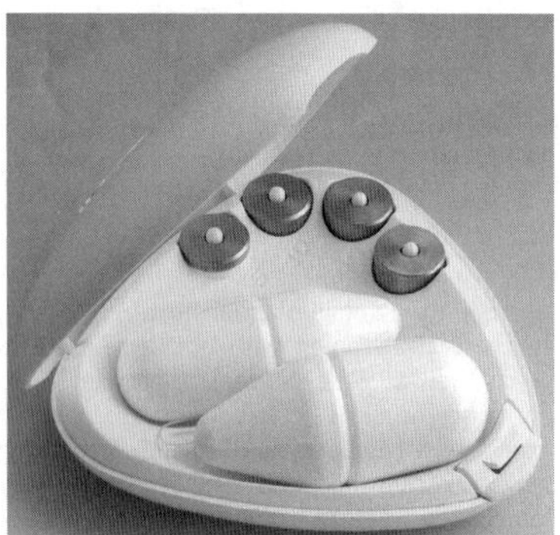

Fig. 10.4 Vaginal cones (Aquaflex). Reproduced with permission from Mobilis Healthcare.

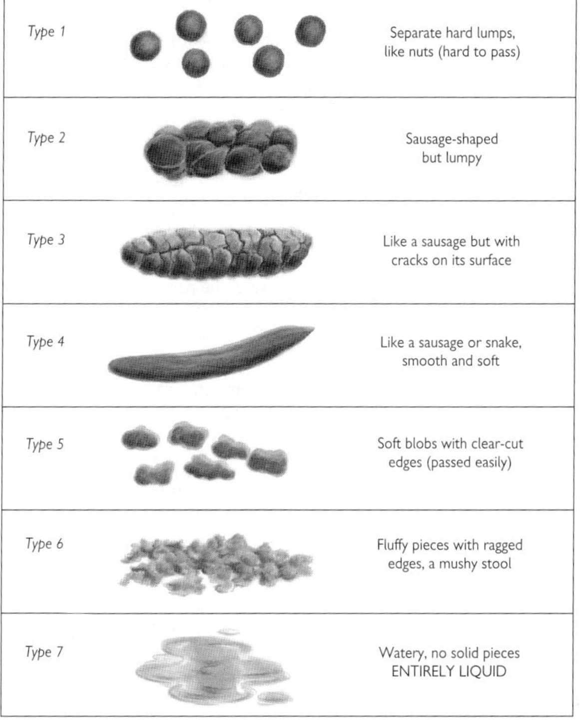

THE BRISTOL STOOL FORM SCALE
Type 1
Separate hard lumps, like nuts (hard to pass)
Type 2
Sausage-shaped but lumpy
Type 3
Like a sausage but with cracks on its surface
Type 4
Like a sausage or snake, smooth and soft
Type 5
Soft blobs with clear-cut edges (passed easily)
Type 6
Fluffy pieces with ragged edges, a mushy stool
Type 7
Watery, no solid pieces ENTIRELY LIQUID
MOVICOL®
macrogol 3350, sodium bicarbonate, sodium chloride, potassium chloride

Fig. 10.5 The Bristol Stool Form Scale. Reproduced by kind permission of KW Heaton, Reader in Medicine at the University of Bristol. Copyright 2000, Norgine Pharmaceuticals Limited.

Cystitis: bacterial and interstitial

Bacterial

Bacterial cystitis is an inflammation of the bladder caused by bacteria entering the bladder via the urethra—also known as a urinary tract infection (UTI). Approximately 50% of women living in the UK will get a urinary tract infection at some point in their lives.

Symptoms

The main symptoms include:

- Dysuria—pain when passing urine.
- Frequency—frequent trips to the toilet.
- Urgency—a strong desire to void even when the bladder is empty.
- Cloudy, offensive smelling urine.

Sometimes there may be blood in the urine, the patient may experience a fever, find sex painful, have a dull ache in the lower back or abdomen and feel generally unwell.

Tests

The urine should be dipsticked for leucocytes and nitrites and sent off for MC&S if these are present. Often women with an infection may also have blood and protein present on urinalysis.

Prevention

Advise those suffering with bacterial cystitis or UTIs to.

- Wipe their bottom from front to back thus preventing the transfer of *E. coli* bacteria into the urethra/bladder.
- Wear cotton underwear and not to wear very tight, restricting jeans/trousers.
- Drink 1.5–2l of fluid a day to help dilute the urine and reduce dysuria, and encourage voiding to wash bacteria out. Consider drinking cranberry juice.
- Pass urine after having sex.
- Use non-perfumed soaps and avoid using bubble baths, talc, and feminine douches.
- Sit on the toilet seat properly when going to the toilet to ensure the bladder has the best chance to empty fully.

Treatments

Bacterial cystitis is often treated with antibiotics. Interaction with oral contraception and propensity for candidal infections should be raised with the patient.

Those at risk

Women who are pregnant, peri- or post-menopausal, those suffering with diabetes or who have a catheter have an increased risk.

Interstitial cystitis (IC)

Interstitial cystitis or painful bladder syndrome is a condition that results in recurring discomfort or pain in the bladder and surrounding pelvic region. People may experience mild discomfort, pressure, tenderness, or intense pain in the bladder and pelvic area. Women with IC usually do not respond to conventional antibiotic therapy but some respond to long-term antibiotic therapy. It can take a very long time for a woman to be diagnosed with IC. IC can affect anyone of any age, male or female, but it is most commonly found in women.

Symptoms

The main symptoms of IC resemble that of bacterial infections and are:

- Frequency.
- Urgency.
- Pain is a cardinal feature.

Diagnosis, treatment, and management

- Because symptoms are similar to those of other disorders of the bladder and as there is no definitive test to identify IC, the diagnosis is by exclusion.
- Diagnostic tests that help in ruling out other diseases include: urinalysis, urine culture, cystoscopy, biopsy of the bladder wall, urodynamic assessment, and distension of the bladder under anaesthetic.
- There is no cure for IC. Symptoms may disappear without explanation or coincide with an event such as a change in diet, or stress. Treatments are aimed at relieving symptoms.
- Analgesics such as ibuprofen and paracetamol or fentanyl patch may help with the discomfort experienced.
- Some sufferers find that tricyclic anti-depressants, such as amitriptyline, may help reduce pain, increase bladder capacity, and decrease frequency and nocturia.
- Many women find that alcohol, tomatoes, spices, chocolate, caffeine, and high acid foods exacerbate their symptoms.
- Bladder retraining may help to increase bladder capacity and reduce frequency and urgency.
- 3-month antibiotic courses have been tried and are likely to help.
- Transcutaneous electrical nerve stimulation (TENS) machines are often offered.
- Botulinum toxin type A may have a role in the management.

Surgery

Surgery should only be considered if all available treatments have failed and the pain is disabling.

Bladder augmentation, sacral nerve stimulation and cystectomy (removal of bladder) are surgical options which may be considered.

Continence products

Pads

The use of an absorbent pad worn or incorporated inside a garment is the most common way of managing incontinence.

Women suffering with urinary incontinence often wear sanitary towels, which are designed to absorb menstrual blood and not urine, so often two or three have to be worn; they are not very effective when the patient has moderate to severe incontinence.

- Light incontinence: small discreet pads, available in a variety of makes and designs.
- Moderate to heavy incontinence: these pads may be rectangular or body shaped. Rectangular pads are generally cheaper than shaped pads. Shaped pads tend to be more comfortable to wear and provide greater security for the patient. They are available in a wide range of sizes.

Washable reusable pads are available and may work out to be more cost-effective for the patient. Some do, however, leak more, which may in turn put a strain on the person doing the washing. Washable pants with an integral pad are also available—people like these because they look like normal pants. They are suitable for people with light incontinence and are often used by people with light or intermittent incontinence to be there 'just in case'.

Catheter valves

The use of a catheter valve in place of a drainage bag is growing in popularity. Catheter valves help to maintain bladder capacity, reduce erosion, and lessen catheter blockage and urine infections by giving the catheter a good flush through periodically throughout the day (📖 see Fig. 10.6).

A valve dispenses the need to wear a bag as the catheter can be emptied straight into the toilet. The valve can be tucked into the woman's underwear or can be held in place with a leg strap.

Catheter valves are cheaper than the traditional drainage systems. They should be changed every 5–7 days as per manufacturer's guidelines.

It is vital that a thorough assessment of the woman is undertaken before using a catheter valve (see Box). Women must be able to manipulate the valve and empty the bladder regularly to prevent overfilling the bladder. If the patient is unaware of the sensation to void, the valve should be opened every 3–4h and a night drainage-bag attached overnight.

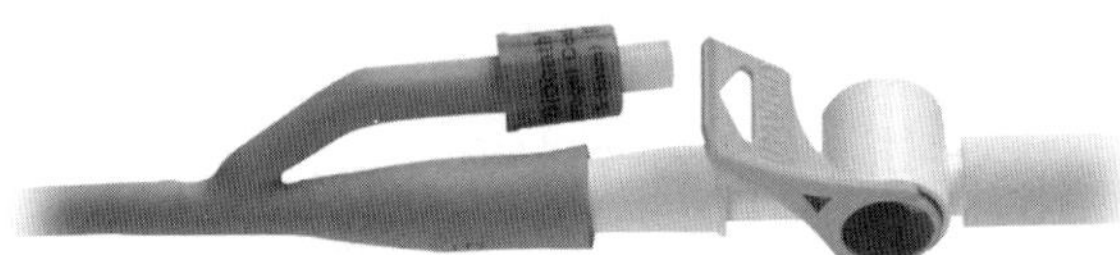

Fig. 10.6 Catheter valve (Flip flo). Reproduced with permission of Bard Ltd.

Contraindications

- Reduced bladder capacity.
- Cognitive impairment.
- No bladder sensation—care should be taken and advice, as above.
- Insufficient manual dexterity to operate the valve.
- Nocturnal polyuria.
- Patient choice.
- If attempting to relieve hydronephrosis due to obstruction.

Female urinals

Handheld urinals are useful for people with severe mobility restrictions and when visiting places or people where the toilet is difficult to use. It is advisable to practice using them in the privacy of the woman's home until she gains the skills and competence to use in public places. A rug or blanket can be placed over the woman's lap when using urinals to maintain dignity and discretion.

The bridge urinal is a popular handheld female urinal. It is slipped in between the legs and has the facility to connect a catheter drainage bag, if needed, i.e. if the urinal is needed on a long car journey or when it is not easy to empty the urine immediately.

Leg straps and holders

Opinion is divided as to whether the catheter itself should be attached to the woman's leg. It may help to reduce pulling of the catheter, which may in turn reduce trauma and decrease the likelihood of developing an infection. Several catheter straps and holders are available commercially (📖 see Figs. 10.7 and 10.8).

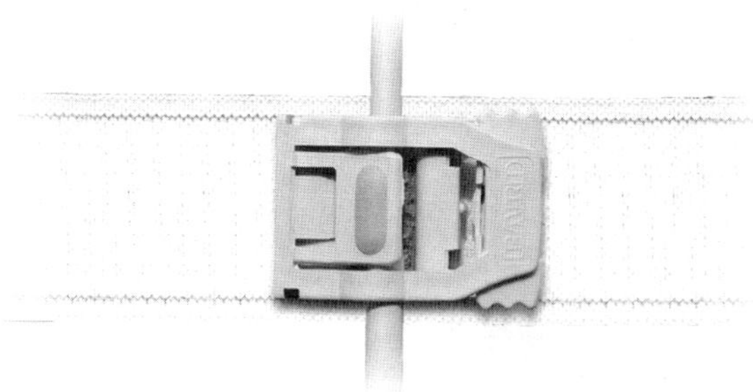

Fig. 10.7 Flame comfasure clamp. Reproduced with permission of Bard Ltd.

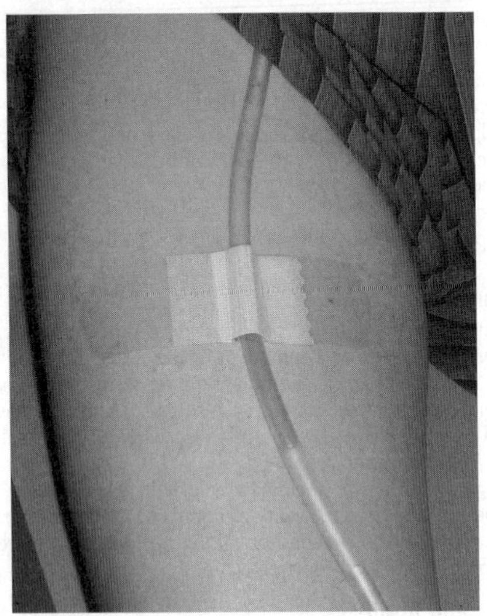

Fig. 10.8 Clinifix. Reproduced with permission of Clinimed Ltd.

Urinary catheters

Urethral catheterization is associated with many potential complications. The highest incidence of hospital-acquired infections is associated with in-dwelling urethral catheters.

Indications for catheterization

- Drainage: acute retention, pre- and post-surgery, accurate measurement of urine output, post-partum voiding difficulty, peri-operative measurement of urinary output.
- Investigation: to establish an accurate post-micturition residual if bladder scanner not available, bladder function tests (urodynamics), obtain a sterile sample of urine.
- Instillation: to introduce intra-vesical medication, use of bladder irrigation post-surgery.
- During labour: if bladder becomes distended and woman unable to void spontaneously, prior to assisted birth.
- Intractable incontinence: as a last resort when surgical and conservative methods have failed. Always consider supra-pubic catheterization as an option.

Types of urinary catheters

Short term

Must be left in for only 7 days—plastic, PVC catheters, i.e. irrigating catheters.

Medium term

These catheters can stay in for up to 28 days—PTFE, coated and uncoated latex, silver alloy coated.

Long term

These catheters can stay in for up to 12 weeks—hydrogel coated latex, 100% silicone, silicone-coated latex, hydrogel-coated silicone.

Intermittent catheters

Used to drain the bladder intermittently (📖 see ISC p.284).

Catheter selection

It is essential that a thorough assessment of the woman's needs is made before selecting the most appropriate catheter. It is important to consider the woman's sexuality—if sexually active and requiring long-term catheterization, consider ISC or a supra-pubic catheter. If the woman is obese and wheelchair-bound, consider a male-length catheter instead of a female length, as this may facilitate emptying and cleaning.

Catheter length and size

- Female: length 25cm, which correlates with the length of the female urethra.
- Male: length 40–45cm.

The golden rule when selecting catheter size is to choose the smallest charriere that will drain adequately. For an adult, this will normally be a size 12ch (bore of the catheter) or 14ch.

Balloon size

- For normal catheterization, a 10ml balloon capacity should be used as indicated on the balloon inflation channel. Follow manufacturer's guidelines and instructions. Never overfill or underfill a catheter balloon.
- Only use sterile water to inflate the balloon NOT saline or air.
- 30ml balloons are usually only used in 3-way irrigating catheters or for transurethral resection of bladder tumours (TURBT), as they can help reduce post-operative bleeding.

Possible complications of catheterization

- Urinary tract infection (UTI).
- Pain.
- Bladder spasm.
- Trauma.
- Stricture.
- Embarrassment, dependence, affecting body image and sexuality.

Use of Instillagel®

Instillagel® may be used prior to inserting the catheter. It provides lubrication, has antiseptic properties, and has an anaesthetic effect that helps to reduce any trauma caused at the time of insertion. It also helps to aid catheterization by opening the urethra, making it easier to insert the catheter.

Documentation

Ensure the following information is documented in the patient's records for each catheterization performed:

- Reason for catheterization.
- Type of catheter used.
- LOT number or the sticker from the back of the catheter with this information on.
- Amount of sterile water in the balloon.
- Urinary residual—measured 15 minutes after catheter insertion.
- Whether a specimen has been sent off for MC&S.

Removal

Catheters should be removed as soon as clinically possible as complications are likely with long-term use.

Advice to give catheterized women

- Ensure that patients open their bowels regularly and that they prevent constipation, if possible.
- Try to encourage an oral intake of 2l of fluid in 24h.
- Train the patient to clean her catheter at the urethral meatus twice a day or more if there is a build up of secretions, with a disposable flannel and ordinary soap.
- Advise the patient to change her leg bag/night drainage bag/catheter valve every 7 days as per manufacturer's guidelines. Show her how to do this before she leaves the ward/clinic/department.
- The patient should wash her hands before and after touching the catheter. She does not need to wear gloves.
- She should only empty the catheter bag when ¾ full to prevent opening the drainage system too often, which, in turn may increase the risk of developing an infection.

Female urethral catheterization

Equipment needed:

- Yellow waste bag.
- Disposable apron.
- Catheter.
- Instillagel®.
- Syringe and sterile water for injection.
- Gloves: x2 sterile pairs.
- Drainage bag/flip flo valve.
- Catheter stand.
- Catheterization pack.
- Cleansing solution.

Procedure

1. Explain procedure to the patient to obtain informed consent.
2. Check for any allergies, i.e. latex, Instillagel®.
3. Clean and prepare a trolley, placing all of the equipment on the lower shelf, checking all expiry dates.
4. Screen the bed to ensure privacy and maintain dignity at all times.
5. Assist patient into the supine position.
6. Ensure adequate lighting is available and that the bed or couch is raised to a comfortable working height. Place the trolley alongside the bed so that the procedure is performed easily and safely.
7. Insert incontinence pad under the patient. Cover her whilst preparing working area.
8. Put on plastic apron and wash and dry hands.
9. Ensure she is lying down with legs abducted and knees flexed. She should be warm and comfortable, not over-exposed.
10. Expose genital area.
11. Remove existing catheter after deflating the balloon first (ensuring you have non-sterile gloves on), if necessary noting size and type and dispose into the yellow bag.
12. Cover the patient once the catheter has been removed.
13. Wash and dry hands again.
14. Open catheter pack, catheter, cleaning solution, drainage bag, sterile gloves, Instillagel®, water for injection with syringe and arrange sterile field.
15. Check expiry date of catheter and type of allergy.
16. Draw up 10ml water for injection for balloon inflation.
17. Wash and dry hands.
18. Put on both pairs of sterile gloves.
19. Pour out sterile saline into gallipot.
20. Using gloved hand, clean vulval area with gauze in saline, using single strokes wiping from the front to the back to prevent bacteria being transferred into the urethral meatus.
21. Isolate the urethral opening and insert the Instillagel® and leave for 3–5 minutes for it to take effect.
22. Remove the first pair of gloves.

23. Place receiver between her legs, separate the vulva, identify the urethra and insert the catheter gently.
24. Once urine has begun to flow, advance the catheter up to the level sufficient to prevent the balloon being inflated inside the urethra.
25. Inflate the balloon using sterile water to the manufacturer's instructions.
26. Once inflated, withdraw the catheter until resistance is felt.
27. Ensure she is comfortable. Gently wipe away any excess gel, front to back strokes.
28. Collect urine sample, if indicated.
29. Connect catheter to the appropriate drainage system (i.e. drainage bag, leg straps and stand, or flip flo valve).
30. Advise the patient to go and have a wash to clean the genital area.
31. Dispose of all equipment as per hospital guidelines, remove apron and wash and dry hands.
32. Document procedure in notes.

Catheter trouble-shooting

(📖 see Table 10.3)

Table 10.3 Catheter trouble-shooting

Problem	Possible cause	Action
Pyrexia Cloudy urine Offensive smell Sediment Haematuria Loin pain* Sudden onset of confusion in elderly patients	Urinary tract infection	• Perform urinalysis, send off CSU if leucocytes, nitrites, blood, or protein are present • Record temperature 4–6 hourly • Inform medical staff • Encourage 2l of fluid daily • Consider cranberry juice therapy • Antibiotics if systemically unwell or positive CSU
No urine draining from catheter	• Kinked tubing • Constipation • Bladder spasms • Blocked catheter • Dehydration • Incorrect placement of catheter • Drainage bag may be too full not allowing further urine into it • Renal failure	• Check tubing is not kinked • Administer laxatives and establish regular bowel motion • Perform bladder washout and/or change catheter • Encourage fluids • Check the catheter and balloon placement • Empty drainage bag • Seek medical advice
Unable to deflate balloon for catheter removal	• Faulty catheter • Collapsed inflation channel	• DO NOT cut any part of the catheter • Inform medical staff—the balloon may require decompression via a suprapubic approach using ultrasound and a spinal needle • DO NOT attempt to put more water in to burst the balloon as the patient will then need a cystoscopy to remove the fragments of the balloon from the bladder • Use needle and syringe to aspirate the inflation arm just above the valve • Insert a few ml, which may help to clear any blockage • Try a different syringe • Leave it attached with the plunger removed, for 20 minutes

Table 10.3 Catheter trouble-shooting (*continued*)

Problem	Possible cause	Action
Spasmodic pain in labia, pelvis usually accompanied by bypassing (leakage around the catheter)	• Blocked catheter • Bladder spasm • Large catheter • Large balloon	• Perform bladder washout, consider changing catheter if no success • Give antispasmodic medication and possible anticholinergic medication (i.e.tolterodine/solifenacin) after discussion with medical staff • Replace with smaller charriere catheter if appropriate • Remove some water if considered appropriate • Increase fluid intake to avoid constipation
Unable to unblock the catheter by performing a bladder washout	• Encrustations • Clot over the eye of the catheter • Accumulation of debris causing the eye to block	• Change the catheter • If encrustation is suspected, cut the catheter once removed and document findings • Consider commencing on a catheter diary to monitor rate of blockage etc.
Difficulties inserting a urethral catheter	• Catheter length • Urethral stricture • Vaginal entry	• Check the correct length catheter has been chosen • If it is difficult to insert a catheter, do not force it in. Get someone with more experience or refer to the urology department for advice. A catheter introducer may be needed to aid insertion, or a supra-pubic catheter may need to be inserted • Occasionally when catheterizing a woman, the catheter may enter the vagina. If this is the case, leave the catheter *in situ*, it will act as a marker. Remove once the woman has been catheterized correctly. The use of Instillagel® will help to reduce the chances of this happening

Intermittent self-catheterization

Definition

Intermittent self-catheterization (ISC) involves the woman inserting a catheter into the bladder via the urethra or cystostomy to drain urine.

Indications for ISC

- Retention—chronic and acute.
- Hypotonic/atonic bladder.
- To measure residual urine in the absence of a bladder scanner.
- Neurological disease, neuropathic bladder—MS, stroke, paralysis with urinary retention/incomplete emptying.
- Administration of intra-vesical chemotherapy and BCG.
- Incomplete bladder emptying.
- Post urethrotomy for stricture therapy.
- Before continence surgery or botox treatment.

For ISC to be successful, four key factors have been identified namely:

- Motivation.
- Mental alertness.
- Mobility.
- Manual dexterity.

Types of ISC catheter

There are many different types of intermittent catheters available on the market. Some are available immersed in a solution, some have bags attached for the urine to drain into, some come with a sachet of water to lubricate the catheter with, some are very small and discreet. There will be a catheter to suit all needs and all women. It may be that a woman has a selection of catheters to use at home, depending upon where and when she may need to perform the procedure.

Teaching ISC

It is natural for the woman to be very anxious about learning the ISC technique. Many women will never have looked at themselves 'down below' before, so may also find it both daunting and scary, and may do everything they can to not have to learn how to do it. It is then up to the nurse to provide her with the time and patience needed and to build up sufficient trust with her to facilitate her learning of the technique. The majority of women cope well if they have a clear understanding of the cause of the bladder dysfunction and the rationale for choosing ISC as a strategy for managing their symptoms. Teaching should always take place in a relaxed, private, and unhurried environment; ideally not in a ward setting behind a curtain. It may be beneficial before the session to provide written information or a video.

The woman must understand that the procedure is a clean procedure, not a sterile one, and also, when teaching the procedure, staff should use an aseptic technique because of the risk of cross infection.

Women may have difficulty locating the urethra when learning, so once the catheter is *in situ*, she should be shown where the urethra is using a mirror. She should also be shown a variety of positions to try to make the ISC procedure easier, e.g. sitting on the side of the toilet, one leg on the toilet, in the bath. Most women, once they have sufficient experience, can learn to catheterize themselves by touch, which will dispense with the need for a mirror.

Women need to be aware of the importance of hand hygiene when undertaking the procedure in the prevention of infection and should be advised to wash the genital area before catheterization if possible.

Potential problems, such as bleeding, urinary tract infections, and the catheter getting stuck, should be explained and a contact number given for patients to call should they have a question or problem.

She should be advised to keep her bowels regular, drink between 1.5 and 2l of fluid a day, and be given information about cranberry juice.

Women should be advised to complete an in and out chart detailing the amount she is passing in the toilet, if any, before catheterization and then the residual. This will help to decide the frequency of catheterization needed.

Most manufacturers producing ISC catheters have a booklet that provides the techniques to use when performing ISC. They have contact numbers and advice for the woman to make their experience as trouble free as possible.

Home delivery

Most manufacturers now provide/offer a home delivery service, whereby catheters can be discreetly delivered to the woman's door whenever they are needed. The companies also often collect the prescriptions from the GPs to make this service very convenient and hassle free for the woman.

Pelvic organ prolapse: overview

Definition

Prolapse means to fall out. Within the pelvic floor it is a condition where a pelvic organ or tissue is displaced from its normal position. Prolapse occurs because of weakened tissues supporting the pelvic organs as a result of poor tissue type and or damage. Prolapse may involve:

- the front wall of the vagina (with the bladder coming down behind) known as a cystocele;
- the back wall of the vagina (with the rectum behind) known as a rectocele;
- or higher up above the peritoneal reflection with the small bowel coming down) as an enterocele;
- or of the uterus as a uterine prolapse.

Prevalence

The exact prevalence is unknown. In the US Women's Health Initiative (WHI) study,[1] the prevalence was 14% and in the UK Oxford Family Planning Association (FPA) study[2] the annual incidence of admission with prolapse was 20.4/10,000.

Symptoms

The symptoms experienced tend to vary depending upon the type of prolapse.

- Local symptoms—many women with a prolapse are aware of a 'bulge' and/or feeling of heaviness or 'something coming down', blood-stained discharge, backache towards the end of the day or after long periods of standing.
- Urinary—frequency, feeling of incomplete emptying, 'digitation' needed to start or complete voiding, weak urinary stream, positional changes required to start or complete emptying.
- Bowel symptoms—feeling of incomplete emptying, digital evacuation and/or digitation to complete defecation, incontinence of flatus or stool.
- Sexual symptoms—dyspareunia, lack of sensation, incontinence during sexual activity.

Examination

- A Sims speculum is often used to help diagnose the type and severity of prolapse. The patient is best examined in the left lateral position, though some clinicians advocate the standing position.
- Start with a cough test to check for stress leakage.
- Uterine descent can be ascertained by traction on the cervix with a single-toothed Vulsellum.
- Bimanual examination.
- Assessment of pelvic tone.

Types of pelvic organ prolapse

Cystocele occurs when the bladder slips down, pushing into the front (anterior) wall of the vagina.

1. Hendrix SL, Clark A, Nygaard I, *et al.* (2002). Pelvic organ prolapse in the woman's heath initiative: gravity and gravidity. Transaction of the Sixty ninth annual meeting of the Central Association of Obstetricians and Gynaecologists. *Am J Obstet Gynaecol.* **186**: 1160–66.

Rectocele occurs when the rectum pushes into the back (posterior) wall of the vagina.
Uterine prolapse. The uterus may drop into the vagina. There may be a mild degree of descent, however, some women experience a total prolapse of the uterus—this is called a procidentia.
Vault prolapse occurs in women who have previously had a hysterectomy. It is where the tissues at the apex of the vagina prolapse. A vault prolapse can contain omentum or small bowel.
Enterocele is the term used if the upper-third of the posterior vaginal wall descends, and a small piece of the bowel or omentum gets herniated into the pouch of Douglas.

The severity of a prolapse can be classified as mild, moderate, or severe or scored according to the International Continence Society pelvic organ prolapse quantification system (POP-Q) into a staging system.

The five stages of prolapse

0: No prolapse.
1: The most distal portion of the prolapse is >1cm above the level of hymen.
2: The most distal portion of the prolapse is <1cm above the hymen.
3: The most distal portion of the prolapse is >1cm below the hymen but protrudes no further than 2cm less than the total length of the vagina.
4: Complete eversion of the vagina.

Risk factors for development of prolapse

- Multiparity.
- Vaginal delivery—possible risk factors are a prolonged second stage, epidural analgesia, macrosomia, episiotomy.
- Ageing and possibly the menopause.
- Obesity.
- Family history.
- Pelvic masses, such as fibroids, cysts, or tumours.
- Previous pelvic surgery, such as hysterectomy.
- Increased abdominal pressure—chronic obstructive pulmonary disease (COPD), chronic cough, constipation.

Prevention

Women should be advised against:
- Heavy lifting.
- Standing for long periods of time.
- Constipation—straining to empty bowels.
- Smoking and obesity.

Investigations

- Mid-stream specimen of urine for culture and sensitivity.
- Urodynamic studies. Potential stress incontinence may be masked by prolapse, so urodynamic studies may be undertaken prior to surgery with the prolapsed reduced.

2. Thakar, R and Stanton, S (2002) Management of genital prolapse. *British Medical Journal* **324**: 1258–1262.

Pelvic organ prolapse: treatment

Advice should be given about increasing fibre intake, and toilet position to help prevent constipation and risk making the symptoms of an enterocele worse.

The treatment chosen for the patient will depend upon the type and severity of the prolapse after a full vaginal assessment has been undertaken. Some women will be able to tolerate their symptoms and so choose to opt for pelvic floor exercises and regular monitoring of their symptoms.

Conservative

Conservative treatment should always be offered in the community and primary care before hospital referral.

Pelvic floor exercises

The role of exercises in managing prolapse is unclear (Hagen 2006).[1] Pelvic floor exercises may prove useful in stage I and 2 prolapse and alleviate symptoms.

Pessaries

Pessaries can be used to support a prolapse in the correct anatomical position. There are many different sizes and shapes of pessaries: the ring pessary and the shelf pessary are the most commonly used in the UK.

The type of pessary chosen will depend upon the type of prolapse, the woman's desire to self-manage or not, and whether or not she is sexually active. Women are generally still able to have intercourse with a ring pessary; however, a shelf pessary is contraindicated in sexually active women.

Indications for pessaries

- Women who do not wish to go for surgery.
- Women unfit for surgery.
- Women who wish to retain child bearing function.
- In pregnancy.

Surgery

Indications for surgery[2]

- Women wanting definitive treatment.
- Failure of conservative measures and pessaries.
- Prolapse with urodynamic stress incontinence.
- Prolapse with faecal incontinence.

Surgery is not suitable for all women, e.g. if a woman has a grade 2 uterine prolapse but has not completed her family, she will be offered a pessary rather than surgery as another pregnancy or vaginal delivery may disrupt the repair. It is essential, therefore, that a thorough assessment has been undertaken before surgery is considered.

1. Hagen, S, Stark, D, Maher, C, Adams, EJ (2006). Conservative management of pelvic organ prolapse in women. *Cochrane Database of Systematic Review* (4): CD0038882.
2. Maher, C, Baessler, K, Glazener, CM, Adams, EI, Magen, S (2007) Surgical management of pelvic organ prolapse in women. *Cochrane database of Systematic Review*: CD004014.

The following operations are performed to correct prolapse detailed above.

Anterior repair. Traditionally the pubo-cervical fascia is placated in the midline with polyglactin 910. Now paravaginal repair is another method where pubo-cervical fascia is sutured to the arcus tendinus. It can be done vaginally, abdominally, or laparoscopically and success rates are higher. If there is concomitant urethral sphincter incompetence, then tension-free vaginal tape may be inserted at the time of the anterior repair.

Posterior repair. A rectocele can be repaired by traditionally placating the rectovaginal fascia in the midline with delayed absorbable sutures, but dyspareunia may be a consequence.

Anterior and posterior repairs using mesh as recurrence with standard anterior repairs can be as high as 40% after the first year of surgery. A mesh can be laid over the pubo-cervical fascia or introduced through the transobturator route. This can reduce recurrences. However, mesh erosion and dyspareunia can occur.

Abdominal sacrocolpopexy is essentially for vault (apical) prolapse and is the gold standard for apical prolapse. In open or laparoscopic sacrocolpopexy, the vaginal vault is attached by a synthetic mesh to the longitudinal ligament over the sacrum. The cure rate is 90%.

Sacrospinous fixation is for vault prolapse, it involves unilateral or bilateral fixation of the vault to the sacrospinous ligament but there is about a 35% risk of anterior wall prolapse after surgery.

Vaginal hysterectomy. This on its own may fail to correct the prolapsed vaginal vault, which should be supported at the time of hysterectomy by vaginal McCall culdoplasty or placation of the uterosacral ligaments. If there is an associated cystocele and/or rectocele, an anterior and posterior repair can be carried out at the same time.

Colpocleisis is reserved for older frail women where sexual function is not desired.

Resources

For women:
www.continence-foundation.org.uk.
NHS direct www.cks.library.nhs.uk.

Vaginal pessaries: conservative treatment for prolapse

Definition

A pessary is a supportive device used for conservative treatment of pelvic organ prolapse including cystocele and rectocele. Two of the commonly used pessaries in the UK are ring and shelf pessaries.

Ring pessaries are used to treat uterine prolapse. They are suitable for sexually active women. A shelf pessary is used when there is poor vaginal support and a ring pessary cannot be supported in the vagina. Shelf pessaries are commonly used to treat a vault prolapse (prolapse after hysterectomy).

When is a pessary used?

A gynaecologist or a specialist may decide to use a pessary to treat pelvic organ prolapse for the following reasons:

- As a temporary measure to relieve symptoms whilst waiting for surgery, or as a trial to ascertain the benefit from surgery.
- As a permanent alternative to surgical treatment for women who do not want surgery, or who are unsuitable for surgery. For example, those with significant co-morbidity, or those women who have not yet completed their family.

Inserting and changing vaginal pessaries

A trained nurse or doctor should fit the appropriate pessary. However, once inserted, it is possible to teach women to remove and insert their own pessary, should they need to. For example, if they find it more comfortable to have sex without it in.

The procedure below is followed for insertion of a ring pessary after informed consent is gained from the patient.

- The patient should be in the lithotomy position and undressed from the waist down.
- The bladder should be emptied prior to removal or insertion of a pessary.
- Conduct a vaginal examination to assess the prolapse and vaginal tissues.
- The appropriate size of ring pessary is ascertained by digitally assessing the length of the vaginal canal (from the posterior fornix to the symphysis pubis). This distance corresponds to the diameter of the ring pessary. The correct size pessary should be able to be rotated whilst *in situ* and remain *in situ* whilst straining. If the pessary is being replaced, ensure the same size is used. Significant changes in a woman's weight may require a change in pessary size.
- To remove the pessary, part the labia to expose the vaginal entrance. Insert a lubricated finger to palpate the anterior rim of the pessary. Then, hook the finger under the rim of the pessary and pull firmly, but gently until the pessary is out.
- A speculum examination should the performed to assess for ulceration, bleeding, and infection.

- If the vaginal examination is normal, remove the new ring pessary from the packet and either run under warm water, or put into a bowl of warm water to make it more pliable.
- Compress the pessary into an oval shape and apply lubricating jelly to the entering edge of the pessary.
- Part the labia and slide the pessary into the posterior part of the vagina. Push it backwards and downwards until it settles into the posterior fornix. The ring will then spring back into a circular shape.
- The pessary should rest behind the symphysis pubis in the anterior part of the vagina. The cervix should sit centrally within the ring pessary.

The patient should be asked if the pessary feels comfortable. She should walk around, go to the toilet, and cough without it falling out. Ring pessaries need to be changed every 6 months. Patients should be given contact details should they experience any problems.

Complications

At pessary change the following is required:

- Inspect vagina for ulceration and excoriations caused by a poorly fitting pessary.
- Look for abnormal vaginal secretions and discharge—this would suggest there is an infection present. This must be diagnosed and treated prior to reinsertion of the pessary.
- Oestrogen deficiency—this will require a prescription for topical oestrogen.

Chapter 11

Gynaecological oncology

Introduction to gynaecological oncology[1]

Gynaecological cancers are associated with the female reproductive organs. This includes the ovaries, fallopian tubes, uterus, cervix, vagina, and vulva. They account for about 15% of cancers in women and about 10% of cancer deaths. The majority of gynaecological cancers are treated in cancer centres by a multidisciplinary team (MDT) approach. The MDT includes surgical gynaecological oncologists, oncologists, pathologist, and nurses. The only gynaecological cancers not treated at cancer units may be stage 1b endometrial cancers and 1a cervical cancers. Many nurses may not see cancer surgery, if not working within a cancer centre and may only be involved with diagnosis and follow-up.

Enhanced cervical screening in the UK has led to a dramatic decrease in the incidence of and deaths from cervical cancer. Abnormal development changes (dysplasia) in cervical cells are diagnosed when the disease is still curable. Unfortunately, ovarian cancer is usually diagnosed at an advanced stage, as it is asymptomatic in the early stages and has a minimal impact on gastro-intestinal systems.

There are additional rare tumours called gestational trophoblastic tumours, which arise from pregnancy and include:

- Pre-malignant complete hydatidiform mole (CHM).
- Partial hydatidiform mole (PHM).
- Malignant invasive mole, gestational choriocarcinoma.
- Highly malignant placental-site trophoblastic tumour (PSTT).

These will not be covered within this book.

1 Adapted with permission from Tadman, M and Roberts, D (2007) *Oxford Handbook of Cancer Nursing*. Oxford University Press.

Overview of cancer of the vulva

Epidemiology

Vulval and vaginal cancers account for <1% of all cancer cases and 6% of gynaecological cancers diagnosed every year in the UK. There are 1022 new cases of vulval cancers diagnosed in the UK and 380 women die of the disease every year.

Incidence

<1 per 100,000 get vulval cancer in the 25–44-year age group.
3 per 100,000 in the 45–64-year age group.
14 per 100,000 in the 65 and over age group.

The incidence rates for young women being diagnosed with vulval cancer have doubled in the last 3 years. Survival rates have improved over the last 30 years. This has resulted in a fall in mortality rates.

Causes

- 15% of vulval cancers are associated with HPV, particularly 16 and 18.
- Smoking is thought to be a risk factor.
- History of pre-cancer of the vulva (VIN 1–3).
- Chronic skin conditions and inflammation, e.g. lichen sclerosis and Paget's disease.
- Past history of genital warts
- It is not related to reproductive factors or exogenous hormones.

Presenting complaints/symptoms

- Itching and burning.
- Lump or ulceration on the vulva.
- Pain or soreness in the area around the vulva.
- Bleeding or discharge.
- Colour change (white, pigment deposition).
- Irregular fungating mass.
- Enlarged groin nodes.

History and diagnosis

- History of chronic skin conditions.
- Previous abnormality.
- Bimanual and speculum examination to rule out abnormalities in the vagina, uterus, and cervix.
- Vulvoscopy though not as specific as colposcopy of the cervix.
- Cervical smear to exclude co-existing CIN.
- Vulval biopsy—multiple punch biopsies should be used to assess the depth of invasion—the device used is a Keyes punch.
- Examination under anaesthesia (EUA).
- Wide, local excision.
- Fine-needle aspiration (FNA) of groin nodes has a specificity and sensitivity of 100%.
- Pelvic ultrasound.
- +/– MRI scan to stage the disease.

Differential diagnosis

Diagnosis made by histology from the biopsy.

Types of vulval cancers

Squamous cell carcinomas (SCC) make up 90% of vulval cancers.
Tumours of the surface epithelium such as Paget's, melanoma, sarcoma, basal cell, and adenocarcinoma make up the other 10%.

Treatment of cancer of the vulva

Depends on staging (see Table 11.1)

Table 11.1 Staging of vulval cancer (this is according to FIGO staging)

Stage	Description
Stage 0	Carcinoma *in situ*, intra-epithelial cancers.
Stage 1	Cancer is found only in the vulva and/or the area between the vagina and the back passage (perineum) and is </= to 2cm wide.
1a	Stromal invasion no more than 1mm.
1b	Stromal invasion greater than 1mm.
Stage 2	Cancer is found in the vulva and/or the perineum. The area affected is > 2cm wide.
Stage 3	Cancer is found in the vulva and/or perineum and has spread to nearby tissue, e.g. lower part of the urethra (tube through which urine is passed), the vagina, the anus (opening of the rectum) and/or groin lymph nodes.
Stage 4a	The cancer has spread beyond the urethra, vagina, and anus into the lining of the bladder or the bowel.
Stage 4b	It may also have spread to lymph nodes in the pelvis or other parts of the body.

Grading of vulval cancer

Grade 1 (low grade) suggests cells that look like the original vulval cells. This type usually grows more slowly and less likely to spread.
Grade 2 (moderate grade) these cells look more abnormal than low grade cancer but not as abnormal as high grade.
Grade 3 (high grade) means that these cells look very different to the original vulval cells. These can grow more quickly and are more likely to spread.

Surgery

Surgery is the main treatment for cancer of the vulva. This is used in early stage disease but can be indicated in more advanced disease also.

- If the tumour is very localized, it may be possible to undertake a wide local excision.
- If the lesion is at one side of the vulva, it may be possible to remove half of the vulva (hemi-vulvectomy).
- If the lesion is in the centre of the vulva or across both sides, it may be necessary to remove both sides (total or radical vulvectomy).
- If the cancer is at one side, the groin lymph nodes at that side will be removed.
- If the cancer is in the centre or across both sides of the vulva, both sets of groin nodes will be removed.

Complications of surgery

- Mortality 1–2%.
- Morbidity in 50% breakdown of groin wound occurs.
- 8–70% chronic lymphoedema of lower extremities.
- Anatomic disfiguration and wound breakdown.
- Sexual dysfunction.

Due to the extensive morbidity associated with radical surgery, there has been increasing support for conservative surgery—removal of small lesions with negative superficial inguinal lymph nodes on frozen section and to omit deep lymph node dissection. However, the groin recurrence rate in such cases is 8%.

Radiotherapy

This can be used after surgery, where the margins were not clear of disease or the lymph nodes were involved. It can be used on its own or with chemotherapy for more advanced disease.

Chemotherapy

This is reserved for:

- Inoperable local disease.
- Recurrent disease.
- Metastatic disease.

Follow-up and prognosis

Careful follow-up is essential to detect recurrent disease, long-term complications, if any, and psychosexual well-being. The prognosis is mainly related to lymph node involvement: 90% 5-year survival rates in node negative and 58% in node positive tumours.

Prevention

If a woman has had previous pre-cancer of the vulva or chronic skin conditions of the vulva, she will require careful monitoring and follow-up.

Prevention may also lie in education and health promotion; cessation of smoking and safe sex and prevention of HPV infection.

Resources

Prendiville, W, Ritter J, Tatti SA, Twiggs L (2003) *Colposcopy: Management Options*. WB Saunders, Elsevier Limited: Chapter 20.

Cancer of the vagina[1]

Epidemiology

Less than 300 women are diagnosed with cancer of the vagina annually in the UK. There are two main types of vaginal cancer: primary vaginal cancer (this originates in the vagina) and scondary vaginal cancer (this spreads to the vagina from elsewhere, e.g. the cervix). This chapter deals with primary vaginal cancer.

Incidence

70% of vaginal cancers occur the over 60–65 age group.

Causes

- It is not clear what stimulates development of vaginal cancer.
- Human papilloma virus (HPV), either of the cervix or in genital warts, have been present in some women with vaginal cancer.
- History of vaginal intra-epithelial neoplasia (VaIN).

Presenting complaints/symptoms

- There may not be any symptoms in early vaginal cancer.
- Chronic itching of the vagina and inflammation.
- Unusual bleeding, e.g. post-coital (after sexual intercourse), in between periods, or after the menopause.
- Excessive or abnormal vaginal discharge.
- Growth/lump in the vagina.

More advanced cancer

- Urinary frequency or pain on passing urine.
- Constipation.
- Lower abdominal pain.
- Swollen abdomen.
- Swollen upper thighs.

Examination/investigations

- Gynaecological examination (full pelvic examination).
- Examination with a speculum.
- Vaginal cytology and cervical smear.
- Colposcopy +/- biopsy.
- Chest X-ray or CT chest (if need to rule out chest involvement).
- MRI to stage disease and lymph nodes.
- EUA.

Types of vaginal cancer

Squamous cell carcinoma makes up the largest numbers of vaginal cancers.

Adenocarcinoma accounts for fewer cancers of the vagina. This usually occurs in younger women. This would be confirmed by biopsy/histology.

Melanoma, small cell carcinoma, lymphoma, and sarcoma are extremely rare types of cancer of the vagina. Usually confirmed on biopsy.

1 Adapted with permission from Tadman, M and Roberts, D (2007) *Oxford Handbook of Cancer Nursing*. Oxford University Press.

Treatment

Surgery

Surgical incision is appropriate management in selected cases, thus surgery will depend upon size, stage (extent), other organ involvement, and general health of the patient.

Surgery may include removing some or the entire vagina, and surrounding tissue. It may be necessary to remove the uterus, cervix, and parametria, as well as some of the vagina.

In more advanced disease, it may be necessary to remove all of the vagina +/- bladder +/- part of the bowel.

Radiotherapy

For many women with cancer of the vagina, radiotherapy will be the treatment of choice. It can be given as external beam radiotherapy on its own or with additional internal beam radiotherapy (brachytherapy). In younger women, chemotherapy can be given alongside radiotherapy to make the radiotherapy more effective.

📖 See Radiotherapy: overview for an explanation of each treatment, p.316.

Treatment decisions

Women with cancer of the vagina are managed in a cancer centre.

Multidisciplinary teams (MDT) made up of medical and surgical oncologists will carry out examinations, request investigations, and have discussions with the women, and devise care plans. Treatments are individualized and can include radiotherapy and/or chemotherapy.

Prevention

As the cause of vaginal cancer is still unclear, it is difficult to advise on prevention.

Special considerations

- Fertility.
- Altered body image.
- Sexuality.
- Psychological care.
- Physical functioning.

Clinicians and nurse specialists are ideally placed to offer support to these women. Onward referrals to other specialists may be necessary.

Cancer of the cervix[1]

Introduction

Rates of cervical cancer vary enormously between countries. It is the commonest female cancer in South-East Asia and Africa. Incidence drops rapidly where national screening programmes have been introduced.

80–90% are squamous cell cancers. Adenocarcinoma is less common but increasing in incidence.

Risk factors

- Early onset of sexual intercourse (before 17 years old).
- Non-barrier forms of contraception.
- HPV—particularly HPV types 16 and 18—is present in approximately 100% of cervical cancers seen in the UK. A vaccination programme has been introduced in 2008 in schools.
- Cigarette smoking.
- Multiple sexual partners.
- Immunocompromise.
- Low socioeconomic group/status.

Presenting complaints/symptoms

- Can be asymptomatic until late presentation.
- Increased vaginal discharge which can be offensive.
- Post-coital bleeding.
- Inter-menstrual bleeding.

📖 For management of screening detected abnormalities see Cervical screening, Chapter 18, p.489.

Examination/investigation

- Speculum examination—there may be a growth and/or ulcer on the cervix in some cases.
- Bimanual examination.
- Colposcopy and targeted biopsies.
- EUA and biopsy.
- Full blood count, renal, and liver function tests.
- Chest X-ray, CT scan of the abdomen and pelvis.
- An MRI scan can define tumour size and any lymph node involvement.
- Cystoscopy is used to assess evidence of bladder disease.
- Sigmoidoscopy may be used if there is evidence of bowel disease.

Staging

Staging is based predominantly on the extent of the primary tumour (📖 see Table 11.2).

The spread is usually from the cervix into the vagina and then into the pelvic wall. Metastatic spread is normally by the lymphatic system and can involve the bladder and rectum.

1 Adapted with permission from Tadman, M and Roberts, D (2007) *Oxford Handbook of Cancer Nursing*. Oxford University Press.

Table 11.2 FIGO staging for cervical cancer

Ia	Micro-invasive disease (max. depth 5mm, max. width 7mm).
Ib	Clinical disease confined to the cervix.
IIa	Disease involves upper one-third of vagina but not parametrium.
IIb	Disease involves parametrium but does not extend to pelvic wall.
III	Disease involves lower two-thirds of vagina and/or pelvic wall.
IV	Involvement of bladder, rectum, or distant organs.

Treatment

Surgery

- Radical hysterectomy is the main treatment option for early stage disease.
- Trachelectomy, where the cervix only is removed or radical tracheotomy is removal of the cervix and 2/3 of the upper vagina and may be offered to women who wish to conserve their fertility. Future pregnancies should be monitored by a consultant obstetrician and caesarean section is generally required.
- Extensive disease may be managed by pelvic exenteration.

Combined chemotherapy and radiotherapy

- Combined chemotherapy (cisplatin) and radical pelvic radiotherapy.
- May be indicated if surgery is unlikely to remove the complete tumour.
- Both external beam radiotherapy and brachytherapy are used routinely within this setting. This can still be a curative treatment.
- Pelvic radiotherapy can also be used in very advanced disease to palliate pelvic symptoms.

Chemotherapy

For advanced disease, platinum-based chemotherapy gives best results.

Prognosis

Survival at five years is typically:

- stage 1a, 100%;
- stage 1b, 70–90%;
- stage 2, 60–80%;
- stage 3, 35–45%;
- stage 4, 10–20%.

These wide ranges reflect the large variation in disease volume seen within the present staging system; it is based on tissue involvement rather than volume of disease. Relapse after 5 years of remission is unusual.

Overview of endometrial cancer

Epidemiology

In the UK, it is the second most common cancer and 4500 new cases occur each year, with the majority being diagnosed in women over 50.

Incidence

Usually menopausal women, average age 63 years. Majority are postmenopausal at diagnosis, 25% are pre-menopausal and approximately 5% are diagnosed under the age of 40.

Risk factors

- Oestrogen exposure—early menarche/late menopause.
- Nulliparity (no children)—no breast feeding.
- Obesity.
- Diabetes.
- Tamoxifen/HRT.
- Endometrial hyperplasia.
- PCOS.
- Unopposed oestrogen therapy.
- Family history of endometrial cancer +/- bowel cancer.
- Women with hereditary non-polyposis colon cancer syndrome have a 50% lifetime risk of developing endometrial cancer.

Presenting complaint/symptoms

- No symptoms—found as a coincidence 5%.
- Post-menopausal bleeding in about 80% of women.
- Abnormal bleeding in the over 35-year-old woman, especially IMB.
- Vaginal discharge—rare about 10%.

More advanced disease

- Pain on passing urine.
- Pelvic/back pain.
- Pelvic lump.
- Pain on sexual intercourse.
- Weight loss.

History and examination/investigations

- Full history looking at risk factors above.
- Bimanual examination and cervical screening.
- Transvaginal ultrasound—this may then lead to a hysteroscopy dependent on the results. A thin endometrium (<4–5mm) in the post-menopausal woman is reassuring and has a high negative predictive value. Further investigations are required in women with thickened endometrium.
- Hysteroscopy and biopsy (📖 see Chapter 12, p.325).
- Ultrasound is less useful in women on Tamoxifen, where hysteroscopy with biopsy is the gold standard.
- Serum tumour markers like Ca125 are generally not helpful for initial diagnosis and/or staging.

- Blood counts, liver and renal function tests when a diagnosis is made.
- Chest X-ray to look for lung metastasis.
- MRI scan—role lies in assessing the depth of myometrial invasion and for cervical involvement. It is increasingly being used in tertiary centres prior to surgery.
- Cystoscopy if bladder involvement suspected.
- CT scanning if intra-abdominal metastasis is suspected.

Differential diagnosis

Histopathological assessment of endometrial biopsy is diagnostic.

Treatment of endometrial cancer

Surgery in most cases to stage and treat.

Staging

Table 11.3 Staging of endometrial cancer (FIGO)

Stage	Description
I	Confined to the body of the uterus.
Ia	Confined to the endometrium.
Ib	Under 50% myometrial invasion.
Ic	Over 50% myometrial invasion.
2	Cervix involved.
2a	Endocervical gland involvement.
2b	Cervical stromal invasion but does not extend beyond the uterus.
3	Spread to serosa of uterus, peritoneal cavity, or lymph nodes.
3a	Involves serosa or adenexae, positive ascites, or peritoneal washings.
3b	Vaginal involvement either direct or metastatic.
3c	Para-aortic or pelvic node involvement.
4	Local or distant metastases.
4a	Cancer involving mucosa of bladder or rectum.
4b	Distant metastases and involvement of other abdominal or inguinal lymph nodes.

Grading of endometrial cancer

Grade 1 (low) cancer cells are not that dissimilar to the original endometrial cells.
Grade 2 (moderate) cancer cells are quite abnormal compared to original cells.
Grade 3 (high) cancer cells are quite abnormal, may grow faster and can spread.

Surgery

Surgery is the mainstay in most women with endometrial cancer. Surgery may be open but there is an increasing trend to laparoscopic procedures. It involves surgical removal of the uterus and cervix, fallopian tubes, both ovaries +/– removal of bilateral pelvic lymph nodes, peritoneal cytology, and inspection of the upper abdominal organs and peritoneal surfaces. Low-grade stage Ib endometrioid tumours are associated with lymph node metastasis in under 5% of cases and lymphadenectomy may have no therapeutic benefit.

📖 The role of lymphadenectomy is discussed further in Chapter 12.

Radiotherapy

This is sometimes used after surgery (as an adjuvant therapy).
Radiation is often used to decrease the chances of the disease coming back. It is usually external or internal radiotherapy.

- External takes place over 5 weeks with one treatment daily so 5 x 5 treatments.
- Internal takes place as an inpatient (low dose over 12–16h) or (high dose) as an outpatient.

Can be useful for women who are not fit for surgery.

Chemotherapy

- Used mostly in recurrent disease, where other treatments have been used already.
- Can be used in advanced cases especially for palliation.

Hormone therapy

Some endometrial cancers are hormone-sensitive and can be treated with hormone therapy. Progestogens are the most commonly used hormones, they have no role in prevention of recurrences, but can be used in recurrences in high doses. Usually this is in the palliative setting.

Prognosis

Prognosis is related to stage. Overall it is about 70% as patients present early with PMB.

- stage I, 72% 5-year survival rate;
- stage II, 56%;
- stage III, 32%;
- stage IV, 11%.

Prognosis is also related to histology type. Endometriod adenocarcinoma has the best prognosis, while papillary and clear cell tumours have a poorer prognosis. Most tumours are oestrogen- and progestrogen-receptor positive, if they are not it is associated with a poorer prognosis.

Prevention

Prevention can be difficult; there aren't any screening methods for endometrial cancer. Monitor closely if there is a family history of endometrial cancer and/or bowel cancer.

Obese women should be advised to lose weight. The combined oral contraceptive pill reduces the risk by up to 50%, lasting up to 20 years post-discontinuation. Depo-Provera® has a similar but smaller effect.

Fallopian tube cancer

Epidemiology

Cancer of the fallopian tube is very rare. Cancer that originates in the fallopian tube is called primary fallopian tube cancer and it accounts for approximately 1% of all gynaecological cancers in the UK.

Incidence

This occurs, for the greater part, in women after the age of the menopause.

Cause

Not known. There is thought to be a risk in women who have a strong family history (more than two direct relatives) of breast or ovarian cancer or both.

Presenting complaints/clinical features

- Vaginal bleeding (not related to periods).
- Vaginal discharge.
- Abdominal pain/colicky (comes in spasms).
- Swollen abdomen.

Examinations/investigations

- Pelvic examination.
- Transvaginal scans.
- CT scan.
- Blood tests.
- Exploratory surgery.

Differential diagnosis

Biopsy looked at under the microscope. Often taken during exploratory surgery. Primary fallopian tube cancer is usually made up of adenocarcinoma cells. Far rarer would be transitional cell or sarcoma.

Treatment

Usually surgery, similar to that for ovarian cancer. Total abdominal hysterectomy, bilateral salpingo-oophorectomy, and removal of omentum (fatty pad).

Chemotherapy may also be recommended. The oncologist is ideally placed in recommending chemotherapeutic agents, if indicated.

Overview of ovarian cancer[1]

- It is the fourth commonest cancer in women in the UK, with peak incidence in the 65–75 age group.
- Less than 5% of cases are clearly hereditary.
- Risk of ovarian cancer is related to an increasing number of ovulatory cycles, thus some protection from the oral contraceptive pill and pregnancy.

Causes/risks

- Nulliparous women.
- Women with high risk of developing ovarian cancer (i.e. women with BRCA 1 or 2 generic mutation).
- Genetic predisposition.
- There has been some suggestion that subfertility treatments might increase the risk of developing ovarian cancer.

Presenting complaints/symptoms

15% of women are asymptomatic at diagnosis. 80% of women present with advanced disease that has spread beyond the ovary to involve the peritoneum and other abdominopelvic organs.
⚠ It often gets mistaken for gastro-intestinal symptoms.

Common symptoms include:
- Abdominal bloating.
- Urinary urgency.
- Constantly swollen stomach.
- Indigestion.
- Ongoing fatigue.
- Back/abdominal pain.
- Weight loss.

Note: primary fallopian tube and peritoneal cancers are rare and behave similarly to ovarian cancer. They can be found on histology when suspicious of ovarian cancer and are treated in the same way.

Examination and investigations

- Ultrasound.
- MRI/CT.
- Chest X-ray.
- Bloods—Ca125 , AFP, FBC, LFT, U&E.
- 80% of women with advanced ovarian cancer have elevated serum Ca125. A raised Ca125 with an abdominal mass or ascites on CT scan are highly suspicious of ovarian cancer.

Ca125 tumour marker testing

Ca125 (cancer antigen), is a protein produced on the surface of cells, including ovarian, uterine, and cervical cells. It is a blood test. It can be a useful tumour marker in diagnosis of ovarian cancer in conjunction with other tests, such as abdominal CT scan. However, it is not elevated in all ovarian tumours. It is also valuable in monitoring response to therapy and in the detection of early relapse.

1. Adapted with permission from Tadman, M and Roberts, D (2007) *Oxford Handbook of Cancer Nursing*. Oxford University Press.

⚠ Ca125 can also be raised in some benign conditions, e.g endometriosis, fibroids, PID, rheumatoid arthritis.

Risk of malignancy index (RMI)

- 21% of PM women have ovarian cysts for which US and Ca125 are not sensitive or specific at detecting malignancy.
- RMI = US x M x Ca125.
- US is a score of 1–3 dependent on the following features: multi-locular, solid area in cyst, bilateral lesions, evidence of metastases and ascetics.
- M is menopausal status and scores 3.
- Ca125 is the number μ/ml.
- A high score is suspicious of cancer.

Treatment of ovarian cancer

Diagnosis and staging (see Tables 11.4 and 11.5)

The two main prognostic factors in ovarian cancer are the stage and the amount of residual disease after surgery.

- Patients with more than a 2cm area of disease after surgery have a poor prognosis, with only 20% surviving 3 years.
- Full histological staging is carried out surgically via total abdominal hysterectomy, bilateral salpingo-oophorectomy, omentectomy, lymph node biopsies, and multiple peritoneal biopsies. Staging is carried out using the tumour node metastasis (TNM) staging system.

Table 11.4 Stage level of spread 5-year survival %

Stage I	**Confined to ovaries 75%.**
1a	Limited to ovary, no ascites, capsule intact, no tumour on surface.
1b	Limited to both ovaries, no ascites, capsule intact, no surface tumour.
1c	Limited to one or both ovaries with a ruptured capsule, surface tumour, and peritoneal washings.
Stage II	**Tumour spread within pelvis 45%.**
2a	Extension to uterus and/or fallopian tubes.
2b	Extension to other pelvic tissues.
2c	Stage 2a or 2b with a ruptured capsule, tumour on the surface, malignant ascites, or positive peritoneal washings.
Stage III	**Peritoneal spread outside the pelvis, e.g. omentum.**
Stage IV	**Distant metastases <5%.**

Table 11.5 Types of ovarian cancer

Epithelial tumours account for 85%	
Serous cystadenocarcinoma	Usually unilocular with solid areas, bilateral in 30%
Mucinous cystadenocarcinoma	Multi locular, mucin-filled, associated with tumours of the appendix or gallbladder
Endometroid cystadenocarcinoma	Resemble endometrial adenocarcinoma and can be associated with it
Clear cell cystadenocarcinoma	Thin-walled unilocular and can be associated with endometriosis
Boarderline tumours of low malignant potential	Can occur in any of the above, more common in mucinous and better prognosis but can reoccur
Other tumours	
1. Sex cord stromal tumours have a low-grade malignancy.	
Granulosa cell tumours	Oestrogen producing
Sertoli-leydig cell tumours	Androgen producing
2. Fibromas	May be associated with pleural effusions and are benign
3. Germ cell tumours	Teratomas—mature (dermiod) are benign and immature are solid, malignant, unilateral
4. Secondary tumours	Most common primary are breast, stomach, and colon

Treatment

Radical surgery

TAH, BSO, and omentectomy. Optimal tumour debulking (no tumour >1cm left). Other than stage 1a, combined surgery and chemotherapy is the best approach. There is uncertainty about the best order for treatment, i.e. surgery before or after chemotherapy. Both offer significant survival improvement.

First-line chemotherapy

Platinum/taxane combinations, normally 6 cycles, are generally regarded as the optimum treatment. Median survival rates are 2–3 years, with some patients cured of their disease.

Treatment at relapse

Patients with a treatment-free interval of greater than 12 months should be re-challenged with a platinum-containing regimen. The longer the treatment-free interval, the greater the likelihood of a worthwhile second response. For those relapsing sooner, a number of new agents, including liposomal doxorubicin, topotecan, and gemcitabine, can be used.

New approaches

Possible new approaches to improve management include:

- Intra-peritoneal chemotherapy.
- High-dose systemic chemotherapy.
- Biological response modifiers.
- Anti-angiogenic agents.

Radiotherapy: overview

This is use of high-energy radiation rays to kill cancer cells, whilst sparing as many healthy cells as possible in the process. Can be used on its own or accompanied by chemotherapy (adjuvant) (see Table 11.6).

Table 11.6 When is radiotherapy used?

Indication	Examples
Primary treatment	Stage 2 or greater cervical cancer, cancer of the vagina.
Adjuvant therapy	Following surgical treatment of cervical cancer. Following surgical treatment of endometrial cancer. Following surgical treatment of vulval cancer. In addition to chemotherapy in cervical cancer.
Recurrent disease	Recurrent endometrial or cervical cancer where recurrence is outside of the site originally treated. Occasionally used in ovarian cancer in cases of localized recurrence.
Symptom control	Vaginal bleeding if the site has not previously been irradiated.
Advanced disease	Vulval cancer.

Dose and duration

Gray (gy) is the unit of measure of absorbed radiation dose. Each dose is called a fraction. Usual treatment for gynaecological malignancies is external beam (45gy over 25 fractions, 1 a day) and/or low-dose internal radiotherapy (as an inpatient) and high-dose internal radiotherapy (as an outpatient). Treatment is usually made up of some of the above.

Pre-treatment planning

Before radiotherapy is given, women need a pre-treatment planning scan. This is done using a machine called a simulator, which allows the radiographers to take pictures of the tumour and pelvis, so that treatment can be planned using the scans. The procedure is painless and can take from minutes to an hour, depending on the complexity of the tumour and the surrounding area. Treatment usually starts 1–2 weeks after the planning scan.

External beam radiotherapy

This treatment usually is given once a day as an outpatient. The treatment itself takes minutes and women will be in the hospital roughly for a half an hour in a day. The treatment is usually given Monday to Friday and usually lasts for 5 weeks or more. The radiotherapy is administered using high-energy rays, and they are directed at the tumour through the pelvis (like strong X-rays). Radiotherapy is not painful (see p.317 on side-effects).

Internal radiotherapy

This is also known as brachytherapy. This is when the treatment is administered directly to the tumour. In the case of cervical and endometrial cancer, this means inserting a rod or rods (applicators) into the vagina and treating the cervix or (in the case of those who have had an hysterectomy) the top of the vagina. This can be administered in a low-dose rate (LDR) overnight and as an inpatient, or in a high-dose rate (HDR) over a few outpatient appointments. This depends on which brachytherapy machines the department has.

Side-effects

The main side-effects of pelvic radiotherapy are:

- Tiredness or fatigue.
- Skin reactions (redness, dryness, blisters, broken skin).
- Irritation to the bowel mucosa (diarrhoea).
- Irritation to the bladder or urethra (cystitis).
- Vaginal fibrosis (scar tissue forming, usually, at the top of the vagina).
- Bone marrow depression (usually red blood cells) resulting in anaemia.
- Ovarian dysfunction.
- Early menopause (in women who were not previously menopausal).

Side-effects can occur during the treatment and many will be temporary. This can mean that they can last for 3–6 weeks up until a few months after the treatment stops. Some side-effects, such as scar tissue in the vagina, can occur in weeks, but could also occur much later in the treatment.

Rare side-effects

Fistulae (holes, abnormal passages forming between organs, e.g. bladder and vagina).

Support

Woman undergoing radiotherapy will be supported by their doctor, clinical nurse specialist, and radiotherapists who administer the treatment. They will be informed of the potential side-effects. They will be advised on how they can minimize some side-effects and offered support and advice on coping with some unavoidable symptoms.

Follow-up

When the radiotherapy treatment is completed, the patient will be followed-up per the cancer centre's protocol by the oncology team. This will usually be 3–4-monthly for the first year and then 6-monthly for the second year and then yearly up to 5 years or longer. Visits include symptom review, detailed history, examination, and investigations including scans.

Chemotherapy: overview

How does chemotherapy work?

Chemotherapeutic agents damage cells that are dividing. Cells in the process of dividing are more sensitive to these drugs. Cancer cells divide more than normal cells. However, because chemotherapy cannot differentiate between cancer and normal cells, some normal cells also get destroyed, but have the capacity to repair and replace themselves.

How often is chemotherapy given?

This largely depends on the regimen and drugs used. In gynaecological cancer, mainly a combination of drugs is given as an outpatient treatment with 3 weeks between courses. This is to give the healthy cells a chance to be restored without the unhealthy cancer cells getting a chance to grow again. Each administration, followed by a rest is known as a cycle of chemotherapy.

When is chemotherapy given?

There are many uses for chemotherapy, it can be:

- After surgery to treat macroscopic (visible) or microscopic disease. When it is given in this way, it is called adjuvant treatment.
- In bulky disease, chemotherapeutic drugs can be given to shrink the disease before surgery is reconsidered—so called as neo-adjuvant treatment.
- Low-dose chemotherapeutic agents can be combined with radiotherapy to make the radiotherapy more effective.
- In recurrent cancer.
- In palliation or control of symptoms.

Drug administration

Chemotherapeutic agents can be given orally, peritoneally (through the peritoneum), and usually in gynaecological malignancy, intravenously.

Chemotherapy in cancer of the ovary

A combination of chemotherapy and surgery is usually used to treat ovarian cancer. Surgery is often used as an initial treatment followed by chemotherapy, but chemotherapy can be the upfront treatment followed by a surgical review interval debulking surgery (IDS). First-line chemotherapy for cancer of the ovary is usually carboplatin and paclitaxel. If a woman's ovarian cancer recurs, she can either be re-challenged with these drugs or there are other drugs (on and off trial) that can be considered.

Chemotherapy in cancer of the cervix

Surgery and/or radiotherapy are the main treatments for cancer of the cervix. Chemotherapy is often combined with radiotherapy, to make the radiotherapy more effective. Cisplatin is the drug used most commonly with radiotherapy to treat cancer of the cervix. Chemotherapy can also be considered in recurrent disease.

Chemotherapy in cancer of the endometrium

Surgery and/or radiotherapy are the main treatments in cancer of the endometrium. Chemotherapy can be used in disease recurrence.

Chemotherapy in cancer of the vulva/vagina

When chemotherapy is used in these rarer cancers, it is usually combined with other treatments such as radiotherapy.

Side-effects of chemotherapy

These depend on the drug and combination of drugs used. Some side-effects include:

- Bone marrow suppression (low white cells usually, less commonly red blood cells), leucopenia, and thrombocytopenia.
- Anaemia.
- Nausea and vomiting—can be prevented with anti-emetics.
- Hair loss—a wig can be given—hair loss normally starts 3 weeks after the treatment and should grow back 6 months later.
- Fatigue.
- Sore mouth/loss of appetite.
- Diarrhoea.
- Peripheral neuropathy (pain in hands or feet).
- Renal toxicity.

Nursing management issues in gynaecological oncology[1]

Treatment support

Many of the treatments available for managing gynaecological cancers are aggressive, and can have profound physical, psychosocial, and sexual impacts on women and their families.

Psychosexual concerns

Loss of fertility, onset of menopause, rectal and bladder dysfunction, and vaginal dryness and tightness are all common difficulties that these women face. Changes in body image, sexuality and fertility may require referral for specialist psychological/psychosexual support.

It is important not to under-estimate the significance of loss of fertility. Even if patients had not planned to have children, or to have more children, the knowledge that this is no longer possible can be devastating.

Concerns regarding sexuality may not emerge until well after major treatment, when women are back at home. Pre-treatment assessment, education, and counselling, often by the clinical nurse specialist, is therefore essential in preparing individuals and their families.

Post-surgery patients need to be informed of what has been removed and the effect this treatment will have on them. It is helpful in planning their care to establish if they are sexually active, planning to have children, or are menopausal.

Appropriate nurse follow-up and assessment is required to ensure any problems are not missed. Primary care involvement may be useful in this area. Early close liaison with the GP and district nursing services is useful.

Other common concerns include the following:

Ascites

This is particularly common in ovarian cancer and can be difficult to manage.

Pain

Perineal and pelvic pain becomes more common in advanced disease. It often has a nerve-based element, making it difficult to completely resolve.

Hormonal symptoms

In most cases where the menopause has been induced early because of treatment (surgery to remove both ovaries or radical pelvic radiotherapy), hormone replacement therapy may be given until the average age of the menopause, i.e. 54 years old. Exceptions to this are hormone-dependent tumours, such as some endometrial or some cervical tumours.

Lower limb oedema

When patients have extensive pelvic disease this is increasingly common. It needs active management including specialist compression bandaging and skin care.

1. Adapted with permission from Tadman, M and Roberts, D (2007) *Oxford Handbook of Cancer Nursing*. Oxford University Press.

Vaginal discharge and odour

This can be offensive and extremely embarrassing. Topical antibiotics, and deodorizing dressings can help.

Bowel obstruction

This is also a problem, especially when the disease is palliative.

Fisulas

To bowel and bladder.

Bleeding

Problems in advanced disease.

In addition:

- Anxiety and depression.
- Fatigue.
- Wound care.
- Rehabilitation.

Resources

Hoskins, WJ, Mitchell, WA, Randall, ME *et al.* (2004) *Principles and practice of gynecologic oncology.* Lippincott Williams and Wilkins, Philadelphia.

Katz, A (2003) Sexuality after hysterectomy: a review of the literature and discussion of nurses role. *Journal of Advanced nursing* **42(3)**: 297–303.

Moore, GJ (ed.) (2000) *Women and cancer a gynaecologic oncology nursing perspective.* Jones and Bartlett, Boston.

NHS Executive (1999) *Guidance on commissioning cancer services: Improving outcomes in gynaecological cancers—the manual.* Department of Health, London.

Smith, JR (1999) *Gynaecological oncology (Fast Facts Series).* Health Press, Abingdon.

White, I (2005) The impact of cancer and cancer therapy on sexual and reproductive health. In: Kearney, N and Richardson, A (2005). *Nursing patients with cancer: principles and practice.* Churchill Livingstone, Edinburgh, pp.675–700.

Living with cancer

In recent years there have been many advances in cancer care. These include earlier detection, screening, improved outcomes, and longer survival. People have to learn to cope following the diagnosis and treatment of cancer. Cancer and cancer treatment can affect people emotionally, physically, spiritually, and socially.

Emotional/psychological/sexual impact

There can be feelings of anxiety, sadness, anger to name but a few. These can be present at diagnosis, but also after the treatment has finished. It can affect the individual with cancer and also partners, families, and friends of the person affected. A woman with cancer/treatments may have fears regarding her personal relationships or single women for their future partners. A diagnosis of cancer and treatment may affect both partners. Doctors or nurses should give the person with cancer the opportunity to bring up this subject or their concerns.

Physical impact

There can be symptoms from the cancer, e.g. nausea, bowel problems, loss of appetite. There is also the risk of side-effects from the treatment,e.g. body image adjustment following surgery for vulval cancer.

Spiritual impact

It is not unusual for someone who has been diagnosed with cancer to fear that they will die from the cancer or the treatment. Some women with gynaecological malignancies may have been diagnosed with a late-stage disease and told that, though their cancer is treatable, it is not curable. Some people will turn to their religious faith for support and others may get their support from friends or family.

Social impact

Women who have been diagnosed with gynaecological malignancies will have to cope with the diagnosis and the treatment. They may have many other roles in their lives. They may be working and need to work during or after treatment, they may be mothers and/or partners and have to support their families and loved ones whilst needing support themselves. They may look after their elderly or ill parents.

Life after diagnosis of cancer

Diagnosis of cancer can lead to a person changing their priorities in regards to relationships, lifestyle, or career. It may enable women to choose what is most important to them.

Some women with gynaecological malignancies may have to live with a physical disability after a cancer treatment, e.g. lymphoedema (swelling with fluid).

A person who has had a cancer diagnosis may be unable to return to work, and yet may have a desire or necessity to do so.

A woman may have to live with some uncertainty as to whether her disease will come back. Her follow-up appointments at the cancer centre or local hospital may fill her with dread but also relief, if there is no evidence of recurrence.

Having a cancer diagnosis can make people feel closer, with a wish to get through it together.

However, this can be a very stressful time and can put pressure on relationships.

There may also be pressure to be positive throughout the cancer journey. This should not mean hiding the tears or feelings. It is very positive to be able to talk about fears and worries.

Support for women living with cancer

What support is out there?

Women who have had a gynaecological malignancy and have to cope with physical changes or difficulties will be offered the support of their hospital doctors and nurse specialists. There are also specialists who deal with specific areas, e.g. lymphoedema nurse specialists and stoma nurse specialists. Some are available at the cancer centre, some in the patient's community. The primary care team will need to be involved in the long-term care and this involves good communication from the cancer centre. A woman's GP and practice nurse will be able to give ongoing physical and psychological support.

Most cancer centres have access to an information and support service. This can provide written information and visual aids. Many offer complementary therapies, such as therapeutic massage and reflexology. There is usually access to dietary information or to see a dietician. Counselling services, support groups, and stress-management courses can be available. Services will vary slightly depending on where one lives. People with cancer should be entitled to these (if available), free of charge.

Organizations

Cancer BACUP provides a website with information on the different types of cancer and the different treatments. It can also signpost people to where they may find help for their specific needs. It also provides a helpline for information and support.

Macmillan cancer relief is a charity that provides information (by way of publications and a website). The charity can provide financial grants to pay for travel to hospital for clients with financial difficulties with no other options. Macmillan also funds palliative care nurse posts in order to offer symptom control or end-of-life care to people with advanced cancer.

Social Services can advise people on their entitlements, e.g. housing benefit or disability. They can help with issues regarding housing or re-housing. They can help with setting up care packages, e.g. home help, meals on wheels, occupational therapy referral, and so on.

Citizens advice bureau can highlight to people their rights and also signpost them to areas that may be more specific to their needs. They can also offer legal advice.

The above are just a few of the organizations or charities that provide support to individuals with cancer. Dependent on the problem or tumour site there are also other support groups, such as:

- Jo's trust for women with cervical cancer who are age 40 and below.
- Ovacome is a charity to support women with ovarian cancer.
- The Daisy Network is useful for all women with premature menopause.

Chapter 12

Nursing care of gynaecological patients in hospital

Introduction to nursing care of women in hospital

The nursing care of women in hospital has changed dramatically over the last decade. The length of stay has reduced and increasingly care is being undertaken in the outpatient/office setting, and more complex laparoscopic surgery is being undertaken in the day case setting. This poses a challenge for nurses caring for women in shorter time-frames and also for nurses in the community who may find that they need to care for post-operative patients. Increasingly this means that the ward will have the more complex operations, complex co-morbidities, and gynaecological oncology.

This chapter looks at:

- pre-operative care;
- post-operative care, including complications;
- psychological care;
- inpatient care and trends in surgery;
- outpatient/office gynaecology;
- specific operations—hysteroscopy, laparoscopy, hysterectomy, major surgery, and urogynaecology.

📖 The care of women undergoing emergency admissions is covered in Chapters 15 and 16.

Pre-operative care

Surgery is a unique experience for each patient. As well as physical aspects of care, psychosocial and physiological factors must be considered. Although some operations are considered minor procedures, surgery is always a major experience for patient and family.

Informed consent

► Patients have the right to self-determination regarding surgical intervention. Consent forms must be signed by the person carrying out the procedure and the patient. First-stage consent should be by a practitioner who is able to undertake the procedure and second-stage consent by the person carrying out the procedure. Nurses, who undertake procedures such as hysteroscopy, are considered competent to undertake consent, as they can undertake the procedure. In other instances, nurses and other healthcare professionals can train to undertake first-stage consent for certain procedures.

Further information on consent and mental capacity can be found at www.dh.gov.uk (search on key word consent).

Allergy status

The patient should be assessed for allergies, especially those to:

- iodine;
- medications, e.g. penicillin;
- latex;
- cleansing solutions;
- adhesive tape and dressings;
- metal.

Medication and substance misuse

Patients with a history of smoking and substance misuse should be highlighted. This is vital as there could be potential adverse effects with some anaesthetic agents and problems with post-operative pain and recovery.

Smoking

Causes an increase in intra-operative and post-operative complications. (See Chapter 16, p.441.)

Drug and alcohol

Alters the effects of anaesthetic agents.

Aspirin/NSAID

These affect the platelet function and may increase risk of intra-operative and post-operative hemorrhage.

Medical history

A full medical history should be taken from each patient by a relevantly trained healthcare professional. This can be a medic, but, more recently nurses have been undertaking further training to undertake this extended role. This includes physical examination, history taking, and assessment of risks.

Outline of history taking

- Patients details and age.
- Presenting complaint and history of the presenting complaint.
    - LMP and contraception.
    - Age at menopause, if applicable.
- Past medical and surgical history.
- Gynaecological/obstetric history.
- Medications, drug history, and allergies.
- Smoking and alcohol history.
- Social, occupational, and family history.
- How the illness has affected psyche, personal and family life, finances, and occupation.
- Previous operations and any problems experienced.
- Systems review.
    - Appropriate blood tests and investigations such as ECG and chest X-ray dependent on history.
- Plan of care.

Pre-assessment clinic

All patients who are to be admitted for elective surgery should be seen in the pre-assessment clinic.

This may be a nurse-led clinic, where the patients are assessed to ensure that they are physically fit for surgery and understand what it involves.

Investigations and blood tests needed pre-operatively will be done at this clinic. It is essential the results are followed up pre-operatively to reduce cancellations of surgery. Patients may also be screened for MRSA, dependent on local policies.

►► For a guide to pre-operative investigations, see NICE website.

Cancellations can be reduced by comprehensive pre-assessment to ensure the patients are physically fit, reducing anxiety by information giving and co-ordination of care.

The clinic helps to identify patients who are more likely to develop complications with surgery or anaesthetics.

Length of stay (LOS) and discharge should be discussed and relevant referrals made if required such as social services or convalescence.

Written information given to patients.

Admission

Many hospitals now have a surgical admissions lounge, where patients can be admitted on the morning of the operation. Otherwise patients should be admitted on the day of surgery, unless there are specific medical reasons that are identified at pre-admission clinic (PAC).

Patients who may need to be admitted prior to the day of surgery are:

- less mobile;
- complex medical problems;
- previous anaesthetic problems;
- lack of social care;
- long journey to the hospital.

In order to reduce risk, the medical notes should be available with consent, blood, and test results. On admission:

- Routine observations should be taken from the patient—BP, pulse, oxygen saturations, and temperature.
- A theatre gown should be given.
- Anti-embolic stockings should be correctly measured and fitted.
- Theatre checklist and correct site surgery checklists should be completed, if appropriate.
- Any questions the patient may have should be answered to ensure informed consent.
- Ensure the patient has the opportunity to see the consultant and anaesthetist.
- The need for a urinary pregnancy test should be considered in all patients, dependent on the patient's history, contraception, and operation.

Post-operative complications

Good quality, evidenced-based nurse care is essential in the post-operation phase to ensure that women have the best recovery from surgery and can return to normal activity and home life as soon as possible. Good nursing care can give reassurance and encouragement, and can also ensure that women with suspected complications can have early access to interventions and medical staff.

Post-operative DVT

The formation of clots (deep vein thrombosis—DVT) in the veins of the pelvis and lower extremities, which impair circulation, is a potentially serious post-operative complication.

Everyone who has an operation is at risk of developing a blood clot. However, some people have certain risk factors that may make them more likely to develop one.

Risk factors for developing post-operative DVT

- Previous history of DVT or family member with spontaneous DVT.
- Cancer.
- Long-standing cardiac history.
- On the combined contraceptive pill.
- Inflamed varicose veins (phlebitis).
- Obese.
- Immobile.
- Long journey in the 4 weeks prior to surgery.
- >60 years of age.
- Pregnancy.
- Pelvic mass.

Preventing DVT

A combination of therapies can be used to prevent post-operative DVT:
- compression stockings;
- inflatable compression devices;
- anticoagulants, e.g. heparin, clexane;
- mobilize the patient early post-operatively.

The symptoms of a DVT include:

- Swelling.
- Pain,which may be made worse by bending the foot upward towards the knee.
- Warm skin.
- Tenderness.
- Redness, particularly at the back of the leg, below the knee.

Symptoms of a pulmonary embolism include breathlessness, chest pain, haemoptysis and, in severe cases, collapse.

Post-operative constipation

Decreased bowel activity can result from surgery and it may take 2–3 days before a patient opens their bowels.

Risk factors for post-operative constipation

- Elderly.
- Malignancy.
- Dehydration.
- Anaesthesia.
- Opioids.
- Decreased activity

Preventing post-operative constipation

- Mobilize the patient as soon as possible.
- Ensure patient is adequately hydrated, whether it be intravenous fluids or orally.
- Consider stool softeners (day 3 for major post-operative patients) or glycerol suppositories.

► Ensure nursing staff ask and document if patient's bowels have been opened.

Post-operative urinary tract infections (UTI)

📖 See Cystitis: bacterial and interstitial, p.270.

In the immediate post-operative period the nursing staff should maintain an accurate fluid-balance chart and ensure that patients have adequate hydration.

Patients with catheters should have good catheter care (📖 see Chapter 10, p.247).

Post-operative wound infections

All patients who undergo surgery have the potential to acquire an infection. Wound infections delay recovery and increase length of stay.

Signs and symptoms for wound infection

- Fever.
- Pain.
- Swelling of wound site.
- Erythema.
- Purulent discharge.
- Raised CRP.
- Raised white cell count (WCC).

Actions

- Wound swab.
- Blood cultures if temp.>38°C.
- Intra-venous antibiotics.
- Refer to tissue viability clinical nurse specialists (CNS).
- Monitor bloods CRP, FBC, WCC.

All women with a wound should have the site monitored frequently in the postoperative period. The dressing should be removed and assessed as needed and the wound assessed for redness, swelling, and discharge. The importance of keeping wounds clean and dry should be stressed to patients and strategies put in place to ensure that this is maintained. The prevention of wound infection starts in the pre-operative phase and through the surgical procedure. Infection control measures should not be under-estimated, e.g. hand hygiene.

Psychological impact of patients in the gynaecological setting

Pre-operatively

Anxiety is a normal adaptive response to the stress of surgery. It commonly occurs in the pre-operative phase, as the woman anticipates surgery, or due to post-operative experiences such as:

- Pain.
- Discomfort.
- Altered body image or function.
- Dependency on others.
- Loss of control.
- Family concerns.
- Changes to lifestyle.
- Threat to sexuality.
- Diagnosis of malignancy/infertility.
- Dying.

Education and information giving is a good way of relieving anxieties. If women feel knowledgeable about their condition and treatment, they often feel empowered and in control.

Sociological response

The usual routine of the patient, even if disrupted for 1 day. This causes disruption to the other family members and friends as they help with issues such as transport, psychological support, and carers to children and other responsibilities.

Inability to work can also cause concern to the patient and her family. Job security may be threatened and financial stress may result.

Referral to social services, Macmillan centres, benefits advice, and psychological support networks are often very useful for women.

Nursing management

Thorough assessment of patients in the pre-operative phase, outpatients, or emergency gynaecology setting is vital.

An holistic approach should be used reflecting the woman's:

- physiological;
- psychological;
- spiritual;
- social needs.

From this, areas for assistance are identified and relevant referrals can be made.

Psychological impact

Within gynaecology there are many sensitive issues that clinicians should be aware of when talking to women. Women are often distressed or anxious with issues such as:

- Menopause and symptoms.
- Malignancy/diagnosis and cancer surgery (📖 see Chapter 11, p.293).
- Loss of fertility.
- Miscarriage and ectopic pregnancy.
- Investigations and receiving results.
- Foetal abnormality.
- Medical termination of pregnancy.
- Emergency admissions.
- Perceived changes to sexuality and sexual functioning.

Nursing staff in all areas of women's health can ensure that there is appropriate support for women by assessment and referral to specialist services if needed. Within gynaecology, this may be a referral onto a specialist nurse. Support can include:

- gynaecological oncology;
- uro-gynaecology;
- stoma;
- fertility;
- liaison nurses;
- nurse consultant;
- bereavement midwife;
- midwife;
- pain management.

Care of the patient: day surgery, trends, length of stay (LOS), and the surgical admission lounge

As trends in healthcare change, women are increasingly having surgical procedures and major operations within a shorter admission time. Women can be discharged in some cases 23h after a hysterectomy. This is leading to an increasing challenge for ward-based nurses and those within the community to ensure that there are the skills *in situ* to transfer the care. The ward staff need to ensure that they are able to impart all of the information that needs to be given to women within a much shorter time-frame, on the background of an increasing throughput of patients.

Day surgery unit (DSU)

Advancements in surgery and anaesthetics have now allowed a range of different types of gynaecological surgery to be safely performed as day cases.

The DSU allows patients to be admitted for surgery as a day case and, therefore, discharged the same day.

Types of surgery performed in DSU

- Evacuation of retained products of conception (ERPC).
- Hysteroscopy.
- Laparoscopy.
- Examination under anaesthetic.
- Sterilization.
- Biopsies.
- Colopscopy/LLETZ, knife cone biopsy.

Not all patients are suitable. Physical health and social circumstances are assessed in pre-assessment clinic.

Occasionally, patients are required to be admitted post-operatively to the ward from DSU. This may be due to the following reasons:

- pain;
- not passed urine;
- nausea and/or vomiting;
- drowsiness;
- not recovered in time;
- vital signs out of range;
- post-operative complications such as perforation of uterus.

In these cases when patients are admitted they are included on the wards admissions and LOS numbers.

Surgical admission lounge (SALS)

SALS is a pre-operative waiting area where patients are admitted on the day of their surgery.

Patients need to be physically fit to be waiting for surgery in a non-clinical area. This assessment will be carried out pre-operatively in the pre-assessment clinic.

Benefits of DSU and SALS

- Reduce LOS.
- Reduce anxiety.
- Reduce risk of hospital acquired infections.
- Reduces staff stress on the ward.
- More convenient for the patient and family.
- Saves money.

LOS

Where a patient stay is required, it is important to minimize the time the patients need to stay, without a shorter stay undermining patient safety or quality of care.

LOS is an important issue and has many benefits:

- Reduces risk of infection.
- Reduces cost.
- Reduces waiting lists.
- Home environment is vital to patients' continual recovery.
- Patients become more mobile.
- Reduces risk of DVT.

5 days is the expected LOS for a patient undergoing laparotomy hysterectomy. If LOS increases, costs are increased and these cases should be investigated to prevent recurrence.

Complex discharges should be addressed from admission and relevant referrals made to prevent extended LOS.

Useful referrals/pathways

- Social services.
- Occupational therapy.
- Palliative care.
- Physiotherapy.
- Delayed discharge team.
- District nurse.

Outpatient/office: ambulatory centres

The gynaecology outpatient department clinics and staffing can be variable—some hospitals have a complete multidisciplinary team, including consultants, nurse consultants, clinical nurse specialists, associate specialists, staff nurses, clerical, and administrative staff. Other hospitals may have smaller outpatient units with medical and nursing staff in small numbers. Staff are important to ensure that the patient has a seamless journey. Alongside general gynaecology, specialist clinics are held. Clinics require referrals from GPs, medical doctor, or practice nurse.

Clinics

Clinics can be set up in a variety of different ways, many have slots for routine and urgent, and patients referred under the 2-week wait system. Most consultants and specialist nurses will have a special interest but there may be a more general feel to clinics in smaller hospitals. In general, new appointments will be scheduled every 20 minutes and follow-ups 10 minutes, but this will vary with the type of clinic. Below are some examples of clinics and the types of women who will be seen in them.

Increasingly, the care of gynaecology patients is transferring into the outpatient setting, with many women never requiring an operation. Women may sometimes require care from more than one health professional, such as in the case of pelvic pain, where there may be a gynaecologist, pain specialist, psychologist, surgeons, and vulva specialists.

- General gynaecology.
- Rapid access clinic.
- Oncology clinics.
- Reproductive medicine.
- Uro-gynaecology.
- Colposcopy.
- Minor procedures/outpatient hysteroscopy.
- Menopause.
- Menstrual dysfunction.
- Laparoscopic sterilization.
- Specialist contraceptive.
- Pre-assessment clinic.
- Pelvic pain.

General gynaecology

Women are referred with general gynaecology problems, such as ovarian cysts, fibroids, menorrhagia, endometriosis, PCOS, or pelvic pain

Rapid access clinic

Referrals are made from GPs and colposcopy. Women present with PMB, PCB, abnormal smears, or a suspected pelvic mass. These women are seen by specialist gynaeoncology doctors and clinical nurse specialists. Ultrasound scans and hysteroscopy, colposcopy, or vulvosocpy can be performed at the same time.

Oncology clinics

Women referred with cancer or women having undergone cancer surgery may be seen in this clinic for immediate and regular follow-up.

Reproductive medicine

These clinics provide advice for women suffering with fertility problems. (📖 See Chapter 17, p.447.)

Minor procedure clinic

This is a one-stop clinic for consultation, diagnosis, and treatment. Indications for referral may include:

- Abnormal/heavy bleeding with or without abnormal scans.
- IMB, PCB, PMB.
- Irregular periods.
- Cervical polyps.
- Heavy/offensive discharge.
- Vaginal/vulval problems.
- IUD/IUS insertions and problems.

Ultrasounds scans, biopsies, hysteroscopy, vulvoscopy, and biopsy, swabs, cauterization of the cervix, cervical polypectomy, or gonadotrophin-releasing hormone (GnRH) injections are some procedures that can be performed in the minor procedure clinic.

Menopause clinic

Women present with menopausal problems, such as severe symptoms, early menopause, difficulty settling down on HRT, abnormal bleeding on HRT.

Uro-gynaecology

Women are referred with continence problems, such as urge and stress incontinence and prolapse (📖 see Chapter 10, p.247).

Colposcopy

Women are referred with abnormal smear tests or a suspicious cervix. (📖 See Chapter 18, p.489.)

Hysteroscopy: diagnostic and operative care

Hysteroscopy

Hysteroscopy allows visualization of the uterine cavity and intra-cavity surgery under direct vision. Using a vaginal approach, an instrument called a hysteroscope is inserted through the cervix. Nurses are expanding their clinical role and undergoing training (see Fig. 12.1).

For more information visit the BSGE website.

Equipment

To ensure that this is undertaken in a safe way, the correct equipment is needed, this includes: hysteroscopes, a method of sterilizng the equipment, camera, light source, insufflating medium, and printer.

- Flexible hysteroscopes—these consist of fibre optics within the main channel. At the distal end is the tip, which can be bent and can aid viewing the cornual areas. They can be associated with less pain, but are expensive, fragile, and difficult to sterilize.
- Rigid hysteroscopes—these have a range of vision from 0 to 30 degrees. Often a 30-degree hysteroscope is used for diagnostic purposes. The diameters vary from 1.2 to 4mm. They can either have a single or continuous flow irrigation in the outer sheath.

All scopes need a distension medium in order to be able to distend the uterus to see and to remove any debris. This can be either normal saline or CO_2, which are used for diagnostic purposes, or non-electrolyte fluids (glycine, sorbitol), which are used for hysteroscopic procedures that involve cutting, as they do not conduct electricity.

The key to ambulatory hysteroscopy is:

- Patient selection.
- Good nursing staff support for the patient and operator during the procedure.
- Good communication and rapport.
- Full description of the procedure.
- Willingness to stop the procedure at the woman's request.

The advantages of ambulatory hysteroscopy are:

- Greater accuracy.
- Faster access to diagnosis and treatment.
- Reduction in delays.
- Faster return to work.
- Increased patient satisfaction.

Nurses working within the hysteroscopy environment can be working in many ways—as chaperones and assistants, nurse practitioners taking histories, or as a fully trained practitioner after specialist training. This training can lead to a rewarding career development for nurses and ensures that hysteroscopy is delivered to an appropriate standard.

Indications for diagnostic/operative hysteroscopy

- Post-menopausal bleeding (PMB).
- Intra-menstrual bleeding (IMB).
- HmB diagnosis and ablation.
- Resection of small submucous fibroids.
- Endometrial polyps diagnosis and removal.
- Subfertility.
- Adhesiolysis—Asherman's syndrome.
- Suspected malignancy.
- Intra-uterine device problems.
- Abnormal scan findings.
- Persistent PCB with no cervical abnormality.
- Sterilization procedures such as Essure®.

Hysteroscopy is routinely carried out as an outpatient procedure. These procedures can be diagnostic or operative dependent on the findings.

However, indications for a GA hysteroscopy include:

- elderly patient;
- virgo intacta;
- cervical scarring and stenosis;
- has concurrent pelvic pain;
- requests general anaesthesia;
- has had a failed outpatient procedure.

In these cases, the women must be aware of the form of anaesthesia planned and given an opportunity to discuss in detail any concerns before the procedure. It is, therefore, necessary for these patients to attend a pre-assessment clinic.

Intended benefits

- Diagnostic hysteroscopy—to find cause of symptoms.
- Operative hysteroscopy—to treat the symptoms/condition.

Hysteroscopy: consent

Consent must be obtained from the patient. Risks and complications should be highlighted to the patient at this time. These include:

- Uterine perforation 8/1000. This is much lower in outpatient procedures.
- Vaso-vagal reflex—this is dependent on the size of the hysteroscope and the dilatation used.
- Cervical trauma—there should be little need to dilate in diagnostic procedures but may be needed in operative procedures.
- Bleeding and discharge—this can vary with either diagnostic or operative. With operative this can be up to 3 weeks.
- Pelvic infection—about 2/1000 women get an infection, acute PID is rare.
- Failure to visualize the uterine cavity.
- Pain.
- Adhesion formation.
- Fluid overload can occur with electrolyte free solutions during hysteroscopic surgery, so, extreme caution is needed.
- Late complications of surgery include thermal damage to bowel, post-operative haemorrhage secondary to haematoma formation.

It is important to explain that if any of the above risks arise, that further procedures may become necessary:

- Laparoscopy—in the event of perforation.
- Blood transfusion—in the event of excessive bleeding.

(a)

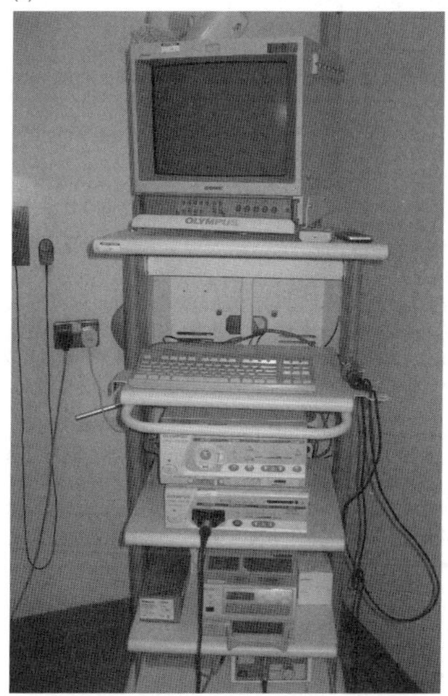

(b)

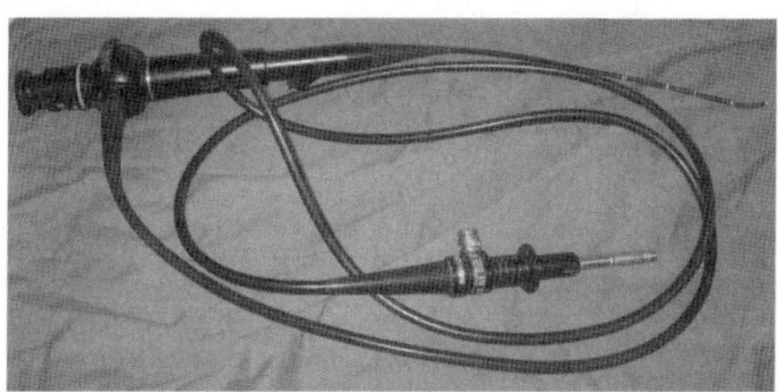

Fig. 12.1 Hysteroscopy equipment: (a) stack for hysteroscopy; (b) flexible hysteroscope.

Hysteroscopy: post-operative care

Recovery

Encourage the patient to mobilize when fully awake and vital signs are stable. If the patient is stable and vaginal bleeding is minimal, she can be discharged within 4–6 hours, except in complicated surgical hysteroscopic procedures carried out under GA.

Within outpatient hysteroscopy, women can be expected to go home as soon as they feel OK, normally within 20 minutes of the procedure.

Vaginal bleeding

If a biopsy is taken or polyps are removed or an outpatient endometrial ablation has been carried out, the patient may need to wear a sanitary towel to absorb any vaginal bleeding. Advise patient not to use tampons to reduce risk of infection. Bleeding can persist for up to 14 days, dependent on the procedure, and the patient should be informed of this.

Pain

This is usually mild period-type pain. Simple analgesia such as paracetamol should be prescribed, if required by the patient, unless allergies. The patient should be advised to report any sharp, continuous pain that is not relieved by analgesics (this may indicate perforation).

Infection

This may cause an unpleasant vaginal discharge or persistent bleeding. Infection is rare but should be treated with antibiotics.

Follow-up procedures

This depends on why the procedure was carried out, and what were the results on direct visualization and of the histology. Some patients may be following the gynaecology cancer pathway. Follow-up appointments should be made, as indicated and appropriate, following the procedure, to reduce anxiety for the patient.

Resources

For health professionals:

Cheong, Y and Ledger, W (2007) Hysteroscopy and hysteroscopic surgery. Obstetrics, Gynaecology and Reproductive Medicine **7**: 99-104.

www.NICE.org.uk

www.BSGE.org.uk

For women:

www.rcog.org.uk

Laparoscopy and laparoscopic surgery: pre- and post-operative care

Laparoscopy is a procedure to look inside the abdomen by using a laparoscope under a general anaesthetic or under conscious sedation. It is performed to diagnose the cause of symptoms such as abdominal pain or pelvic pain. It may also be performed as an operative procedure, e.g. if an X-ray or ultrasound scan has identified a problem within the abdomen or pelvis, such as ovarian cysts. It can be an elective or emergency procedure.

📖 See Table 12.1 for gynaecological indications.

Table 12.1 Gynaecological indications

Indication	Type of laparoscopy
Suspected endometriosis	Laparoscopy and ablation/diathermy
Acute pelvic pain	Laparoscopy and removal of ectopic/ tubo-ovarian mass
Chronic pelvic pain	Laparoscopy and division of adhesions
Ectopic pregnancy	Laparoscopy and salpingectomy/salpingostomy
Ovarian cyst	Laparoscopy ovarian cystectomy/oophorectomy
Unwanted fertility	Laparoscopic sterilization
Fertility problems	Assessment of the pelvis, tubal patency

Pre-operative care

Other treatment options should be considered before laparascopy. For example:

- GnRH analogues can be used in the treatment of endometriosis. GnRH analogues can alleviate symptoms, including pain, and reduce the size and number of endometrial lesions. They act by switching off the ovaries, thus reducing the oestrogen and progesterone levels, as in post-menopausal women. Ultrasound scans should be carried out pre-operatively to provide more information and help to diagnose the cause of her symptoms.
- Surgery is a unique experience for the patient. Psychosocial and physiological factors must be considered. Although a laparoscopy is considered a minor procedure, surgery is always a major experience for the patient and family. Gynaecological procedures, where fertility and womanhood are indicated, can be an emotional and difficult time for the patient. Informed consent must be taken, explaining the procedure, risks involved, and what it is likely to achieve.

Pre-operative checklist

- Medical history assessment.
- Allergy status.
- Medication.
- Bloods tests FBC, U+Es, G+S, cross-match.
- ECG (in some women).
- Chest X-ray (in some women).
- Ultrasound scan.
- Observations.
- Pregnancy test, if indicated.

Post-operative care

- Cardiovascular observations—blood pressure, pulse.
- Respiratory—oxygen saturations, respirations.
- Temperature (in case of post-operative infection).
- Pain—ensure adequate analgesia prescribed using analgesic ladder.
- Wound care—observe laparoscopy sites for bleeding.
- Observe vaginal bleeding.
- Micturition.
- Discharge advice.
- Discharge letter and any medication.
- Explanation of findings to the woman.
- Follow-up procedure/appointments.

Resources

For patients:

Patient information on laparoscopy and checklist for health professionals: www.rcog.org.uk

Major gynaecological surgery

Women undergo major gynaecological surgery for various reasons, depending on what symptoms they are experiencing.

There are various procedures performed in specific sub-specialties of gynaecology. These are:

- General gynaecology.
- Uro-gynaecology.
- Gynaecological oncology.
- Fertility.

General gynaecology

Myomectomy

Definition

A myomectomy is the removal of uterine fibroids. All other structures are left intact. This can be performed via a laparotomy, laparoscopy, or hysteroscopy, if it is sub-mucosal.

Symptoms

Fibroids are benign growths that form in the uterine wall (📖 see Fig. 7.1). They cause symptoms such as menorrhagia, dysmenorrhoea, pressure symptoms, and pain in pregnancy. (📖 See Chapter 7, p.126.)

There are three types of fibroids:

- **Serosal**—fibroids grow just under the outside surface of the uterus.
- **Intramural**—fibroids grow within the muscle wall of the uterus.
- **Submucous**—just under the inside surface of the uterus.
- **Pedunculated**—grown on a stalk.

Procedure

The procedure is performed under a general anaesthetic and the time taken will depend on the route, number, and size of the fibroids to be removed.

With all myomectomy operations, there is a risk of hysterectomy, if there is bleeding that cannot be stopped and all women must be warned of this prior to operation. The nursing care will depend on the route of the operation, but, most women will return to the ward area with a catheter and a drain and need careful monitoring and analgesia.

Hysterectomy

📖 See Abdominal, vaginal, and laparoscopic hysterectomy, p.352 and Chapter 11, p.293.

Laparotomy

Definition

A laparotomy is a surgical procedure to investigate or remove certain intra-abdominal structures. A laparotomy is referred to as a surgical procedure by itself. However, when a specific operation is already planned, a laparotomy is considered the first step of the procedure, e.g. laparotomy may proceed to TAH BSO.

A laparotomy is performed in general gynaecology for conditions such as ovarian cysts and adhesions.

Occasionally, a mini laparotomy is required in emergency operations such as ectopic pregnancy and ruptured ovarian cysts.

Uro-gynaecology

📖 See Chapter 10, p.247.

Gynaecology oncology

📖 See Chapter 11, p.293.

Nursing care after gynaecological operations

This is specialized and each patient should receive individualized care that relates to the exact operation and follows any post-operation instructions from both the surgeon and the anaesthetists.

General care will ensure the patient is supported in activities of living, while she is recovering, until she is able to return to self-care.

- Monitoring of observations.
- Maintaining fluid balance via an intravenous infusion.
- Introduction of fluids and diet.
- Pain control.
- Hygiene.
- Care of wounds, drains, dressing, sutures.
- Care of catheter, bladder and bowels.
- Advice, support and information.
- Liaison with family.

Abdominal, vaginal, and laparoscopic hysterectomy: types and indications

What is a hysterectomy

A hysterectomy is a major surgical procedure to remove the uterus. It is used as a treatment for a variety of reproductive tract conditions. These may include:

- Gynaecological cancers.
- Menorrhagia not responsive to treatment.
- Dysmenorrhoea.
- Chronic abdominal pain—caused by endometriosis, pelvic adhesions, fibroids.
- Utero-vaginal prolapse.

With the exception of cancers, hysterectomy may be indicated if none of the initial treatments for these conditions have been successful.

Risks involved

- Bleeding.
- Chest, urine, and wound infection.
- Blood clots (DVT/PE).
- Pain.
- Making a slow recovery.
- Problems caused by having a general anaesthetic.
- Impact on body image and sexuality.

Types of hysterectomy

There are different types of hysterectomy depending on the patient's gynaecological problem. 📖 Table 12.2 and Fig. 12.2 show the different types of hysterectomy performed and why.

Table 12.2 Types of hysterectomy and indications

Type of hysterectomy	What is removed	What is left behind
Subtotal hysterectomy	Uterus	Fallopian tubes, ovaries, vagina
Total hysterectomy	Uterus, cervix	Fallopian tubes, ovaries, vagina
Total hysterectomy with bilateral salpingoophorectomy	Uterus, cervix, ovaries, and fallopian tube	Vagina
Radical hysterectomy	Uterus, cervix, top part of vagina, fallopian tubes, ovaries, supporting tissues, and lymph nodes	Vagina
Radical hysterectomy and conservation of the ovaries	Uterus, cervix, top part of the vagina, fallopian tubes, supporting tissues, and lymph nodes	Ovaries
Vaginal hysterectomy	Uterus, cervix	Ovaries, fallopian tubes
Laparoscopic assisted vaginal hysterectomy	Uterus, tubes, ovaries	
Laparoscopic subtotal hysterectomy	Uterus	Cervix, fallopian tubes, ovaries, and vagina
Laparoscopic assisted robotic hysterectomy	Uterus	

Hysterectomy: post-operative care

Depends on the type of hysterectomy performed. The following provides a guideline of expectations.

Vaginal hysterectomy

Patients usually return to the ward from recovery after 2–3h. They will have:

- Catheter.
- Intravenous fluids.
- PCA or epidural.

Laparotomy/hysterectomy

Patients usually return to the ward from recovery after 2–3h. They will have:

- Catheter.
- Redivac drain.
- Intravenous fluids.
- PCA or epidural.
- Oxygen.
- Naso gastric tube (sometimes).
- NBM.

Laparoscopic assisted hysterectomy

- Catheter.
- +/– redivac drain.
- Intravenous fluid.
- Patient controlled analgesia (PCA) or spinal anaesthesia.

Length of stay (LOS)

📖 See Table 12.3 for LOS.

Table 12.3 LOS

Type of hysterectomy	Length of stay (LOS)
Vaginal hysterectomy	3 days
Laparoscopic hysterectomy	3 days
Laparotomy total hysterectomy	5 days

*With the exception of radical hysterectomy as these patients usually have a catheter for 5 days, so LOS may be a day longer.

Post-operative recovery

- All patients should be mobilized out of bed from day 1.
- Proceed onto oral analgesia when eating and drinking.
- Remove attachments as soon as appropriate to reduce risk of infection and encourage mobilization.
- Seen by physiotherapist to be taught pelvic floor exercises before discharge.

The normal recovery time is 6 weeks, although this will depend on the patient. Recovery time may take longer for the patients with a malignancy or co-morbidities.

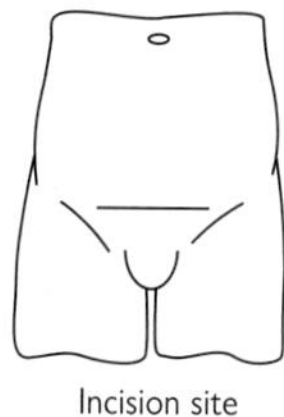

Incision site

Total hysterectomy

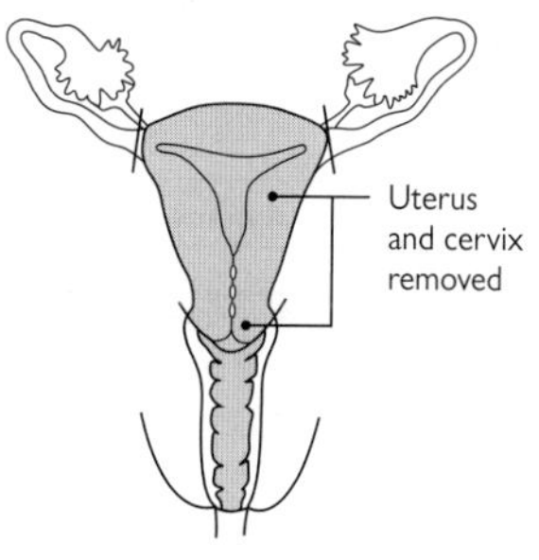

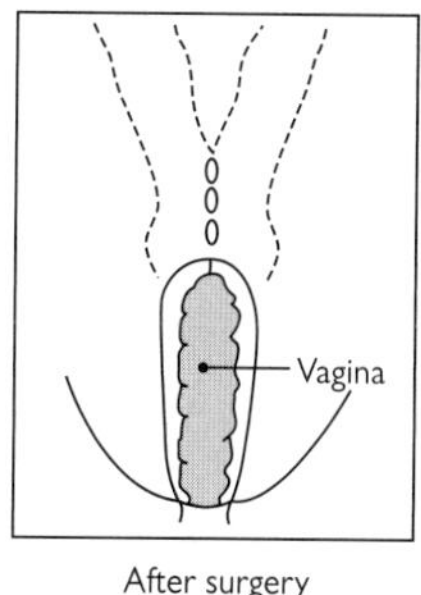

After surgery

Subtotal hysterectomy

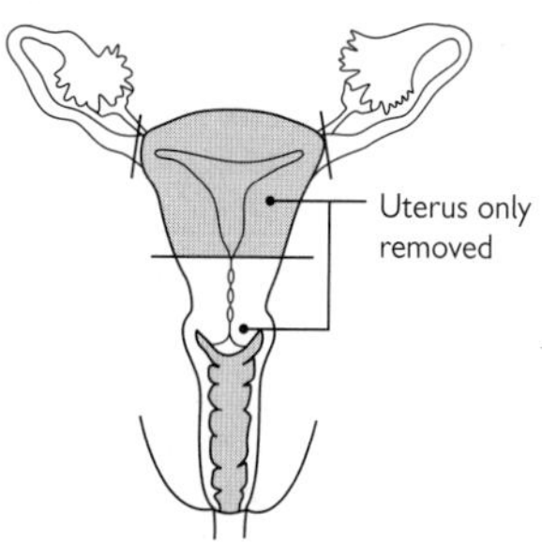

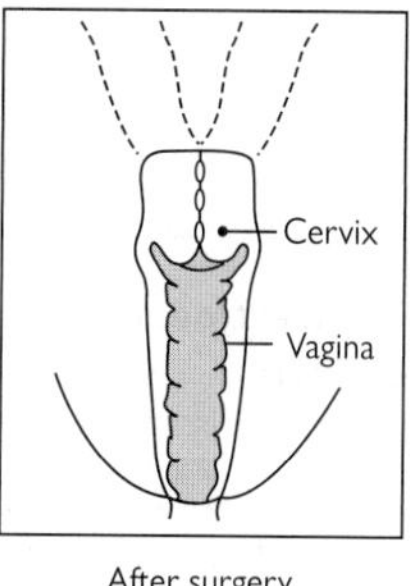

After surgery

Fig. 12.2 Types of hysterectomy. Reprinted with permission from Patient Pictures: Gynaecology, © 1996. Oxford: Health Press Limited.

Uro-gynaecological surgery

Uro-gynaecological surgery specializes in treatment of women with pelvic floor disorders. These include:

- Urinary incontinence.
- Prolapse.

These symptoms affect the quality of life for the women suffering. It can cause embarrassment, anxiety, and limit a woman's daily activities.

This section focuses on the surgical treatment for these conditions and how the procedures are performed. Generalized nursing care for operations is in the section on hysterectomy.

Types of prolapse

A prolapse occurs when the pelvic floor muscles (and other supportive ligaments) weaken or stretch. When this happens one or more of the organs within the pelvis lose their support and drop down. (📖 See Chapter 10, p.247.) 📖 Also see Table 12.4.

Table 12.4

Types of prolapse	Causes	Symptoms
Cystocele	Occurs when the bladder slips down.	Urinary incontinence. Difficulty emptying bladder.
Rectocele	Occurs when the rectum slips down.	Difficulty in emptying bowels. Causes or worsens constipation. Lower back pain.
Uterine prolapse	Occurs when the womb drops into the vagina.	Depending on severity, the womb may be felt or seen in the vagina.
Vault prolapse	Occurs when the superior vaginal support mechanism is disrupted at the time of abdominal or vaginal hysterectomy.	

Surgical treatment

Anterior repair

The anterior repair is a procedure traditionally used for moderate or severe stress urinary incontinence. A cut is made through the lining of the front (anterior) wall of the vagina. The supports to the bladder are shortened with stitches and the bulging part of the vagina cut away. This repairs the weakness. The wound in the vagina is then stitched.

Posterior repair

A small cut is made through the lining of the back (posterior) part of the vagina. The supports to the rectum are shortened with stitches and the bulging part of the vagina cut away. This repairs the weakness. The wound in the vagina is then stitched together.

Vaginal hysterectomy

A vaginal hysterectomy may be performed alongside surgery to repair a prolapse. The uterus and cervix are removed through the vagina rather than through an abdominal incision. The bladder and rectum are restored to their normal positions. Ovaries are left intact.
(📖 See Abdominal, vaginal, and laparoscopic hysterectomy: types and indications for care, p.352.)

Abdominal sacrocolpopexy or vaginal sacrospinous fixation for vault prolapse

In sacrocolpopexy, the reconstructed vaginal tube is attached to the anterior longitudinal ligament of the sacral promontory using a mesh. Can be done as an open abdominal or laparoscopic procedure.

Tension-free vaginal tape

A piece of mesh is inserted through a small cut in the front wall of the vagina. It is then passed under the middle of the urethra to support it. The mesh is secured through two small cuts in the abdominal wall or through two small cuts on the inner thigh. A cystoscope (small camera) is inserted in the bladder to check for any bladder injury during the procedure. A catheter is inserted into the bladder and is left in until the next day. This can be performed under a spinal or a general anaesthetic.

Transobturator approach for insertion of a sub-urethral tape can be an outside-in (TOT) or an inside-out (TVT-O) procedure. Cystoscopy should be performed after completion of both procedures, as bladder injuries have been reported.

Colposuspension

The operation is performed through a cut in the lower part of the abdomen. Stitches are inserted alongside the bladder closure mechanism to support it and make it stronger. Following the operation, the catheter should be on free drainage for 72h. On the third day, the catheter should be clamped to allow the patient to pass urine normally. This must be measured each time and documented.

⚠The patient should only be allowed to drink 2l/day.

Chapter 13

Contraception

Principles of contraception

The 10 Cs

- ***Control*** of fertility during different stages of female and male reproductive lives preventing an unwanted pregnancy.
- ***Consideration*** and assisting in reducing world population.
- ***Counselling*** about the risks, side-effects, and circumstances when suitable contraceptive technology can provide added health benefits.
- ***Comfortable*** and acceptable to individuals and their culture and faith.
- ***Convenience*** to suit female and male lifestyles.
- ***Confidentiality*** and respect with young women less than 16 years.
- ***Compliance*** of the 13 methods available.
- ***Clinical*** judgement for medical eligibility.
- ***Condoms*** to prevent STIs/HIV.

Measures of effectiveness

- Efficacy is defined as being the inherent protection the method offers in perfect use cycles only.[1]
- Effectiveness is based on clinical studies and presented as a failure rate, which is given as the % of women who might experience an unintended pregnancy in a year (assuming 13 menstrual cycles per year). This includes data on all usage, which includes instances where compliance may not be perfect.
- The risk of conceiving from a single unprotected intercourse anytime in the cycle is 1 in 24.

Choice: factors to be considered

- Availability of method, suiting the individual, with appropriate effectiveness.
- Lifestyle and life-stage, planning pregnancy/spacing a family.
- Effects on sexual activity.
- Long-acting reversible contraception associated with fewer adverse effects.
- Possible additional health benefits.
- If a method fails, access to termination of pregnancy (TOP) or feasibility of continuing with the pregnancy.
- Return to fertility once method stopped.
- Never wanting to conceive.

Community access to contraception

- Free from contraceptive clinics (UK). Many are walk-in.
- Requires a prescription from a GP/doctor.
- Over the counter (OTC) for emergency contraception, barrier methods, fertility devices.
- Small provision by private sector.
- Information through: internet, telephone advisory services, texting.
- Convenience, suitability, accessibility of venue.
- Provider's role.
- Privacy and confidentiality, especially for the young.

1. Stenier, M, Dominik, R ,Trussell, J and Herzs-Piccioto, I (1996) Measuring contraceptive effectiveness: a conceptual framework. *Obstetrics Gynecology* **88:** 24S–30S.

Risk/benefit analysis of contraception

Health professionals are required to discuss the risks and non-contraceptive benefits for men, women, and couples, when deciding on the appropriate contraception.

Most people are healthy and able to decide on a method of their choice. Some methods have minor side-effects, rarely life-threatening.

Couples counselled may choose a highly effective method with accepted risks, whilst others want one with lower efficacy but no risks.

Decisions about risks and benefits are not technical but value decisions. Certain conditions are associated with increased health risks when a particular method is used.

Using expert opinion and evidence-based systematic reviews, the WHO (2008) made recommendations categorizing medical eligibility criteria (MEC).

Medical eligibility criteria categories

1—No restriction on use.
2—Benefits outweigh risks.
3—Risks outweigh benefits.
4—Unacceptable risk.

Concommittant diseases such as diabetes and epilepsy should be considered when prescribing contraceptives.

Absolute risk

This is the number of individuals in a group who will experience a discrete event: e.g. of 100,000 women on gestodene/desogestrel combined oral contraception pill (COCP), 30 will develop VTE per year (30 per 100,000 woman-years). This should be distinguished from relative risk, and care taken when quoting especially percentages (particularly with regard to change).

Women are far more likely to die from pregnancy-related complications, from automobile accidents or from a fall than they are from using hormonal contraception or having undergone either a medical or surgical abortion.

Factors to consider in counselling

- Different developmental stages of reproductive life.
- Educational and literacy levels.
- Culture and religion.
- Tendencies to misunderstand risk (optimism–pessimism bias).
- Chronic disease.
- Risk factors: obesity, smoking, alcohol.
- Influence of media—unfortunately, the media often give a poor representation of risks, leading to failed compliance, avoidance of a method, and unwanted pregnancies occurring.

Contraception not only protects against unwanted pregnancy, but may have additional health benefits. The 'benefit' side of the risk/benefit analysis should include non-contraceptive benefits and 'added value' aspects such as anti-androgenic pills improving acne or Mirena® IUS treating menorrhagia. While *women* often take the major responsibility, the wishes and needs of male partners must be considered, if contraception is to be used effectively. Many *women* are tending to delay childbearing and having fewer children; therefore, the need for safe and effective reversible methods are required for most *women* during their reproductive lives.

Resources

James T and Jordan B (2006) Reproductive health risks in perspective. *Contraception* **73:** 437–439.

Principles of contraception: eligibility

Medical eligibility

The provision of contraception is guided by recommendations from World Health Health Organization Medical Eligibility Criteria.[1] Healthcare professionals have a responsibility for ensuring both male and female medical suitability for all available methods, and assessing the safety for individuals.

The information required to make an informed choice include: efficacy, risks, side-effects, advantages and disadvantages, and non-contraceptive benefits based on evidence.

📖 See Box 13.1.

Practice in UK has been adapted from the above, and produced by a consensus process, the UKMEC.[2]

Definitions for UK categories for barrier methods, intra-uterine devices, and hormonal contraception

Box 13.1 MEC categories

- UK 1: A condition for which there is no restriction in the use of the contraceptive method.
- UK 2: A condition where the advantages of using the method generally outweigh the theoretical or proven risks; follow-up may be required.
- UK 3: A condition where the theoretical or proven risks usually outweigh the advantages of using the method: Expert clinical judgement/ referral to a specialist provider required.
- UK 4: A condition which represents an unacceptable health risk if the contraceptive is used.

Categories relating to fertility awareness based methods (FAB)

- UK A: Accept there is no medical reason to deny the particular FAB methods to women in these circumstances.
- UK C: Caution that the method is normally provided in routine setting, but with extra preparation and precautions. For FAB methods, this usually means that special counselling may be needed to ensure correct use of this method by women in these circumstances.
- UK D: Delay use of this method until the condition is evaluated or changes (e.g. breastfeeding stops). Alternative temporary methods of contraception should be offered.

Categories relating to male and female sterilization

In addition to the three categories above, a fourth category also applies: non-reversible methods of contraception.

- UK S: Special. The procedure should be undertaken in a setting with experienced surgeon and staff, equipment to provide general anaesthesia, and other backup medical support. For these conditions, the information to decide on the most appropriate temporary methods of contraception should be provided, if referral is required or there is otherwise any delay.

Terms in UK MEC different from or additional to the WHO document: additional items (📖 see p.364)

- Inflammatory bowel disease (IBD) is considered UK 2 for COCP, POP, and 1 for other progestogen-only contraceptives.
- Subheadings given for existing conditions:
  - BMI 30–34 UK 2 for COCP, UK 1 for all other methods.
  - BMI 35–39 UK 3 for COCP, UK 1 for all other methods.
  - BMI >40 UK 4 for COCP, UK 1 for all other methods.
- Family history of VTE in first-degree relatives aged <45 years UK 3 for COCP and UK 1 for all other methods.
- Immobility unrelated to surgery UK 3 for COCP and UK 1 for all other methods.
- Long past-history of migraine with aura UK 3 for COCP; UK 2 for POP, DMPA, implant, IUS and UK 1 for IUD.
- Carriers of known gene mutations associated with breast cancer risk (e.g. BRAC1) UK 3 for COCP; UK 2 for POP, DMPA, implant, IUS and UK 1 for IUD.

The specific changes different from WHO categories in the UKMEC

- Women who are partially breastfeeding (between 6 weeks and 6 months post-partum) UK 2 for COCP.
- Hypertension UK 1 for POP.
- Current VTE UK 2 for POP; UK 3 for DMPA, implant, IUD, IUS and UK 4 for COCP.
- Nulliparity and intra-uterine methods is UK MEC 1.

1 WHO (2004) *Medical eligibility criteria for contraceptive use* (3rd edn). Geneva: Reproductive Health and Research. World Health Organization.

2 *UK Medical Eligibility Criteria for Contraception Use*. Faculty of Family Planning and Reproductive Healthcare and Royal College of Obstetricians and Gynaecologists July 2006 (to be reviewed 2009).

Emergency contraception (EC)

This may be required following:

- Unprotected consensual sexual intercourse.
- Sexual assault or rape.
- A barrier method failure.
- Missed COCP or POP, incorrect use of patch or vaginal ring.
- Partial or complete expulsion or mid-cyle removal of IUD/IUS if unprotected sexual intercourse occurred in last 5 days.
- Late injectable contraceptives.
    - >14 weeks for medroxyprogesterone acetate.
    - >10 weeks for norethisterone enantate.
- Interactions of liver-enzyme inducers including St John's Wort, advised to have an IUD EC (copper).
- Post-partum LNG EC from 21 days if breastfeeding.
- Post-partum IUD from 28 days.

In some clinics, demand for emergency contraception may be seasonal (post holidays or 'celebrations').

Methods

- Oral hormonal method using levonorgestrel (LNG EC).
- Copper intra-uterine device (EC IUD).

Mode of action

- ***LNG EC:*** interferes with ovulation and fertilization, and, rarely, also implantation, depending when taken during the menstrual cycle.
- ***EC IUD:*** evidence indicates that IUDs act primarily by impairing gamete viability before fertilization.

Effectiveness

LNG EC

1.5mg single dose: The sooner taken after sexual intercourse the better the efficacy. Within 72h (3 days).

- 0–24h up to 95% pregnancies prevented.
- 25–48h up to 85% pregnancies prevented.
- 49–72h up to 58% pregnancies prevented.

LNG EC can be taken more than once in a cycle, if clinically indicated.

IUD

With over 300mm^2 and ideally 380mm^2 of copper is optimal, as can be inserted up to 120h (5 days) after the first episode of unprotected sexual intercourse (UPSI) or, if necessary, up to 5 days after the earliest expected date of ovulation (day 19 in a regular 28-day cycle). It has over 99% efficacy and can be used as an ongoing method of contraception.

Verbal information of failure rates and FPA leaflets on other methods of contraception increase compliance.

History

- Sexual history to assess date of LMP.
- Day of the cycle at presentation.
- Date and time of exposure to sexual intercourse.
- Indication for EC.
- Any other risk in the cycle.
- Possibility of malabsorption (e.g. small bowel resection).
- Liver-enzyme inducers (St John's Wort/drugs).
- Risk of STIs.

Management

- Advise to take LNG EC after food. Should vomiting occur within 2h, repeat dose or offer EC IUD.
- Disturbance of menstrual cycle possible; if next period >1/52 late, PT advised.
- Counselling re normal contraception or abstinence until next period, and future method(s).
- Discuss risks before insertion of IUD. In at risk population (age <25 years, change in sexual partner, more than two in last year) should be offered testing for Chlamydia trachomatis and gonorrhoea, contact tracing and prophylactic antibiotics.
- Ectopic pregnancy risk—similar risk as in IUD users.
- Offer follow-up 3–6 weeks for IUD (removal can be any time after next period, providing no UPSI). 3/52 for LNG EC.
- For girls under 16 years, Fraser criteria must be applied.

Hormonal EC supplied free from

- GP.
- Contraceptive clinics.
- Young person's clinic.
- Brook Advisory centres.
- Sexual health or some GUM clinics.
- NHS walk-in centres and some minor injuries centres.

Can buy over the counter from most chemists, private clinics (Marie Stopes or British Pregnancy Advisory Services), and on the internet.

Resources

National Institute for Health and Clinical Excellence (NICE) (2005) *Long-acting reversible contraception: the effective and appropriate use of long-acting reversible contraception.* RCOG Press, London, UK.

Combined oral contraceptive pill (COCP)

Formulations

Contains synthetic oestrogen (ethinylestradiol) and various progestogens. Natural oestrogen formulations are likely to become available in the UK soon.

Mode of action

Suppresses ovulation, thickens cervical mucus, alters endometrium so that sperm transportation is impaired.

Preparations

- 21 days for monophasic same dose daily, then 7 days hormone-free period.
- Everyday (ED) combined (monophasic) + 7 inactive placebos.
- 21 days biphasic and triphasic preparations variable oestrogen and progestogens doses, 7 days hormone-free.

Oestrogen

20, 30, or 35, or 40μg of ethinylestradiol (EE).

Progestogens

- norethisterone (NET).
- levonorgestrel (LNG).
- norgestimate.
- gestodene (GSD).
- desogestrel (DSG).

recent developments

- drospirenone.

Lower strength

- 20μg EE + NET acetate 1mg.
- 20μg EE + DSG 150μg.
- 20μg EE + GSD 75μg.
- 20μg EE + drospirenone 3mg

Standard strength

- 35μg EE + NET 500μg.
- 35μg EE + NET 1mg.
- 30μg EE + NET acetate 1.5mg.
- 35μg EE (biphasic) + NET 500μg/1mg.
- 35μg EE (triphasic) + NET 500μg/1mg/500μg.
- 35μg EE (triphasic) + NET 500μg/750μg/1mg.
- 30μg EE + LNG 150μg.
- 30μg/40μg/30μg EE (triphasic) + LNG 50μg/75μg/125μg.
- 35μg EE + norgestimate 250μg.
- 30μg EE + GSD 75μg.
- 30μg/40μg/30μg/ EE (triphasic) +GSD 50μg/70μg/100μg.
- 30μg EE + DSG 150μg.
- 30ug EE + drospirenone 3mg.
- 50μg mestranol + NET 1mg.

Starting COCP

- Day 1 of period immediate efficacy.
- Days 2–5 of period also use condoms 7 days—new guidance does not mandate this and can be started up to 7 days.
- Same day as a miscarriage/TOP immediate efficacy.
- Day 21 post-partum, if not breastfeeding.
- Instant switch to lower dose COCP.
- Switch to higher dose COCP after 7 days hormone-free.
- Day 1 period if changing to POP.

Quick starting

Any method of contraception can be started any time in the cycle, provided two conditions are satisfied:

- Clinician must exclude pregnancy.
- Patient advised to use backup contraception for 7 days.

Practical usage

⚠ Stop immediately if sudden chest pain, severe or prolonged headaches, calf pain + swelling, severe stomach pain, first fit or collapse, sudden neurological deficit, breathlessness, haemoptysis, BP>140/90mmHg with repeated reading, acute jaundice.

- Starters: low oestrogen normally 30μg LNG monophasic pills.
- Breakthrough bleeding: exclude problems. Increase progestogen content or change to a potent progestogen.
- If oestrogen excess side-effects such as weight ↑, nausea, bloating, breast engorgement, increased vaginal discharge. Exclude infection, then increase progestogen, use more potent progestogen or reduce oestrogen.
- In progestogen excess (moody, PMS, dry vagina, breast pain, reduced libido, acne, hirsutism) increase oestrogen or reduce progestogen.

Combined oral contraceptive pill (COCP): risks, benefits, and side-effects

Risks

Careful assessment/case history required to exclude absolute and relative contraindications. (📖 See Box 13.1, MEC category 3 and 4.)

The potential risks:

- Venous thrombosis (VTE/PE).
- Rare stroke ↑ with age and MI (smoking is an important risk factor).
- Migraine with aura and migraine in age >35 increase the risk.
- Hypertension.
- Small risk of breast cancer: an association with early detection and is reduced to no increased risk 10 years after stopping the pill.
- A small increase in cervical cancer risk with use > 5 years. Further duration of use effect is seen for longer use.
- Rare benign hepatic adenoma.

Benefits

- Protects against unwanted pregnancy.
- 12% decrease in the risk of developing cancer overall.[1]
- ↓ ovarian, endometrial, colorectal cancer (50%, 50%, and 30%).
- Improves acne vulgaris.
- ↓ rheumatoid arthritis, though data for this is rather weak.
- ↓ in PID.
- ↓ in ovarian cysts.
- ↓ in dysmenorrhoea, menorrhagia and PMS.
- Improves cyclical breast pain.

Side-effects

- Headaches, migraine, and dizziness.
- Breast tenderness.
- Nausea and vomiting.
- Breakthrough bleeding.
- Weight gain and fluid retention.
- Mood changes.
- Loss of libido.
- Greasy skin.

Most occur within 3–6 months of commencing the pill and disappear. If not, a change of pill may be required.

1. Hannaford, P, Selvarja, S, Elliot, A, Angus, V, Iversen, L and Lee, A (2007) Cancer risk among user of oral contraceptives: cohort data from the Royal College of General Practitioner's oral contraceptive study. *British Medical Journal* (September) **335:** 621–622.

Absolute contraindications of the COCP

- Past or present circulatory disease.
    - Multiple risk factors for cardiovascular disease.
    - Ischaemic heart disease or angina, VTE.
    - Known thrombogenic abnormality of coagulation/fibrinolysis.
- Hypertension, stroke.
- Other conditions predisposing to thrombosis:
    - before and after major elective surgery;
    - immobilization after trauma, varicose vein treatments;
    - Raynaud's disease with lupus anticoagulant.
- Cardiomyopathies.
- Transient ischaemic attacks even without headache.
- Congenital and valvular heart disease complicated by pulmonary hypertension, atrial fibrillation, sub acute bacterial endocarditis (SABE).
- Otosclerosis.
- Trophoblastic disease with raised hCG.
- Current breast cancer.
- Migraine headaches with aura at any age.
- Smoking above age 35.
- Obesity (BMI >40).
- Breastfeeding under 6 weeks post-partum.
- Long-standing diabetes mellitus.
- Diseases of the liver: active liver disease, recurrent cholestatic jaundice or a history of cholestatic jaundice in pregnancy, Dubin–Johnson and Rotor syndromes, liver adenoma, cirrhosis, gallstones (but not after cholecystectomy) and some porphyrias.

Combined oral contraceptive pill (COCP): missed pills

The possibility of pregnancy when pills are missed depends on how many and where in the packet.

- Missed <24h take missed pill ASAP, and then take next pill at the normal time and continue pill taking.
- If missed any of the last seven pills of the packet, omit the pill-free interval and start the next packet without a break.
- Efficacy is reduced when pills are missed at the beginning or end of the packet, extending the hormone free interval.

Using EC when COCP missed

- Consider the need for EC (see Table 13.1).

Table 13.1 EC guidance for missed COCP

Where pills missed	Need for EC if unprotected intercourse
First 7 pills	Yes, if 3 or more 30–35μg EE pills are missed. Yes, if 2 or more 20μg EE pills are missed.
8–21 pills	Yes, if 4 or more missed regardless of dose.
15–21 pills	No need for EC if PFI omitted (starting next packet without a break).

- Use condoms or abstinence 7 days.
- Discard the pills for the days that EC was taken and restart the pill next day.
- Resume pill-taking at normal time, but not more than 12h after EC.
- Some authorities recommend the 2 missed pill trigger for all types of pills.

Combined hormonal contraception: transdermal 'patch' (Evra®)

Definition

Beige 20cm^2 matrix patch delivers an average of 33.9μg ethinyloestradiol and 203μg norelgestromin over 24h (manufacturer's SPC) into the systemic circulation, producing changes similar to the COCP (📖 see Combined oral contraceptive pill, p.368).

Mode of action

Similar to the combined hormonal contractive pill (📖 see Combined oral contraceptive pill, p.368).

Medical eligibility

As for COCP (📖 see p.364).

Effectiveness

>99% similar to COCP and similar menstrual cycle control.

Advantages

- Simplicity in use.
- Convenient compared to COCP with similar safety.
- May reduce menstrual problems.
- Change weekly, which increases compliance.
- Still effective should diarrhoea and vomiting occur.
- No interference with lifestyle.

Disavantages

- Visible.
- Cosmetics, oils, creams, etc., should not be applied near the patch.
- Can cause skin irritation.
- No protection against STI/HIV.
- Breakthrough bleeding, nausea, breast tenderness, headaches common in first 3 months of use.
- Less effective when weight 90kg and over.

Starting regime

As for the COCP but:

- If >48h after normal start day, apply new patch and additional precautions for next 7 days.
- Consider adopting 'patch change day', e.g. Sunday, to increase compliance.
- Apply same day weekly for 3 weeks then 7 days patch-free.
- Recommended areas: upper outer arm, torso, or buttocks, but not breasts.

Combined hormonal contraception: intra vaginal ring (NuvaRing®)

Definition

A flexible, transparent, soft plastic ring, which releases 15μg ethinylestradiol and 120μg etonogestrel into the vagina daily (📖 see Fig. 13.1). Outer diameter 5.4cm and 4mm thick. The ring is *in situ* for 21 days and removed for 7 days when a withdrawal bleed occurs.

Mode of action

Similar to the combined hormonal contractive pill.

Efficacy

- When applied consistently, 99% effectiveness.
- If the ring is removed, accidentally expelled, or left outside the vagina for more than 3h, a barrier method must be used for 7 days.
- The exact position *in situ* is not critical for its action. The ring has adequate hormone content to be effective for 4 weeks.

Advantages

- Self-administered once a month.
- Easy to insert.
- Less nausea and breast tenderness than COCP.
- Less risk of weight gain.
- Improved cycle control with long-term compliance.

Disadvantages

- Psychological aversion or inability to touch the genital area.
- Not suitable where no running water available.
- Increased risk of vaginal discharge
- Health professional required to instruct use.
- Does not protect against STI/HIV.

Contraindiactions

As for COCP (📖 see p.368).

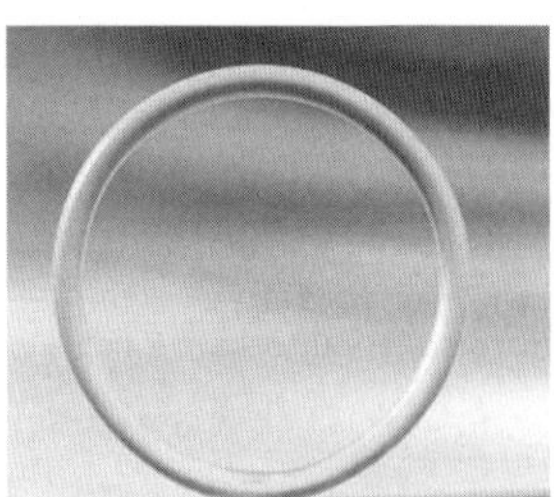
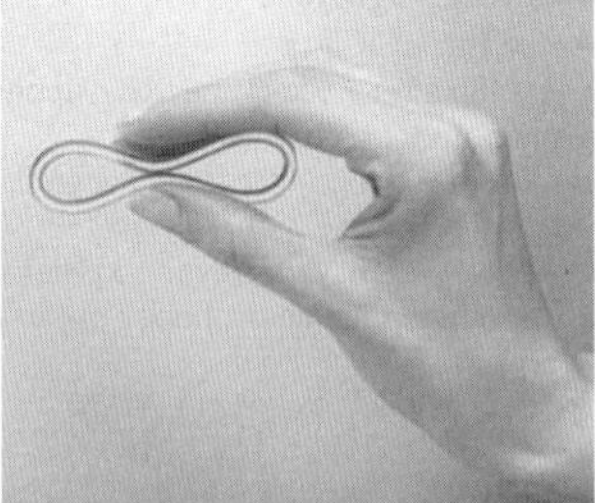

Fig. 13.1 NuvaRing®. Reproduced with permission of Schering-Plough.

Progestogen-only pill (POP)

POP or 'mini-pill'.

Definition

The POP is a small dose of progestogen taken daily. Cerazette® is a desogestrel pill with a mode of action similar to the COCP.

Indications

An alternative method to COCP, when oestrogens are contraindicated.

Mode of action

- Inhibits ovulation (Cerazette® only).
- Thickens cervical mucous, thus hampering the penetration of sperm.
- Suppression of luteal activity and follicular growth (traditional POPs).
- Some endometrial modification preventing implantation.

Efficacy

- 98–99% when taken correctly.
- Higher in breastfeeding mothers and women over 35 years.
- Lower efficacy in teenagers.

Contraindications

- Pregnancy.
- Undiagnosed vaginal bleeding.
- Severe arterial or cardiac disease.
- Functional ovarian cysts (relative).
- Active liver disease.
- Post-hydatidiform mole (until normal gonadotrophin values)—applies to combined hormonal contraception.
- Porphyria—applies to combined hormonal contraception.
- Breast cancer, current or within last 5 years—applies to combined hormonal contraception.
- Drugs that affect liver enzymes.

Advantages

- Unrelated to sexual intercourse.
- No medication cycle to remember, as taking 1 pill a day all the time.
- Can be started immediately following early medical or surgical TOP.
- No adverse effect on breastfeeding.
- Alternative for smokers over 35 years.
- No effect on efficacy if taking broad-spectrum antibiotics.
- Sickle cell disease unaffected.
- Hypertension unaffected.
- Allowed in migraine.
- Can be continued up to major surgery.

Disadvantages

- Loses effectiveness with severe diarrhoea or vomiting.
- Not suitable for the young with poor compliance.
- Menstrual irregularities.

Forgotten pills

- If a pill is missed or delayed >3h (12h for Cerazette®) extra precautions for 48h.

Progestogen-only subdermal implant (Implanon®)

This is a long-acting, slow-releasing progestogen implant. Counselling is needed prior to insertion and a trained health professional is required to insert and remove.

Mode of action

Inhibits ovulation and increases viscosity of cervical mucous, inhibiting sperm penetration.

Delivery mechanism

A non-biodegradable flexible single rod (40cm long and 2mm diameter) that contains 68mg etonogestrel, inserted in the subdermal plane on the inner aspect of the upper arm, 8–10cm from the medial epicondyle. 📖 See Fig. 13.2.

Effectiveness

>99%, lasting 3 years.

Indications

- For unreliable or problematic pill takers.
- Erratic lifestyles or travellers.
- Oestrogen contraindications.
- Reduces dysmenorrhoea and possibly PMS.
- Spacing children.

Advantages

- Independent of sexual intercourse.
- No user failure/misuse.
- Rapidly reversible (by removal of implant).
- No relevant effects on lipids.
- A long-acting reversible 'fit and forget' method.

Disadvantages

- Changes in menstrual pattern: prolonged or frequent bleeding, infrequent bleeding and/or amenorrhoea.
- Does not protect against STI/HIV.
- Irregular bleeding is the commonest cause for removal.

Contraindications

- Current VTE (on anticoagulants), or history of cerebrovascular accident (CVA).
- Undiagnosed vaginal bleeding.
- Known or suspected pregnancy.
- Breast cancer: current disease or within last 5 years.
- Current hepatic disease with abnormal liver function.
- Liver enzyme inducing drugs.
- Hypersensitivity to any components of the implant.

Common side-effects, mostly transient

- Acne.
- Breast tenderness.
- Headaches.
- Mood swings.

Nurse training Implanon® fitting/removal

- Must hold a valid family planning training certificate.
- Competent in administration of local anaesthetics.
- A nurse-independent prescriber qualification or training in use of Patient Group Directions.
- Attend theory training on implants.
- Take model arm training followed by live patient training.
- Two or more supervised fittings and removals under an instructing doctor.
- Recertification every 5 years.

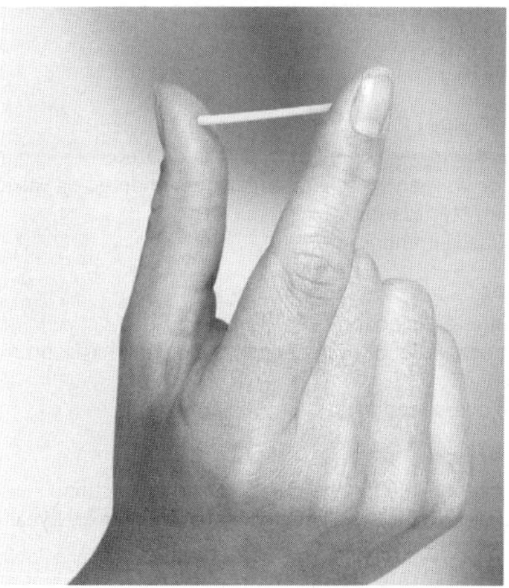

Fig. 13.2 Implanon®. Reproduced with permission of Schering-Plough.

Progestogen-only injectables

Definition

- Long-acting IM depot medroxyprogesterone acetate (DMPA) 150mg every 12 weeks with 1–2 weeks extra effectiveness.
- Shorter-acting oily injection norethisterone enantate (NET EN) 200mg may be repeated once after 8 weeks. Licensed in UK for short-term use only.

Mode of action

Inhibits ovulation and increases viscosity of cervical mucous inhibiting sperm penetration.

Effectiveness

Over 99% if starting within 5 days of cycle, any time post-partum, but 3 weeks post-partum if breastfeeding, 1–5 days post-miscarriage or TOP.

Indications/special cases

- Sickle cell disease—fewer crises.
- Endometriosis.
- Epilepsy.
- Difficult pill takers.
- Where synthetic oestrogens are contraindicated.
- NET EN for women waiting their partners undergoing vasectomy or post-partum sterilization.
- Prior to rubella immunization.

Advantages

- Only requires an injection every 12 weeks.
- Amenorrhoea, relief of dysmenorrhoea, menorrhagia, premenstrual syndrome.
- Suitable in breastfeeding.

Disadvantages

- Effects not reversible for the duration of the injection.
- Menstrual disturbance, weight gain up to 2–3kg over 1 year and progressive.
- Return of fertility can take up to 1 year.
- Not first choice for adolescents unless other methods not suitable or acceptable, because of anxiety about reversible delay in attaining peak bone mass.
- All users experience a small (6%) reduction in bone density, which reverses within 2 years of discontinuation.
- No protection STI/HIV.
- Vaginal dryness, mood swings.

Contraindications to injectable progestogens

- Decompensated cirrhosis or active hepatitis.
- Liver tumours.
- Undiagnosed genital tract bleeding.
- Past breast cancer (<5 years ago, or recurrence).
- Current DVT—implant/injection (but pregnancy is a greater risk).
- Arterial vascular disease/multiple risks.
- Diabetes with vascular complications.
- Ischaemic heart disease/stroke.
- Migraine with aura developing on the method.

Clinical history

- Re-evaluate risks and benefits if the method is to be continued for more than 2 years. Promote good bone health strategies.
- With lifestyle or medical risk factors for osteoporosis, other methods should be considered.
- Not seen as first option for >45 year olds.

Intra-uterine contraception/ intra-uterine system

Factors to discuss at counselling

- Parity—can use in nullipara (UK MECI).
- Mode of delivery, i.e. post-partum, can fit at 4 weeks regardless of mode of delivery.
- Known tubal disease or previous ectopic pregnancy is a point for counselling but, not on the list of absolute contraindications.
- Epilepsy to be considered as potential reaction at insertion.
- Current or recent STI should be investigated.
- Menorrhagia, abnormal bleeding should be investigated.
- Allergy to copper—applicable to IUDs only.

Management

- Pre-insertion counselling (discuss failure, change of bleeding pattern, ectopic pregnancy, PID, displacement and perforation).
- STI screening of risk factors.
- Advise oral analgesia and food 1h prior to insertion (preferably NSAID).
- Each IUD type has specific insertion technique.

Fitting

- An IUD can be fitted any time within days 1–12 of cycle, any other time of the cycle if risk of pregnancy is excluded, immediately post-TOP, >4 weeks post-partum.
- IUS insertion within first 5 days of cycle, immediately post-TOP, >4 weeks post-partum, any other time if risk of pregnancy is excluded and precautions used for 7 days after the fitting.
- Resuscitation equipment must be available in case of vasovagal attack, epileptic fit, or anaphylaxis.
- Two health professionals must be present: one for fitting the IUD and the second for reassurance and assistance in case of emergency.
- Specific sterile equipment for the non-touch technique—single use preferred.
- 10–15 minutes rest and observation recommended post-insertion.
- Teach feeling of threads and return if unable to.
- 3–6 weeks follow-up to exclude infection, expulsion according to local protocol. Threads to be seen (through speculum)—if too long, cut.
- No need for further timed follow ups, if no problems.

Removal

- IUD/IUS within first week of cycle, if pregnancy desired, if not, establish another method or abstinence for 7 days prior to removal.
- If urgent (e.g. infection) oral EC required, if intercourse occurred in last 72h.
- After age 40, copper-bearing IUDs can remain *in situ* until 1 year after last period.
- After age 45, Mirena® IUS can remain *in situ* to menopause unless used as part of HRT, then it is changed 4-yearly.

Nurse training for IUD fitting/removal

Eligibility

- Must have recognized post-registration qualification in contraception and sexual health and at least 2 years post-qualification experience, with current CPR/ALS anaphylaxis training.
- Competent in pelvic-bimanual examination and use of local anaesthetic.
- A nurse independent prescriber qualification or training in use of Patient Group Directions.
- Knowledge of IUD/IUS: attendance of recognized theoretical training.

Practical training must be overseen by FSRH registered trainer holding a current Letter of Competence (Loc IUT) or a nurse accredited by RCN and having fitted additional 25 devices and qualified to train nurses in the procedure.

Observe a minimum of 5 insertions, fit a minimum of 10 (using more than 1 type) and training must be completed within 1 year.

Maintain competence with a minimum of 12 insertions per year.[1]

Nurses who are also qualified nurse hysteroscopists can be trained to fit IUS as part of their training with accreditation from the BSGE.

1. Royal College of Nursing (June 2006) Fitting intra-uterine devices. Training guidance for nurses and midwives. London: RCN.

Intra-uterine device (IUD)

Small T-shaped plastic devices, with metallic copper wire or band on the stem (see Fig. 13.3).

Mode of action

Disrupts sperm transportation and fertilization and rarely interferes with implantation of any fertilized ovum.

Efficacy

98–99% over first year of use. Choice depends on availability: IUDs with at least 300mm^2 of copper have the lowest failure rates </= 1%.

Indications

- Long-acting, reversible method, ideal for spacing a family, deferring decision about sterilization in the young.
- First choice when in monogamous relationship and nulliparous.
- Available for emergency contraception.
- Contraindications to hormonal methods.

Advantages

- Suitable for forgetful pill-takers.
- From 40 years IUD can remain *in situ* until 1 year after last period (menopause).
- Suitable for breastfeeding mothers.
- Fertility returns once removed.
- No interference with sexual activity.

Disadvantages

- High STI risk is a contraindication.
- Menstrual disturbance, spotting 2–3 days pre- and post-menses.
- Heavier and painful periods first 3–4 months.
- Spontaneous expulsion/displacement varies from 1 to 10% within the first year of use.
- Uterine perforation/transmigration, but rare (1/1000)—presents as lost IUD strings—possible reasons for lost IUD strings are:
    - Thread curled up into cervix.
    - Expulsion.
    - Perforation at the time of insertion.
    - Important to rule out pregnancy.
    - Advise barrier methods.
- Ectopic pregnancy occurs in around 5% of IUD pregnancies but is lower than the risk in the non-contracepter population.
- Small increased risk of pelvic infection in the first 20 days after the insertion.

Medical eligibility: category 4 contraindications

- Pregnancy, puerperal sepsis, post-septic abortion.
- Unexplained vaginal bleeding before evaluation.
- Cervical cancer awaiting treatment.
- Endometrial cancer.
- Uterine fibroids and anatomic abnormalities that distort the cavity.
- Current PID.
- Current STI.
- Known TB.[1]

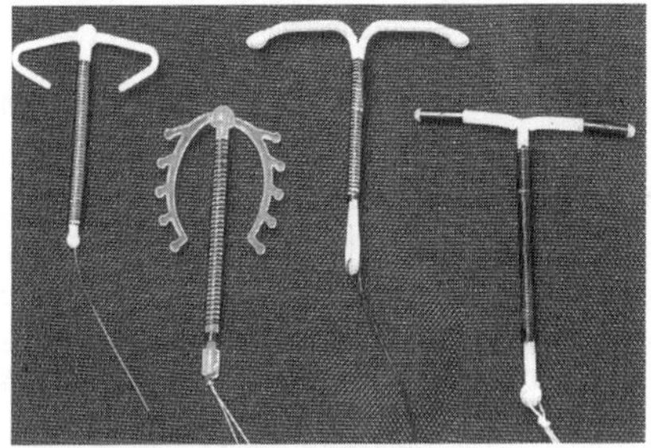

Fig. 13.3 Copper IUD. Reproduced with permission from Sunanda Gupta.

Resources

NICE LARC Guideline 2005 ☞ www.nice.org.uk (Accessed on March 2008.)

1. WHO (2005) *Medical eligibility criteria for contraceptive use*. Reproductive Health and Research, World Health Organization, Geneva.

Intra-uterine system (Mirena®)(LNG-IUS)

Definition

This is a T-shaped device 19mm long with a thread, which has a reservoir of slow-releasing progestogen (levonorgestrel).

Mode of action

The reservoir diffuses 20µg of levonogestrel into the uterine cavity per day over 5 years, producing endometrial atrophy and thickening of the cervical mucous, disrupting fertilization. Menstruation is short and light or non-existent. Suppression of ovulation occurs in some women.

Efficacy

Over 99% effective, increasing with age.

Indications

- Long-term, reversible contraception.
- Progestogen component of HRT (license for 4 years only).
- Treatment for menorrhagia/DUB (reduced need for hysterectomy) and to manage bleeding secondary to endometriosis and fibroids.
- Alternative to surgical sterilization.
- Treatment for endometrial hyperplasia.

Contraindications

As for IUDs and additionally breast cancer, liver disorders, and allergy to progestogens.

Advantages

- Menstrual blood loss reduced by up to 90%.
- Last for 5 years.
- Suitable for breastfeeding mothers, can be inserted 4 weeks post-partum.
- No liver-enzyme induction or drug interaction.
- No upper age limit for use.

Disadvantages/side-effects

- Menstrual bleeding irregularities/spotting first 3–4 months, can last up to 6 months and may be worse in women with menorrhagia prior to fitting.
- Psychological effects—mood changes as for other progestogens.
- Headaches, breast tenderness, facial acne can happen in first 3–4 months.
- Amenorrhoea is 20–30% at year 1 and creates difficulties in some cultures.
- No protection in STI/HIV.
- Small risk of functional ovarian cysts which are asymptomatic.

Barriers: male and female condoms

Mode of action

Prevents spermatozoa gaining access to the female upper genital tract.

Effectiveness

- If used correctly and consistently: 96–98% male, 96% female but 12% failure in 'typical' use.
- Failure higher in the young and inexperienced.
- Latex is vulnerable to oil based lubricants.
- Inform all users about emergency contraception.

Indications

- When a couple use a reversible method.
- Following pregnancy, miscarriage, or abortion before another method is adopted.
- For protection from STIs/HIV and practising 'safer sex'.
- When an additional method is required, e.g. forgotten to restart a new packet of hormonal pills, or missed some pills.
- If hormonal methods unsuitable or have contraindications.

Contraindications

- Allergy to latex rubber—polyurethane condoms are alternatives.
- Malformation of the penis or female genital tract.
- Psychologically unacceptable.

Female condoms

Advantages

- Available over the counter or the internet and supermarkets.
- Stronger than latex condoms.
- Less disruption of the sexual act as can be inserted hours before.
- Controlled by the female.
- Can be used with oil based products.

Disadvantages

- Appearance unattractive.
- A 'rustling' noise and altered sensation during intercourse.
- Sometimes inserted incorrectly, completely into the vagina, and penetration can occur outside the condom.
- Not suitable for women who dislike touching their genitalia.
- Initial difficulty with insertion can be experienced, but this improves with practice.

Male condoms

Advantages

- If used consistently and correctly, an effective method.
- Inexpensive or freely available from a wide range of sources.
- Simple to use.
- No advice required from healthcare professionals but instruction should be encouraged for the young.
- No local or systemic side-effects.

- A very high level of protection against STIs/HIV infection: studies indicate that consistent use of condoms results in 80% reduction in HIV incidence.[1]
- Protection against human papilloma virus, therefore pre-malignant disease and carcinoma of the cervix.
- Some improvement of performance in males with premature ejaculation.

Disadvantages

- Requires application before coitus and quick removal thereafter, which can be unacceptable interruption to sexual activity.
- Appearance can be distasteful to some.
- For some males, reduced sensation during sexual intercourse.
- Oil-based lubricants (e.g. baby oil, petroleum jelly, Vaseline®, and some vaginal medications) reduce the efficacy and may cause breakage.
- Before use, check for valid expiry date and safety markings on the packets.

1. Weller, S and Davis, AR (2006) Condom effectiveness in reducing heterosexual HIV transmission. (Review) The Cochrane Libary.

Vaginal barriers, caps, and diaphragms

Oldest method that prevents spermatozoa from entering the female upper genital tract and reaching ovum. Vaginal barriers are used with a vaginal spermicide.

Caps

- Cervical: (Prentif® cavity rim cervical cap) similar to a thimble designed to fit closely over the cervix.
- Vault: (Dumas®) hemispherical bowl designed to fit in to the vaginal vault, remains *in situ* by suction covering the cervix.
- Vimule®: a variation of the vault with thimble-shaped prolongation of the dome. All made of opaque rubber.
- Recent cervical caps: Lea's Shield® silicone, re-usable, one–size with a removal loop, can be left *in situ* for 48h, available over the counter in USA and some European countries.
- Femcap®: flexible silicone dome-shaped cup shaped like a US sailor's hat, held in position by the vaginal walls (only disposable cap now available in UK).

Diaphragms

📖 See Fig. 13.4.

- Flat-spring: transparent rubber (Reflexions®).
- Coil-spring: opaque rubber (Ortho®) or silicone (Milex Omniflex®).
- Arcing spring: opaque rubber (All-Flex®) or silicone (Milex Arcing Style®).

Effectiveness

- Concurrent spermicide recommended.
- If used correctly, 92–96% depending on the experience of the user and frequency of intercourse.
- The FemCap is less effective.

Advantages

- Reusable and depending on usage, durable.
- Does not interfere with breastfeeding.
- Can be inserted up to 3h prior to intercourse.
- No systemic side-effects.
- Reduction in the risk of PID.
- Reduction in risk of cervical cancer.

Disadvantages

- Requires a health professional to fit, teach, and follow-up.
- Can cause loss of some cervical/vaginal sensation.
- Discomfort to female or male during sexual activity.
- No protection STI/HIV.
- Use of spermicide can be 'messy'.
- Increased incidence of cystitis, candidiasis.
- Requires premeditation, losing the spontaneity of intercourse.

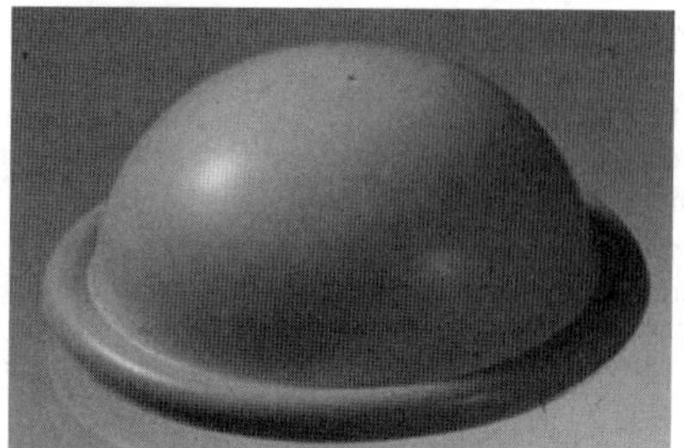

Fig. 13.4 Diaphragm. Reproduced courtesy of Mrs. Walli Bounds.

Male methods

Coitus interruptus

Oldest practice widely used in Muslim and Christian communities. Known as 'withdrawal', 'being careful', or 'lucky'.

Mode of action

The withdrawal of an erect penis from the vagina before ejaculation. Sometimes, however, pre-ejaculatory secretions containing sperm can escape from the urethra during penetration, resulting in conception.

Effectiveness

Depends on the experience and age of the couple but tends to be poor.

Advantages

- Free, no health professional required for teaching.
- No side-effects.
- Complete privacy for the couple's sexual relationship.
- Accepted by many cultures and religions.

Disadvantage

- No protection from STI/HIV.
- High failure rate especially in the young and inexperienced.
- Reduces complete enjoyment of intercourse.
- This method is only used by 4% of sexually active population in the UK.[1]

Male condoms

📖 See Barriers: male and female condoms, p.388.

Vasectomy

📖 See Vasectomy: male sterilization, p.399.

Currently no systemic methods available. Development of the male equivalent of oral, injectable, and implantable hormonal contraception has been researched for many years.

1. Taylor, T, Keyse, L and Bryant A (2006) *Contraception and sexual health 2005/2006*. Office for National Statistics. Department of Health, London.

Spermicides

Definition

- Nonoxinol-9 is a non-ionic detergent incorporated in an inert base capable of destroying sperm.
- UK cream formulation is 2% nonoxinol-9, which liquefies at body temperature and disperses rapidly through the vagina.
- Gels, suppositories, and foams are available in some countries.

Mode of action

Base material of the cream blocks sperm progression whilst nonoxinol-9 is toxic to sperm.

Effectiveness

Used alone, failure rate of 6–8% within first year.

'Any method is better than none'.

Indications

It is recommended for use with a diaphragm or cervical cap.[1]

Contraindications

- Not to be used for protection against STI/HIV.
- Not appropriate for frequent repeated use.

Advantages

- An extra lubrication when vaginal dryness is a concern.
- Available over the counter.
- No partner co-operation.
- No evidence of topical vaginal toxicity.
- Possible protection against cervical cancer (transmission of HPV). This, however, is not evidence based.

Disadvantages

- Impaired vaginal sensation.
- Irritation of vagina or penis by nonoxidol-9, and allergy.
- High failure, if used alone.
- Some degree of 'messiness' depending on the preparation and unpleasant odour.
- Not for use for anal sex.
- Increased urinary tract infection (unproven).
- May be increased risk of HIV among sex workers (frequent use—now not recommended).
- A full applicator of cream must be inserted into the vagina prior to intercourse.
- If more than 1h between insertion and intercourse, second application required.

1. Cook, I, Nanda, K and Grimes, D (2003) Diaphragm versus diaphragm with spermicide for contraception (Cochrane Review). *Cochrane Databases Systematic Review* **1**: CD002031.

Natural family planning

Fertility awareness can be used to help women conceive or not to conceive.

Ova are only viable for 12–24h. Sperm can live up to 7 days in the reproductive tract, leaving 8–9 days of fertility per cycle. This is the biological principle for fertility awareness (FA).

Three methods based on the fertile phase of the menstrual cycle

1. In the calendar method, estimating time of ovulation and avoiding unprotected sexual intercourse or abstinence for 1/3–1/2 of cycle. On the whole, the last week or so of the cycle is deemed safe.
2. Temperature method—using rise of temperature after ovulation as green light not to use contraception (the safe period is 3 days after the rise of temperature).
3. Mucous method—checking for 'wet days' due to oestrogen-driven increase in mucous production. Wet days are deemed the risky fertile days.

These three methods are known to be less reliable. Effectiveness rates are variable, depending on regularity of cycles, the age of the couple, frequency of sexual intercourse, and whether taught by a health professional. Effectiveness rates are:

- Following instructions, up to 98%.
- Computerized monitor up to 94%.
- Lactational amenorrhoea method up to 98%.

Lactational amenorrhoea method (LAM)

- Only applicable post-partum.
- Fully breastfeeding with feeding interval less than 4h.
- Amenorrhoea since lochia stopped.
- Baby under 6 months old.

Ovulation devices

These work by monitoring hormone alterations in urine or saliva, combining data with data on the length of cycle.

A computerized handheld monitor Persona® with a set of disposable dipsticks, which measure oestrone-3-glucuronide (E3G) to indicate the start of the fertile period and LH concentrations to assess when it is safe to stop using contraception in early morning urine. The monitor reads unsafe days (red light) and safe days (green light): computer stores data from the user's last 6 cycles.

Fertility indicators

Temperature

Take prior to rising or drinking using ovulation thermometer, charting from first day of period. A rise of 0.2–0.4°C indicates ovulation has occurred. When temperature has been raised for 3 days, then may be safe until next cycle.

Cervical mucous (Billing's method)

'Dry days/wet days', monitoring daily vaginal secretions. Following menstruation, mucous scanty for 3–4 days, then increasingly clear, profuse, stretchy up to 4 days 'peak fertility' followed by 3–4 days scanty, sticky, and opaque, after which the safe 'period' begins to next menses.

Calendar/rhythm method

Monitor the length of 6 cycles. To calculate fertile days, subtract 18 from the length of the shortest cycle and 11 from the longest, the two resulting numbers indicate the start and end of fertile days.

Advantages

- Increases awareness of body physiology, either to conceive or prevent pregnancy.
- No hormones or 'foreign bodies'.
- Familiarization with body changes may enhance sexuality.
- Accepted in many religions and cultures.
- Little cost (except devices).

Disadvantages

- Requires charting/recording over 3–6 months.
- Difficult for cycles <23 days or >35 days and in anovulatory cycles, such as women over 40.
- Less reliable peri-menopausal or post-partum.
- Indicators affected by illness, stress, erratic lifestyles, travel.
- Abstinence from intercourse 15–17 days of cycle.
- No protection from STI/HIV.
- Requires learning from a trained teacher.

Laparoscopic sterilization of women

- A surgical operation to block the fallopian tubes, stopping sperm and ova from fertilizing/conceiving.
- GA, LA, or epidural/spinal anaesthesia required.
- Pneumoperitoneum is produced by insufflation of carbon dioxide gas into the peritoneal cavity.
- Through a subumbilical incision, a trochar and canula are inserted into the gas–filled abdomen. Trochar then replaced by the laparoscope with fibre-optic light source. Pelvic organs examined. Operating forceps introduced through a second cannula, performing the procedure by application of titanium clips. Falope rings or diathermy have also been used in the past, but are now rarely used in the UK.

Effectiveness
- A failure rate of only 0.2–0.33% using Filshie® Clip.
- Depends on experience of operator.

Advantages
- No effect on menstrual cycle or sexual function.
- Usually performed as day case.
- Effective immediately after the operation.
- Partner not required to sign consent form but advised to attend for counselling prior to operation.
- Permanent.
- Free on NHS.

Disadvantages
- Risk of ectopic pregnancy post-op, if recent intercourse (1: 2000) or procedure fails.
- Reversal difficult—success not guaranteed. Not free on NHS—expensive in private sector. Success is better with IVF, not on the NHS.
- No protection against STI/HIV.
- Counselling appointments prior to operation.
- Will have a return to normal menstruation if been on hormonal methods and may then complain of menorrhagia.

Essure® sterilization of women

- Performed under LA or intravenous sedation as an outpatient procedure.
- The procedure is carried out through a hysteroscope, inserting micro-inserts into each fallopian tube using a thin catheter (see Fig.13.5).
- The micro-inserts are made of polyester fibre, nickel-titanium, and stainless steel, causing scar tissue to develop and block the fallopian tubes.
- A hysterosalpingogram (or X-ray/ultrasound) is required at 3 months to confirm tubal occlusion with correct placement of the micro-inserts.

Effectiveness

Preliminary data showed bilateral placement was achieved in 90% and no pregnancies were reported over 4 years in these women.

Advantages

- Less invasive than other techniques.
- No incision or external scarring.
- Short procedure.
- Less severe post-operative pain and better tolerance of the procedure compared to laparoscopic sterilization.[1]
- Suitable for the obese/previous pelvic surgery.
- No interference with sexual pleasure.

Disadvantages

- Requires effective contraception for 3 months after, with follow-up hysterosalpingogram to confirm tubal occlusion.
- Not suitable post-partum, miscarriage, or TOP. Can be done after 6 weeks.
- Contraindications include PID (active or recent) and uterine abnormality.
- Allergy to nickel.
- Not reversible.
- No STI/HIV protection.
- Long-term data available from recent trials, where bilateral placement was achieved in 90% and no pregnancies were reported over 4 years.[2]
- Ectopic pregnancy is a theoretical risk.

1. Duffy, S, Marsh, F, Rogerson, L, Hudson, H, Cooper, K, Jack, S, Hunter, D and Philips, G (2005) Female sterilisation: a cohort controlled comparative study of Essure versus laparoscopic sterilisation St James's University Hospital, Leeds, UK. *British Journal of Obstetrics and Gynaecology* Nov. **112**(11): 1522–1528.
2. Bradley, LD. Long term follow up of hysteroscopic sterilisation with the Essure micro-insert. Abstract. *Journal of minimally invasive Gynaecology* **15**: S1–S159.

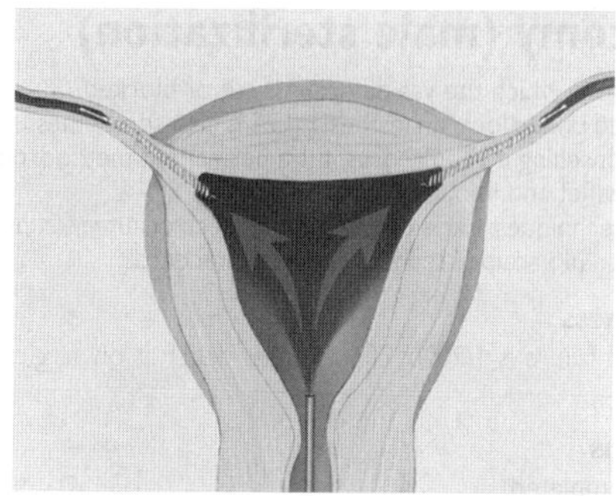

Fig. 13.5 Essure®. Reproduced with permission from Conceptus, Inc.

Vasectomy (male sterilization)

- Procedure in which the vas deferens is cut or blocked.
- Performed under local anaesthesia (GA is also sometimes used).
- Initial counselling is required, as it is a permanent method: needs information leaflet and informed consent signed.
- Various techniques: excision or ligation, electrocautery, clips, use of chemicals. 'No scalpel' technique is now standard.

Effectiveness

The quoted failure is 1/2000: Effectiveness depends on surgical technique applied.

Indications

- Family completed.
- No children desired.
- A carrier with a high risk of transmitting an inherited disorder.
- Suffering from chronic ill-health, which contraindicates pregnancy and a couple's ability to raise children.

Advantages

- Can be performed at GP surgeries, private sector, and outpatient clinics.
- No interruption to sexual intercourse.
- Simple and quick procedure.
- Less invasive than female sterilization and more effective.
- Mortality and operative morbidity extremely rare.

Disadvantages

- Continue alternative method until checked for two negative sperm counts (at 2 and 3 months).
- Low success rate, if reversal is required.
- 48h rest recommended after procedure.
- No STI/HIV protection.

Chapter 14

Unwanted fertility

Overview of abortion and legal aspects

Unwanted pregnancy (or unwanted fertility) affects many women worldwide. A woman's chance of experiencing an unwanted pregnancy at some point during her reproductive life is approximately 1 in 3. For many women the only option is to undergo an abortion, otherwise known as termination of pregnancy (TOP). Approximately 200,000 women per year undergo abortion in England and Wales with a further 13,000 in Scotland. Therapeutic abortion is the commonest gynaecological procedure performed in the United Kingdom.

Definition of abortion

The artificial removal or expulsion of a pregnancy using medical or surgical methods.

Legal aspects

Background

The law in relation to abortion is found in statute. The Abortion Act (1967), with some provisions amended by the Human Fertilization and Embryology Act (1990), defines grounds upon which an abortion can take place in a lawful manner. The law covers England, Scotland, and Wales but does not apply to Northern Ireland, where the Offences Against the Person's Act (1861) applies. The legal time-limit for the majority of abortions is 24 weeks; however, there is no gestational limit when the indications are risk to the life of the woman, grave permanent damage to the physical or mental health of the woman, or foetal abnormality.

Essentially two doctors have to agree, in good faith, that an abortion can take place under one of the grounds of the Abortion Act (1967):

1. The continuance of the pregnancy would involve risk to the life of the pregnant woman greater than if the pregnancy were terminated.
2. The continuance of the pregnancy would involve risk of injury to the physical or mental health of the pregnant woman greater than if the pregnancy were terminated.
3. The continuance of the pregnancy would involve risk of injury to the physical or mental health of the existing child(ren) of the family of the pregnant woman greater than if the pregnancy were terminated.
4. There is substantial risk that if the child were born it would suffer from such physical or mental abnormalities as to be seriously handicapped.

The Abortion Act (1967) provides a right of conscientious objection, which allows healthcare professionals to decline to participate in an abortion. This right is limited only to the active participation in an abortion where there is no emergency with regard to the physical or mental health of the pregnant woman. A conscientious objector would normally refer the woman to a colleague.

Consent and confidentiality

Consent can be defined as:[1]

'A voluntary, uncoerced decision, made by a sufficiently competent or autonomous person on the basis of adequate information and deliberation, to accept rather than reject some proposed course of action that will affect him or her'.

- Every woman with an unwanted pregnancy has the right to decide and to determine the outcome of her pregnancy—including those under 16 years of age (see Consent, p.36).
- All women undergoing an abortion procedure need to sign a written consent form.
- All women (including those under 16 years of age) seeking an abortion have a right to confidentiality from all healthcare and ancillary staff. Only in exceptional circumstances (e.g. where the health, welfare, or safety of the woman, a minor, or other persons is at risk) should a third party be informed.

Legal age and capacity in relation to consent

In England, Wales, and Northern Ireland, young women aged 16 and 17 years are presumed competent to give consent. The legislation is slightly different in Scotland, but, the age of consent is still the young person's sixteenth birthday. In the UK, young people under 16 years of age can give consent if they fully understand what is involved, although ideally their parents/guardians should be involved. Although specifically relating to contraception, guidance can be found in the House of Lords ruling in the Gillick case (HC(FP)(86)1) (DH 1986),[2] which is widely used with abortion services. This guidance is now superseded by the Department of Health professional guidelines for health professionals (DH 2004,[3] FFPRHC 2004).[4]

► Fraser guidelines

Although originally these guidelines were established for medical and nursing staff dealing with young people under the age of 16 years requesting contraception, they are also applicable to requests for abortion. A doctor is justified in proceeding without the parents' consent or knowledge if:

- the girl will understand his/her advice;
- he/she cannot persuade her to inform her parents or allow him/her to inform her parents that she is seeking contraceptive advice;
- she is likely to begin or to continue having sexual intercourse with, or without, contraceptive advice;
- unless she receives contraceptive advice or treatment her physical or mental health, or both, are likely to suffer;
- her best interests require him/her to give her contraceptive advice, treatment, or both, without parental consent.

1. Gillon R (1985) Philosophical medical ethics. *British Medical Journal* **291**: 1700–1701.
2. HCFP (86) 1 Department of Health (1986) Original guidance relating to the provision of advice and treatment to young people under 16 years of age on contraception—now cancelled. Relates to the House of Lords ruling in Gillick vs West Norfolk and Wisbech Health Authority (1986) AC112.
3. Department of Health (2004) Best practice guidance for doctors and other health professionals on the provision of advice and treatment to young people under 16 on contraception, sexual and reproductive health.
4. FSRH (2004) Contraceptive choices for young people. Faculty of sexual and reproductive healthcare. Clinical Effectiveness Unit. *Journal of Family Planning and Reproductive Healthcare* **30**: 237–251.

Nurse's role in abortion provision

The authorization and provision of abortion is the legal responsibility of a registered medical practitioner, and the strict requirements are set out in the Abortion Act (1967). The role of the nurse has historically been to provide general nursing care. Recent advances in abortion methods, particularly medical abortion, have led to the development of innovative nursing roles and an enhanced nursing role in the actual process of abortion. Nurses are now caring for a significant proportion of women undergoing medical abortion under the guidance of a registered medical practitioner.

Nurses undertaking role development should ensure that they are competent and have the appropriate knowledge, skills, education, and training. Once competency has been achieved, the nurse should be able to practise independently within agreed protocols and under the guidance of a registered medical practitioner. Examples of role development following appropriate training and competency assessment may include:

- Performing a pregnancy test and communicating the results to the patient.
- Pre-admission medical assessment.
- Pre- and post-abortion counselling.
- Obtaining consent for abortion procedures.
- Administration of abortifacient drugs.
- Vaginal (bimanual) and speculum examination.
- Screening and/or testing for sexually transmitted infections.
- Ultrasound assessment of gestational age, implantation site, chorionicity, and viability.
- Assessment and provision of contraception via nurse-independent prescribing or patient group directions (PGDs).
- Discharge following medical and surgical procedures.

To develop such roles, nurses need:

- To be accountable for their own practice.
- To identify a medical champion who will supervise and support the development of the nursing team.
- A sound knowledge base and be appropriately educated and trained. (This may include undertaking an accredited training course, e.g. sonography, counselling, family planning/reproductive and sexual health course, faculty of sexual and reproductive health abortion modules).
- Up-to-date knowledge of evidence based practice.
- Competency assessment, ensuring confidence in performing practical skills (e.g. pelvic examination, sonography).
- A thorough working knowledge of the law on abortion.

What nurses cannot do within the current legislation:

- Sign the Department of Health legal documents relating to the Abortion Act (1967) (forms HSA1 and HSA4).
- Perform surgical abortions.

- Prescribe the abortifacient drugs, which are used in medical abortions, or to prime the cervix prior to surgical abortion.
- Provide abortion services alone without a doctor being on call and remaining responsible for the woman.

Nurses need to be mindful that they are only working lawfully in the limits of the Abortion Act (1967), providing that they are delivering treatment in accordance with delegated instructions from a registered medical practitioner. The registered medical practitioner must at all times remain responsible for patient care throughout any treatment.

Pre-abortion assessment process

All women requesting an abortion should have a pre-abortion assessment. This should include the following:

- A discussion regarding the implications of their decision and reason(s) for the abortion request, which should consider all options (e.g. continuing with the pregnancy, adoption). Women will vary in the level of support and counselling that they require.
- A detailed medical assessment to include:
  - Date of last menstrual period (LMP) and menstrual history.
  - Past gynaecological, obstetric history, and sexual health history.
  - Past and current medical history.
  - Current medication.
  - Awareness of any allergies, including assessment of contraindications to abortifacient drugs.
  - Use of substances, e.g. nicotine/alcohol/recreational drugs.
- Physical assessment to include:
  - Confirmation of pregnancy by urine pregnancy test.
  - Assessment of gestational age, ideally by ultrasound.
  - Prevention of post-abortion sepsis—ideally services should offer screening for chlamydia and gonorrhoea (either via urine, endocervical swabs, or self obtained swabs) and/or prophylactic antibiotics.
  - Obtaining blood for haemoglobin concentration/studies, blood group, and rhesus status. Rhesus prophylaxis post-abortion for those women who are rhesus negative is essential. The recommended treatment is anti D immunoglobulin 250 units intramuscularly up to 20 weeks gestation and 500 units thereafter.
- Explanation of methods of abortion dependent upon gestational age and local policy/availability. This should include a full explanation of the risk of potential complications (including percentages of risk). Written information should be available.
- Obtain consent for chosen procedure, including assessment of competence to consent in the case of a mature minor based on Fraser Competencies.
- Assessment and discussion of past, current, and future contraceptive needs.
- Appropriate and speedy referral to other agencies as required.
- Completion of the legal requirments of the Abortion Act (HSA1 form).
- Prescribe any necessary medication (e.g. mifepristone, misoprostol) before treatment is commenced.

Surgical termination of pregnancy

The majority of abortions are carried out as surgical day cases under a general anaesthetic at between 6 and 14 weeks gestation. Most NHS abortion providers in England and Wales only provide suction termination of pregnancy (STOP) up to 12 weeks gestation. There are a growing number of abortions carried out in early pregnancy (below 12 weeks gestation) under local anaesthetic (with or without conscious sedation). This is commonly known as manual vacuum aspiration (MVA). MVA under local anaesthetic is known to be a safer option than conventional STOP. The method of surgical procedure is determined by the gestation of the pregnancy.

The operative technique below 15 weeks gestation

The uterine cervix is dilated to approximately the number of millimeters that is equivalent to the gestation in weeks. The pregnancy tissue or products of conception (POC) are then evacuated from the uterus using a transparent cannula. This can either be attached to an electric pump generating a vacuum of between 500 and 600mmHg (in the case of conventional STOP) or a vacuumed syringe (in the case of MVA). The transparent cannula allows the POC to be identified easily. There is no need to send the POC for histological examination. Cervical preparation approximately 2–3h prior to the surgical procedure with a prostaglandin analogue (e.g. misoprostol) is recommended for surgical abortion beyond 10 weeks gestation and for women aged under 18 years. In practice, most units will administer cervical preparation to all women undergoing STOP.

If the MVA technique is used under local anaesthetic, then it may be useful to prepare the woman prior to the procedure with:

- Rectal analgesia, e.g. diclofenac suppository.
- Mild sedative, e.g. oral temazepam.

⚠ Repeated instrumentation of the uterus should be avoided in order to reduce the risk of infection or perforation. Sharp metal curettes should **not** be used.

⚠ Conventional STOP should be avoided at under 7 weeks gestation, as it is three times more likely to fail to remove the gestation sac compared to STOP performed above 7 weeks gestation.

The operative technique above 15 weeks gestation

For 15 weeks gestation and above, dilatation and evacuation (D&E) is used. This involves the removal of the pregnancy with forceps, through the cervix. For gestations 19 weeks and above, osmotic dilators (e.g. dilapan) are used to dilate the cervix prior to the evacuation. Beyond 21 weeks and 6 days gestation, some abortion providers inject intra-amniotic medication (e.g. potassium) the day prior to a surgical abortion. This is known as foeticide and is required to be performed by a registered medical practitioner. This causes autolysis of the foetus, thus enabling an easier evacuation. This is not a practice routinely undertaken by all providers and it is not described in the latest RCOG (2004) guidelines.[1]

1. Royal College of Obstetricians and Gynaecologists (2004). The care of women requesting induced abortion. Parthenon Press, London.

⚠ Surgical procedures above 12 weeks gestation should only be performed by experienced operators.

Cervical priming agents and regimen

- Misoprostol 400µg (2 x 200µg tablets) administered vaginally 2–3h prior to surgery. (❶ Misoprostol is unlicensed for use as an abortifacient). Or
- Gemeprost (a prostaglandin E1 analogue) 1mg administered vaginally 3h prior to surgery. Or
- Mifepristone 200mg administered orally 36–48h prior to surgery.

Medical termination of pregnancy (MTOP)

MTOP is carried out using drugs called abortifacients. The introduction of the anti-progesterone mifepristone in the early 1990s made this technique readily acceptable. MTOP is also known as medical abortion or early medical abortion (EMA) if carried out under 9 weeks gestation. Mifepristone is a competitive inhibitor of progesterone, which acts at the receptor site in the nucleus of the cells of the end organ—in this case, the uterus and cervix. The anti-progestogenic steroid effectively blocks the action of progesterone, preventing the pregnancy from progressing. It also facilitates the process of medical abortion by sensitizing the uterus to the prostaglandin, which induces uterine contractions, and also by softening and dilating the cervix. By itself, mifepristone has limited use as an abortifacient, therefore, mifepristone should be used in conjunction with a prostaglandin analogue (e.g. misoprostol or gemeprost). The dose of mifepristone depends upon the gestational age.

❶ Misoprostol is known to be teratogenic (harmful to the developing foetus); therefore, if MTOP fails, it is imperative that the woman has already been counselled fully. There is insufficient evidence to suggest that mifepristone alone is teratogenic

Early medical termination is the most effective method of abortion below 7 weeks gestation.

Contraindications and cautions

- Uncontrolled severe asthma.
- Suspected ectopic pregnancy.
- Chronic adrenal failure.
- Porphyria.
- Long-term corticosteroid use—mifepristone is mildly anti-glucocorticoid.
- Older women who smoke heavily—although the evidence on which this is based probably does not apply to current UK regimens.
- Known allergy to mifepristone or prostaglandins.

MTOP regimen up to 13 weeks gestation

- **Licensed regimen up to 63 days gestation**—mifepristone 600mg orally, followed 36–48h later by gemeprost 1mg vaginally.
- **Unlicensed regimen (recommended by the Royal College of Obstetricians and Gynaecologists)**—mifepristone 200mg, followed 1–3 days later (gestation up to 9 weeks) or 36–48h later (gestation between 9 and 13 weeks) by misoprostol 800μg vaginally. In women at 49–63 days gestation, if the abortion has not occurred 4 hours after misoprostol, a further dose of vaginal or oral misoprostol 400μg may be given. For gestation between 9 and 13 weeks, a maximum of 4 further doses of misoprostol may be required at 3-hourly intervals if the abortion is incomplete. This is the most frequently used regimen.

MTOP regimen 13–24 weeks gestation

- **Licensed regimen**—mifepristone 600mg, followed 36-48h later by gemeprost 1mg vaginally 3-hourly to a maximum of five doses.
- **Unlicensed regimen (recommended by the Royal College of Obstetricians and Gynaecologists)**—mifepristone 200mg orally, followed 36-48h later by misoprostol 800μg vaginally. Further doses of vaginal or oral misoprostol 400μg given 3-hourly may be required if the abortion is incomplete, to a maximum of four doses. This is the regimen that is used most frequently

► Points:

- Oral administration of misoprostol tends to cause more gastro-intestinal side-effects but is considered to be less invasive.
- Vaginally administered misoprostol is more invasive from the woman's point of view but it does enable the carer to regularly assess the dilatation of the cervix and the progress of the abortion process. Moreover, misoprostol is better absorbed when given vaginally.

Complications and risks associated with abortion

Regardless of method, abortion is extremely safe and effective, and is safer than continuing a pregnancy to term. However, as with all medical and surgical procedures there are potential complications that should be explained to the patient during the pre-assessment process. The main complications are discussed below.

Infection

The rate of *chlamydia trachomatis* carriage associated with an unwanted pregnancy is greatest in young unmarried women and is at least 10%. Women undergoing TOP with an untreated chlamydial infection have a significant risk of pelvic inflammatory disease (PID). Long-term consequences of PID are chronic pelvic infection, subfertility, and risk of ectopic pregnancy.

Management options:

- **Prophylactic antibiotics** given to all women undergoing abortion. Either a single dose of azithromycin 1g orally or doxycycline 100mg twice daily for 7 days (plus metronidazole 1g rectally for both regimes). This option ensures that all women are treated. However, it does not allow for referral to genitor-urinary medicine/sexual health clinics for partner notification, and women may not take or complete the course of treatment.
- **Screen then treat policy**—all women undergoing abortion are screened for STIs and treated if the results are positive. This allows for partner notification and a full explanation of the implications of the infection. However, it is more expensive and open to administrative errors.
- **Screen and treat prophylactically**—this is a combination of the first two options.

Haemorrhage

Significant primary haemorrhage at the time of abortion is rare at ~1 in 1000 cases. The risk is lower for early abortions at less than 13 weeks gestation (0.88 in 1000 cases), and higher for gestations above 20 weeks (4.0 in 1000 cases). The need for blood transfusion is rare. Significant secondary haemorrhage occurs occasionally with retained products of conception (RPOC) and infection. Women should be advised that prolonged minor bleeding following abortion is common.

Failed abortion and continuing pregnancy

All methods of first-trimester abortion carry a small risk of failure to terminate thus requiring a further procedure. The risk for surgical abortion is ~2.3 in 1000 and can be associated with early gestation, undiagnosed septate uterus, uterine perforation, or the creation of a false passage during the cervical dilatation process, and missed ectopic pregnancy. The failure rate is 1–14 in 1000 for medical abortion, dependent upon the gestation, drug regimen used, and the experience of the service. If an abortion is thought to have failed, an urgent ultrasound scan should be carried out and further management offered if necessary. Scanning prior to abortion can overcome some of these problems.

Incomplete abortion

Incomplete abortion occurs in ~2–3% of surgical abortions and is directly associated with experience of the surgeon, but can still occur with very experienced surgeons. Incomplete abortion occurs in ~4–5% of medical abortions dependent upon gestation. If a small amount of RPOC is found, then a conservative approach may be justified as this will probably be expelled spontaneously. Otherwise oral or vaginal misoprostol or surgical evacuation may be necessary

Uterine trauma

The risk of uterine perforation at the time of STOP is 1–4 in 1000 and is directly associated to the experience of the surgeon and with advancing gestations. This can be significantly reduced by pre-treating the cervix with vaginal prostaglandins. As a minimum standard, nulliparous women and those over 10 weeks gestation should be treated. If perforation does occur during the dilatation process, then, the abortion should be completed under ultrasound or laparoscopic guidance. If bleeding is not excessive, then further intervention may not be required, but the woman should be given antibiotic cover and observed for 48h.

If perforation is suspected, damage can occur to the intra-abdominal organs. It is, *therefore,* essential to investigate further via laparoscopy or laparotomy. Uterine rupture has been associated with mid-trimester medical abortions with a low risk at less than 1 in 1000.

Cervical laceration

Damage to the external cervical os during dilatation occurs in ~1 in 100 cases. Again, the risk is reduced if the cervix is pre-treated with prostaglandins, and the operation is performed early in pregnancy and by an experienced surgeon.

Psychological sequelae

There is conflicting evidence regarding the rate of psychological response to abortion. Up to 50% of women may experience a transient grief reaction following abortion, while the majority (80–90%) will ultimately experience feelings of relief. Approximately 10% will experience adverse psychological outcomes. However, it is worth noting that this may not be related to the abortion, but a continuation of pre-existing conditions.

Long-term complications and future reproductive outcomes

There are no proven associations between induced abortions and subsequent ectopic pregnancy, secondary subfertility, and subfertility. However, abortion may be associated with a small increase in miscarriage and pre-term labour. Rarely, uterine adhesions may result in Asherman's syndrome (amenorrhoea). This is possibly linked to higher gestation abortions and repeat abortions.

Resources

Abortion Act (1967): http://www.opsi.gov.uk/acts/acts1967/pdf/ukpga_19670087_en.pdf
www.bpas.org
British National Formulary: www.bnf.org
Department of Health: www.dh.gov.uk
Medical Foundation for Aids and Sexual Health: www.medfash.org.uk
Office of Public Sector Information: www.opsi.gov.uk
Royal College of Obstetricians and Gynaecologists: www.rcog.org.uk
British Pregnancy Advisory Service: www.bpas.org

Chapter 15

Early pregnancy problems

The role of the early pregnancy assessment unit (EPAU)

The role of the EPAU is both specialist and special. It is mainly to confirm viability and determine the location of existing pregnancies. Many of the women who attend are young and unfamiliar with hospital attendance or indeed health problems in general. These women are often extremely anxious and, therefore, the utilization of high-quality counselling and communication skills within the EPAU workforce is extremely important. The role can potentially include investigations and support of women with recurrent miscarriage and a systematic approach to registering and follow-up of women with trophoblastic disease.

The aim of EPAUs is to provide immediate access to appropriate care for women experiencing an early pregnancy problem. By approaching the woman holistically, both physical and psychological needs are identified and addressed. Through information, reassurance, and counselling, any fears and anxieties are alleviated as swiftly and effectively as possible.

Women should be able to access their nearest EPAU directly, but in some departments, a GP referral is required.

The EPAU should have access to specialized staff and equipment to safely investigate and manage any woman with a problem in early pregnancy.

Although some departments will have extended acceptance criteria, particularly with the recent evolution of emergency gynaecology units, primarily, the responsibility of the EPAU is to determine the location and viability of a pregnancy, and to manage the woman safely through the process of investigation, diagnosis, and management.

The majority of EPAUs are open for specified hours during the week, it is, therefore, important the patient group have an alternative route to care out of hours and that appropriate communication channels are maintained.

The role of staff in the EPAU

Each EPAU will be staffed differently and different roles are allocated to staff members, depending on the opening hours, patient numbers, skills and competence, etc.

Many EPAUs are nurse-led, with support from a dedicated consultant. Medical cover should be available on a daily basis from the on call gynaecology team. The following are general descriptions that may vary, dependent on the size and opening times of the unit.

Healthcare assistant (HCA)

The front desk is staffed by an administrator and a HCA. HCAs may be able to perform a basic triage assessment on the women when they arrive, referring anyone who does not obviously fall within the acceptance criteria, or who in any way appears to be unstable/in pain/distressed/bleeding heavily, to the nurse co-ordinator for the day. The HCA will perform baseline observations, urinalysis, and a pregnancy test on every patient.

Care of women with bleeding in early pregnancy

Bleeding in early pregnancy is one of the most common reasons f women to present to hospital. There are several possible causes f bleeding in early pregnancy and it is important to establish a diagno quickly, as the patient will invariably believe she is miscarrying and w be extremely anxious. Bleeding should be investigated, whether one in dent of spotting or heavy bleeding, also do not dismiss a history of ame orrhoea and brown discharge, as this is often an indication of a delay miscarriage.

Possible causes of bleeding in early pregnancy

- Miscarriage (delayed/incomplete/complete).
- Ectopic pregnancy.
- Molar pregnancy.
- Implantation/subchorionic bleed.
- Cervical erosion.
- Post-coital bleed.
- Cervical polyp.
- Sexually transmitted infection (STI).
- Other causes.

History

A thorough history can help establish a diagnosis and guide management

History should include:

- When bleeding started.
- Type/pattern of bleeding.
- Any associated factors such as recent sexual intercourse.
- Associated pain and description.
- Recent cervical smear history.
- Any history of STIs.
- Obstetric history.

⚠ Often a history will guide you to what seems to be a clear diagnosi e.g. if a woman describes heavy vaginal bleeding with large clots and ass ciated crampy lower abdominal pain, this is a strong indication of misca riage, however it is vital to confirm this diagnosis with βhCG and sca findings as history alone can never give a conclusive diagnosis.

Examination

Examination includes speculum, vaginal, and bimanual assessment.

Note whether the cervical os is open or closed, the presence of an products of conception, any discharge/odour, cervical ectropion, cervic polyp, cervical tumour, amount of bleeding, including colour and flo (clotted, etc.).

If products of conception are visible in the os, their careful removal wi often alleviate the pain and bleeding.

The HCA also has the important role of monitoring the patients on a trolley or waiting room, if appropriate, again calling the co-ordinator when needed.

The HCA and administrator have the difficult job of keeping the patients informed of expected waiting times and ensuring all patients are seen within a timely manner.

Band 6: senior staff nurse

This group of nurses makes up the main complement of staff in most departments. They will see, assess, and plan the ongoing care of all the patients who attend the EPAU. The ongoing care may include a referral on to the on-call medical team, however approximately 80% of EPAU patients can be managed holistically by the nursing team.

The nurse is responsible for the management of their patient on the day and will follow up their own blood results, make their own referrals, and arrange their own admissions or follow-up appointments.

Although the patient may see a different nurse at each visit due to shift patterns, etc., all care is dictated by structured and clear guidelines, and all documentation is recorded electronically or in notes; this includes any telephone advice given, therefore the patient is assured of consistency of care throughout their patient journey.

All results should be reviewed on a daily basis with the medical staff, to ensure that all patients have a diagnosis or are kept under review until one is made.

Band 7: unit manager

The unit manager also works within the compliment of nursing staff, carrying out the role outlined above. In addition, the unit manager is responsible for the overall management and development of the staff; the overall running of the department, and ensuring adherence to trust-wide and government directives.

Unit consultant

The unit consultant works with the unit manager and team to ensure development and overall smooth running of the department. The unit consultant is involved in the development of guidelines and ensures their implementation by the other hospital gynaecology consultants, nurses, and junior doctors. The unit consultant also plays an important role in the development and support of the EGU team, offering regular teaching, as well as being an accessible source of skilled specialist medical expertise.

Sonographer

In a typical EPAU, the unit sonographer performs the ultrasound assessment and reports the findings to the nurses who explain the findings in detail and organize ongoing care. The benefit of a dedicated sonographer for the department is that they become expert in providing a diagnosis and are sensitive to the sensitive and specific needs and requirements of this patient group.

Many nurses are now undertaking and obtaining scanning qualifications, and in many EPAUs a nurse or doctor will replace or complement the sonographer. In these instances responsibilities will differ.

On-call doctors

The medical team on-call will attend the EPAU when requested. They will be asked to review a patient who perhaps is unstable and needs urgent medical intervention, a patient who may require admission, or a patient who may require a review of medication. The on-call doctors are also extremely useful as they offer immediate access to advice and information when needed by the nurses.

Vaginal and bimanual examination will assess the size of the uterus, identify any localized pain, including cervical excitation (pain on touching and moving the cervix from left to right) that can indicate ectopic pregnancy or adnexal irritation due to other causes. Any masses will also be palpable and noted during bimanual assessment.

Investigations

After history and examination, a scan should be performed (if the gestation is expected to be >6/40) to view an intra-uterine gestation either viable or non-viable. Policies on crown-to-rump length (CRL) measurement and expected foetal heart beats will vary between trusts. If no intra-uterine gestation can be confirmed, serial serum βhCGs taken 48h apart will be needed to confirm the diagnosis and exclude the possibility, however unlikely, of an extra-uterine pregnancy.

Care of women with pain in early pregnancy

Pain in early pregnancy is the second most common reason for women to present to hospital. The most significant concern with this presentation is ectopic pregnancy and this must always be investigated as the priority, regardless of the patient's symptoms or history. There are, however, several possible causes for pain in early pregnancy and frequently the symptom is a result of a normal pregnancy.

If the patient is unstable on presentation and the pain is severe, then an ectopic pregnancy should be assumed and urgent laparoscopy arranged.

Possible causes of pain in early pregnancy

- Ectopic pregnancy.
- Miscarriage.
- Corpus luteal cyst.
- Other ovarian pathology.
- Infection.
- Fibroids.
- Endometriosis.
- Related to vomiting/hyperemesis.
- Constipation.
- Urinary tract infection (UTI).
- Surgical cause.

History

- A thorough history should be taken with regard to the pain presentation: location, duration, type, and contributing factors.
- Any relevant risk factors for ectopic—previous pelvic inflammatory disease (PID), IUD, tubal surgery, as well as any history of gynaecological problems, as listed above.
- Any related vaginal bleeding, constipation, urinary symptoms, or vomiting should be identified.
- Often an answer may appear obvious once a thorough history has been taken; however, it is always vital that once a patient has reported pain in early pregnancy, the location of the pregnancy is quickly and conclusively diagnosed.

Examination

Examination should obtain an overall assessment of the patient condition:

- BP, pulse, temperature, respiratory rate, and oxygen saturation level.
- Urinalysis to confirm pregnancy and exclude infection.
- Pain behaviour.
- Visual assessment of the abdomen to identify any previous surgical scars.
- Gentle abdominal palpation to assess and localize pain, guarding, rebound or masses, and assess the fundal height.
- Bimanual examination should be performed to assess the uterus and adnexa further and also to assess for cervical excitation.
- Speculum assessment should be performed to allow assessment of any vaginal discharge and/or bleeding, and enable swab taking.

It is vital that any palpation of the abdomen is gentle for if an ectopic pregnancy is present, this might rupture by forceful palpation to the area.

Investigations

- BP, pulse, temperature, respiratory rate, and oxygen saturations.
- βhCG and progesterone.
- FBC and Group and Save.
- HVS and endocervical swabs.
- MSU for urinalysis.
- Transvaginal USS—if patient stable and symptoms minimal, await βhCG and perform scan if >1000IU/l.

⚠ However, if patient condition unstable or symptoms severe, but laparoscopy not arranged urgently, then admit the patient and perform scan as soon as possible.

Management

Management will depend on the findings of investigations. Even if a cause is found, such as fibroids or ovarian cyst, it is still vital that the location of the pregnancy be established before discharge.

Treat those conditions that are treatable, such as infections, constipation, hyperemesis; manage conservatively with analgesia those that cannot be treated during pregnancy, such as fibroids.

Miscarriage: definitions and causes

Miscarriage refers to pregnancy loss before 24 weeks gestation, previously referred to as abortion; however, this terminology should be discouraged. Although miscarriage is a major life event, it is rarely life-threatening in the way an ectopic pregnancy can be. Approximately 1 in 4 pregnancies will end in miscarriage, therefore, it will be a common diagnosis within early pregnancy management.

There are many different presentations of miscarriage, these will be outlined further. It is vital, however, that strict protocols are in place that determine the definition of miscarriage. Evacuation should never be performed if there is any doubt about the diagnosis and, therefore, any possibility of viability. Patient certainty of LMP should not be relied upon.

Spontaneous miscarriage

Spontaneous miscarriage refers to the expulsion of the products of conception before 24 weeks gestation.

The causes of spontaneous miscarriage can be divided into maternal and foetal (📖 see Table 15.1 for causes). However, the most common cause is thought to be chromosome abnormality; the incidence of chromosome abnormality increases with maternal age.

Table 15.1 Causes of miscarriage

Foetal causes	Maternal causes
Congenital malformations	Acute febrile illness/infection
Genetic abnormalities	STI
Multiple pregnancies	Trauma or injury to the abdomen
	Antiphospholipid syndrome
	Clotting disorders
	Diabetes
	Hypertension
	Hypothyroidism
	Hormonal irregularity such as PCOS
	Abnormality of the uterus such as fibroids
	Cervical incompetence
	Smoking, alcohol, drugs
	Extreme stress can be a contributing factor but it is not known whether isolated stress can cause miscarriage

Complete miscarriage

This refers to a miscarriage where all the products of conception are expelled and none retained.

Bleeding is normally minimal at the time of diagnosis, but, heavy PV bleeding with clots and abdominal pain would have been experienced prior to the presentation.

A diagnosis of complete miscarriage at first presentation or first scan must always be confirmed with a falling βhCG level; otherwise, if no intra-uterine pregnancy has ever been confirmed, an ectopic pregnancy cannot be excluded without βhCG confirmation.

Incomplete miscarriage

This refers to a miscarriage when some of the products of conception are retained in the uterine cavity.

Missed miscarriage (delayed miscarriage)

This refers to a pregnancy that has failed but has not yet been expelled from the uterus. This may be an empty gestation sac (sometimes referred to as a blighted ovum), a gestation sac with a yolk sac that does not develop further, or a foetus with no foetal heart activity.

Recurrent miscarriage

This is when a woman has had three consecutive miscarriages.

The causes are most commonly:

- Antiphospholipid syndrome.
- Clotting disorders.
- Abnormality of the uterus, such as fibroids.
- Cervical incompetence.
- Hormonal irregularity, such as PCOS.
- Maternal medical complication such as diabetes.

Molar pregnancy

This refers to a pregnancy affected by gestational trophoblastic disease (GTD). GTD can be categorized into complete, partial, or invasive hydatidiform mole or choriocarcinoma.

- Molar pregnancy is rare, occurring in approximately 1.5:1000 UK pregnancies.
- Molar pregnancy is characterized by either a generalized or localized swelling of the villous tissue, diffuse or focal trophoblastic hyperplasia, without embryonic tissue in a complete mole or with embryonic tissue for a partial mole.
- Maternal age and a previous history of GTD are risk factors for molar pregnancy. There is some evidence that suggests a 'possible' link between GTD and the dietary habits of different ethnic groups.
- There is some suggestion that maternal blood groups could be a factor in the incidence of GTD. Women with blood group A are more likely to have a molar pregnancy than those with blood group O.

Miscarriage: assessment and diagnosis

It is very important that a miscarriage is not diagnosed on history or symptoms alone. Any patient presenting to hospital with pain or vaginal bleeding in a pregnancy that has not yet been identified as certainly intra-uterine on USS, the possibility of an ectopic pregnancy must always be conclusively excluded.

⚠ Nothing can be assumed, everything must be proved.

For instance, a patient may present at 7 weeks gestation reporting heavy vaginal bleeding with associated crampy abdominal pain. However, this patient may be miscarrying a demised twin and still retain a viable foetus; this patient may also be experiencing a resolving haematoma, again retaining a viable foetus. Therefore, investigation in conjunction with examination and history is the only safe and reliable method of reaching a diagnosis.

Assessment

Assessment should begin with a thorough history taking, specifically relating to the presenting symptoms, duration and type of bleeding, discharge, and/or pain. Questions should explore LMP and normal cycle, identify when a positive pregnancy test was performed, whether the pregnancy was planned and if the pregnancy is a result of failed contraception. Past parity should be ascertained, as should a full past medical history with specific reference to gynaecological problems.

Examination

- Examination should obtain an overall assessment of the patient condition.
- BP, pulse, temperature, respiratory rate, and oxygen saturation level.
- Urinalysis to confirm pregnancy and exclude infection.
- Visual inspection of bleeding on pad or sheet.
- Pain behaviour.
- Visual assessment of the abdomen to identify any previous surgical scars.
- Gentle abdominal palpation to assess and localize pain, guarding, rebound or masses, and assess the fundal height.
- Bimanual examination should be performed to assess the uterus and adnexae further, to assess the cervix as open or closed, and also to assess for cervical excitation.
- Speculum assessment should be performed to allow assessment of bleeding, to identify any products of conception being passed, to visually assess the cervix as open or closed, and to identify any vaginal discharge and enable swab taking.

Investigations

- BP, pulse, temperature, respiratory rate, and oxygen saturation.
- FBC, Group and Save, βhCG, and progesterone.
- MSU for urinalysis.
- HVS and endocervicval swabs.
- TV USS to assess the uterus, location and viability of the pregnancy. If the pregnancy is <6 weeks gestation await βhCG result, as scan will most likely be inconclusive if <1000IU/l.

Diagnosis

Delayed miscarriage

- Foetal pole of 6mm or more with no foetal heart activity. Absent foetal heart movements should be confirmed by two qualified operators.
- Empty gestational sac with mean sac diameter of 20mm or more.
- Gestational sac with yolk sac that has not changed in appearance at rescan at least 1 week later.

Incomplete miscarriage

- If the pregnancy has previously been seen on scan and now only RPOC are seen.
- If retained products of conception (RPOC) are seen on scan and failed pregnancy is confirmed with significantly falling or static βhCG levels when repeated over 48h.

Complete miscarriage

- If the pregnancy has previously been seen on scan and now an empty uterus is seen.
- If the patient has had a previous positive pregnancy test that has been verified and now presents with a negative pregnancy test following an episode of PV bleeding.
- If an empty uterus is seen on scan with significantly falling βhCG levels over 48h.

Molar pregnancy

- Normally described as visible cystic changes on scan, sometimes a 'snow storm' appearance is noted.
- Typically the βhCG will be higher than expected for the gestational age.
- Conclusive diagnosis of molar pregnancy is only obtained through histological confirmation.

Miscarriage: treatment

There are three options: expectant, medical, and surgical. It is very much the woman's preference and the circumstances that will influence the decision, although there are sometimes medical reasons to advise one management over the other.

Expectant management

Expectant management is when the patient decides to wait for the miscarriage to complete naturally without any intervention. It is likely to be successful in symptomatic women. If expectant management is chosen, it is important the patient is given information about how to access medical help in the instance of severe symptoms, and to agree a time-scale of review of management. For advantages and disadvantages 📖 see Table 15.2.

Table 15.2 Expectant management

Advantages	Disadvantages
Likelihood of infection is lower than with surgical management.	Patients will not be able to know when the miscarriage will complete.
Symptoms are similar to those experienced with medical management, although without the occasionally reported side-effects to the medication.	Uncertainty of the expected unpleasant symptoms often dissuades the woman from choosing this option.
Does not require an inpatient stay.	Can be very unpredictable.

If the demised foetus is very large (CRL >45mm), then expectant management would not be advised.

Medical management

Medical management can be offered to women who wish to avoid surgery but want to know when the miscarriage will occur.

Medical management can also be offered to women when the foetus is too large for an ERPC; however, in this instance the procedure must be performed as an inpatient. The usual regimen is a combination of the anti-progesterone mifepristone followed 36–48h later by a prostaglandin. There is agreement that a dose of 200mg mifepristone is appropriate, higher doses are likely not to confer any major advantages.

Medical management is suitable in the following patients:

- Does not want or not progressing with expectant management.
- Prepared and capable of self-administering misoprostol vaginally (not necessary if managed as inpatient).
- No contraindications to mifepristone or misoprostol.
- Observations within normal limits.
- Possibility of molar changes has been excluded through USS.

The women must be thoroughly counselled in the method of medical management with clear information about expected symptoms, and fully consented for medical management by a doctor.

Clear instruction must be given to the patient for administration of misoprostol vaginally.

Patient should be reviewed and rescanned 10 days later.

The prescription should be given to the patient for:

- 800μg misoprostol per vaginum (PV).
- Paracetamol and dihydrocodeine PRN (as required).

Surgical management

Table 15.3 Surgical management

Benefits	Disadvantages
Rapid	Requires GA
Predictable	Risk of cervical trauma
Woman does not experience miscarriage	Risk of perforation
Karyotype is possible	Requires admission

Surgical management is evacuation of retained products of conception (ERPC). Dependent on the gestation and the amount of retained products on scan, the cervix can be primed with a prostaglandin.

⚠ Surgery is the only option when molar pregnancy is suspected, to ensure the products can be sent to histology. Other determinants will be patient choice, failure to progress with conservative or medical management, or unsuitability for conservative or medical management.

An ERPC will sometimes be necessary if the patient presents with heavy bleeding and the condition is unstable. For advantages and disadvantages, 📖 see Table 15.3.

Care of women with miscarriage

Women attending the EPAU with any problem in early pregnancy will undoubtedly be concerned about the possibility of miscarriage. Every woman will respond to the threat of miscarriage individually, although in the majority of cases the emotional response will be that of bereavement. Regardless of whether a pregnancy was wanted or planned, the woman's emotional response will be her own and no assumptions should ever be made on this matter.

The incidence of miscarriage in the UK is about 1 in 4 pregnancies. The majority of women who experience a miscarriage are surprised by this statistic. Reassurance should be offered that miscarriage is common and recurrence is rare.

It is important that information given during the care pathway of the woman being investigated for miscarriage is honest and factual throughout. As full an explanation as possible about the management and diagnosis should be given to the patient and partner, and exploration of any possible causes should not be avoided, although they are rare to find. If a treatable cause is found, then referral and management should be arranged.

Recurrent miscarriage

The standard definition for recurrent miscarriage is three consecutive miscarriages under 20/40 gestation with foetuses weighing less than 500g, normally with the same partner. Recurrent miscarriage occurs in 1–2% of women of child bearing age.

Assessment is primarily through:

- History of pregnancy losses, whether first- or second-trimester loss, determine any cause and/or association for the pregnancy loss. Neural tube defects, bicornuate uterus, was any cytogenetic analysis carried out.
- Detailed menstrual history important as PCOS can be associated with recurrent miscarriages.
- Past gynaecological history of subfertility followed by miscarriages is relevant.
- Full medical history.
- Personal and family history of thrombosis to assess possibility of inherited thrombophilias.
- Social history—of caffeine intake, smoking, alcohol, cocaine, cannabis, other drugs relevant, as have been associated with recurrent miscarriage.
- Investigations include:
  - Chromosomal karyotype from both parents and/or foetal products.
  - Maternal blood for lupus anti-coagulant and anti-cardiolipin antibodies. Two tests are required 6 weeks apart, as viral infections are known to cause false-positive results.
  - Maternal blood for inherited thrombophilias.
  - Consider hysterosalpingogram and/or ultrasound to assess fibroids, bicornuate uterus, cervical incompetence, and ovaries for PCOS.

If an abnormality is found this can be offered as a probable diagnosis for the cause of the recurrent miscarriages. However, if no abnormality is found, as is often the case, a diagnosis of unexplained recurrent miscarriage is given.

Causes

- 90% of women with this condition will be unable to maintain a pregnancy without medical intervention and management.
- Anti-phospholipid syndrome accounts for approximately 15% of women who have been investigated for recurrent miscarriage.
- Chromosomal abnormality accounts for approximately 5% of women who have been investigated for recurrent miscarriage.
- Cervical incompetence is often diagnosed in later pregnancy losses, where the weight of the developing pregnancy is not supported by a cervix weakened, often through multiple pregnancies, colposcopy treatments, or other surgical interventions.
- Clotting disorders appear to be more prevalent in women who experience recurrent miscarriage.
- Anatomical uterine abnormality, such as large uterine fibroids or subseptate uterus, can be associated with recurrent miscarriage.

Treatments

Treatments for recurrent miscarriage, as with any other condition, will depend on the diagnosis of cause.

If chromosomal abnormality is discovered, then a referral should be made to a geneticist.

Those patients found to have lupus anti-coagulant or anti-phospholipid syndrome are now regularly treated with low-dose aspirin daily, combined with subcutaneous heparin throughout the pregnancy, as this has been shown to be effective in RCTs.

If cervical incompetence is diagnosed, then a cervical suture can be considered. The effectiveness of the suture is likely to be determined by whether it is placed transabdominally or transvaginally. This is normally inserted around 14/40 pregnancy gestation and remains *in situ* to term.

Immunotherapy paternal leucocyte transfer has been subjected to multiple RCTs and has not been shown to be effective.

If no cause for recurrent miscarriage is found, many women find complementary therapies helpful, particularly when related to relaxation and reduction of stress. Counselling, hypnotherapy, and acupuncture are widely recognized as helpful for managing this diagnosis.

Resources

Rai, R and Regan L (2006) Recurrent miscarriage. *Lancet* **368**: 601–611.

Royal College of Obstetricians and Gynaecologists (RCOG) (2006) The management of early pregnancy loss (25) October.

Royal College of Obstetricians and Gynaecologists (RCOG) (2003) The investigation and treatment of couples with recurrent miscarriage (17) May.

www.earlypregnancy.org.uk

www.ectopic.org.uk

www.miscarriageassociation.org.uk

Ectopic pregnancy: definition, assessment, diagnosis, and causes

Definition

An ectopic pregnancy is the diagnosis given for any pregnancy that is extra-uterine. They can be ovarian, cervical, or intra-abdominal, but the majority of ectopic pregnancies will be located in the fallopian tube.

In rare cases an intra-uterine pregnancy will have a co-existing ectopic pregnancy (heterotopic pregnancy). The incidence is 1:7000.

The incidence of ectopic pregnancy is about 1 in 200 in the UK; however, this is quickly rising with the increased prevalence of STIs, particularly chlamydia.

Assessment

The classic presentation of a patient with an ectopic pregnancy is amenorrhoea and pain, and/or bleeding. It is a one-sided abdominal pain that is sharp and worsening, sometimes with associated shoulder-tip pain (indicating blood may have tracked to the diaphragm and stimulated the phrenic nerve), and sometimes with ongoing dark PV spotting.

With increasing expertise in diagnosing ectopic pregnancy, it is actually quite rare to find this historically classic presentation associated with a diagnosis of ectopic. It is, therefore, important that women who present to hospital with either pain or bleeding—no matter how these symptoms are described—or a risk factor for ectopic (see below) is present, then an ectopic is always a considered diagnosis until it has been conclusively excluded.

History taking

Assessment should include a thorough history taking, identifying any risk factors for ectopic pregnancy.

Risk factors for ectopic:

- Previous ectopic.
- History of chlamydia or PID.
- Failed oral contraceptive pill or IUD.
- Endometriosis.
- Pelvic surgery.

Tests

Blood pressure and pulse rate can indicate vascular instability, most commonly if the ectopic has ruptured and intra-abdominal bleeding is occurring.

A positive urine pregnancy test directs the possible diagnosis towards ectopic.

Examination

Speculum examination is useful to assess any bleeding and obtain chlamydia and gonorrhoea swabs. With increasing use of self-taken vulvovaginal swabs and urine PCR for chlamydial screening, there may be less need for speculum examination.

Bimanual examination performed gently will allow assessment for cervical excitation, localized tenderness, rebound tenderness, guarding, and possible masses. Examination must be gentle, as palpation has a risk of association with tubal rupture.

Blood should be taken for βhCG and progesterone, full blood count (FBC), and Group and Save. A transvaginal ultrasound scan should be performed as soon as possible.

Diagnosis

Serum βhCG

This is produced by the trophoblast and in a normal intra-uterine pregnancy it reaches peak levels at 9 weeks gestation.

- βhCG levels will normally double every 48h in a viable intra-uterine pregnancy.
- In a miscarriage the level will fall.
- In a delayed miscarriage, βhCG will remain static.
- In an ectopic the level normally increases but does not double. However, there are exceptions to this rule, with approx 15% of ectopic pregnancies exhibiting a doubling in serum βhCG level.

Progesterone level

- A progesterone level below 20nmol/l normally indicates a failing pregnancy.
- Above 60 normally indicates an ongoing pregnancy.
- Between 20 and 60 generates slight concern for an ectopic pregnancy. However, it is quite possible to have a failing or ongoing ectopic pregnancy, therefore progesterone is a useful addition to the assessment process, not a definitive marker.

FBC

This is useful for assessing the Hb, which may indicate bleeding and possible rupture of an ectopic.

USS findings

With a βhCG of >1000 it is expected that a gestational sac (GS) will be visible on USS; this indicates there is probability of an intra-uterine pregnancy. However, unless a yolk sac (YS) is also identified, it is important not to exclude the possibility of a pseudo-sac presentation. Therefore, unless a GS and YS are both seen, an ectopic pregnancy cannot be truly excluded. Due to a variety of assays and reagents used, there is no agreement on a particular discriminatory zone level.

The adnexae

This should also be assessed during an USS, noting any masses. If an adnexal foetal heart/yolk sac is seen, it is diagnostic of ectopic pregnancy. Presence of free fluid in the pouch of Douglas is a pointer to an ectopic pregnancy.

A large proportion of ectopic pregnancies will be diagnosed by either blood results or scan indication. With accessibility of services and increased knowledge, a large proportion of ectopic pregnancies are treated before they reach the level of rupture or the size of visibility on scan.

A suboptimal elevation of βhCG over 3 or 4 readings is often able to direct towards a diagnosis of ectopic pregnancy.

As already stated, a βhCG of >1000 with no evidence of an intra-uterine gestation sac is diagnostic of ectopic pregnancy, even though often the adnexae will be reported as normal. Exceptions to this may be if the patient has experienced heavy bleeding directly before the scan, whereby a complete miscarriage may also be a diagnosis, βhCG levels should be used to confirm this diagnosis.

Causes

There are several risk factors that may predispose a woman to an ectopic pregnancy.

Once the ovum is fertilized, it reaches the uterus in approximately 5 days. The ovum is normally fertilized within the fallopian tube. The trophoblast is, however, able to implant before it reaches the uterus, therefore anything that obstructs or delays the fertilized ovum in its journey along the fallopian tube, will result in an ectopic pregnancy.

Often, however, the cause of an ectopic pregnancy is unknown and no risk factors are identified.

PID

The most common and accepted cause of ectopic pregnancy is pelvic inflammatory disease (PID). This is a broad term to cover upper genital tract infection, such as endometritis, salpingitis, and oopheritis. These infections usually spread from the vagina or cervix through the uterine cavity. Many different organisms can cause PID but approximately 80% are a result of an STI, usually chlamydia or gonorrhoea. PID causes tubal damage and subsequently interrupts the passageway of a fertilized ovum through the fallopian tube, often resulting in ectopic pregnancy.

📖 See Chapter 8, p.167.

Failed oral contraception

Failed oral progestogen-only emergency contraception is another widely known cause for ectopic pregnancy. Progestogen works by creating hostile cervical mucous, and by making the endoemtrium thin and atrophic, preventing sperm transport and fertilization.

Failed IUD

Pregnancy that occurs with IUD *in situ* is also a cause of ectopic pregnancy. Implantation in the uterus is prevented by the contraceptive device, therefore alternative implantation sites are chosen.

Endometriosis

This can cause narrowing of the tube, it can also cause adhesions that can cause alterations to the tubal structure as well as tubal damage. Pelvic surgery can also lead to adhesions.

Other causes

- Previous caesarean section can sometimes lead to an ectopic pregnancy within the scar.
- There may be congenital malformation of the reproductive organs, resulting in problems with implantation.
- There is some suggestion that as the fallopian tube is under hormonal control, with the cilia activity increasing after ovulation, this could suggest the reason for a notable increased incidence of ectopic pregnancy when the woman has had treatment for subfertility.
- Finally, contra-lateral implantation is a suggested cause of ectopic pregnancy. The theory being that the fertilized ovum may be carried from one ovary towards the opposite tube, the journey therefore taking longer, allowing the trophoblast to develop further and seek implantation before the uterine cavity can be reached. In this instance the ectopic pregnancy will be on the opposite side to the corpus luteum.

Ectopic pregnancy: expectant and surgical management

Once ectopic pregnancy is diagnosed, the method of management has to be decided. There are three main categories of management, expectant medical, and surgical (see Table 15.4).

Table 15.4 Categories of management

Expectant	Surgical	Medical
Monitoring hCG	If unstable	Must be stable
Decreased admissions	Can be laparoscopy or laparotomy	Must commit to follow up
No risk of surgery	Removal of ectopic from tube or removal of tube	Needs monitoring βhCG
Open access, if pain increases	Hospital stay	Contraindications as below
May progress to surgical if βhCG not falling	GA required	Multiple hospital visits

Expectant management

Some ectopic pregnancies can be treated conservatively if a tubal abortion is expected. However, close monitoring of these patients with serum βhCG is needed as even a failing ectopic pregnancy can rupture. Close monitoring of the patient and beta βhCG levels is important.

Surgical management

The clinical picture determines the need for surgical management. If the patient presents haemodynamically compromised, in shock, collapsed with a positive pregnancy test, immediate resuscitation and surgery is required.

If the patient is clinically stable, then further diagnostic measures can be used, alongside patient preference, to determine between surgical expectant and medical management of ectopic pregnancy.

Surgical management is in the form of laparoscopy and removal of ectopic pregnancy. This can be by salpingostomy, if the ectopic pregnancy is located near the fimbria, but most commonly salpingectomy. The evidence that conserving the tube confers any advantage in terms of the woman's future fertility is poor, but, it is clear that it increases the risk of a future ectopic pregnancy.

Criteria for surgical management

- If the ectopic has ruptured and the patient is severely compromised, then laparotomy may be required, although this is rare.
- If a live ectopic pregnancy is seen on scan, surgical management is always necessary.
- The presence of free fluid indicates potential rupture of an ectopic pregnancy, it also excludes suitability for medical management.
- Due to the length of follow-up required, and inability to pursue another pregnancy for at least 3 months after completion of medical management, patient choice will also often lean towards surgical rather than medical management of ectopic pregnancy.

Ectopic pregnancy: medical management

If an ectopic pregnancy is diagnosed early, and the diagnosis falls within specified criteria, the option of medical management can be given. However, if the patient is in a significant amount of pain, this option will be inappropriate.

Methotrexate is an established and effective treatment option in this instance. In addition, it is specifically indicated where conservative tubal surgery has failed. Patient selection and thorough counselling are vital.

Protocols will differ between hospital trusts so outlined below is an example of a protocol.

What is methotrexate?

It is a drug that interferes with cell growth and will prevent the ectopic pregnancy-related tissue from growing. Although the manufacturer's licence does not specify use in ectopic pregnancy, it is effective, and used widely for this purpose as an unlicensed preparation.

Methotrexate is effective in about 90% of cases. Most women only require a single dose but, on occasions, a second dose is required.

Criteria for medical management

- The patient must be clinically stable with no active bleeding.
- An ongoing intra-uterine pregnancy must be excluded.
- Adnexal mass of <4cm.
- Absent foetal heart activity.
- NO haemoperitoneum.
- βhCG <5000IU/l (can be given up to 15,000IU/l with consultant agreement).
- Patient consent to medical management, which involves several weeks weekly follow-up.
- NO acute infection.
- NO severe anaemia.
- NO renal or liver impairment.
- NO active peptic ulcer or colitis.
- NO blood disorders.
- NO active pulmonary disease.
- NO immunodeficiency.

Administration

- Appropriate dose prescribed by consultant.
- Anti D immunoglobulin to be prescribed, if patient is rhesus-negative.
- Patient to be counselled and supportive literature given.
- Written consent obtained.
- Patient height and weight.
- Methotrexate 50mg/m^2 given intramuscular (IM). An appropriate method to convert to surface area must be used and great care must be taken when calculating the dosage level.
- Information leaflet to be sent to GP.

Follow-up with medical management

- The patient should be advised to return immediately if she experiences significantly worsening abdominal pain, dizziness, collapse, or heavy vaginal bleeding.
- Separation pain can be expected between days 2 and 6. However, surgery should be considered with careful clinical assessment if the patient reports pain following methotrexate administration.
- The patient will return for a βhCG on day 7 and this should decline by at least 15%. If not, then a second dose will be needed.
- Patient to avoid sunlight, alcohol, vitamins including folic acid, aspirin, NSAIDs, and sexual intercourse.
- Patient must use adequate contraception for at least 3 months after treatment is completed and advised of a 1:10 chance of a future ectopic pregnancy.
- The patient should be monitored with weekly βhCG levels until non-pregnant levels are reached and the woman advised that risk of haemorrhage remains until this has been achieved.

Psychological care in early pregnancy loss

Miscarriage should be considered as bereavement for the woman and her partner, regardless of how early the pregnancy was or whether the pregnancy was planned or not. It should not be expected that the patient will not have any psychological needs surrounding her miscarriage just because the pregnancy was unwanted.

Women will display a wide variety of reactions to miscarriage: some will be demonstrably devastated, others will seem completely unfazed by the news, while others may appear relieved.

It is important not to simply accept the initial response from the patient and possibly ignore her psychological needs. Often a dismissive response will be a coping strategy or defence mechanism employed by the patient at the moment of receiving the news. It is very common in all stages of emotional response for the response and reaction to evolve over a length of time as the news is fully absorbed and dealt with.

A woman who may have voiced her intention to terminate the pregnancy will then feel she does not deserve sympathy or compassion once a miscarriage is diagnosed. In reality this woman may only be able to draw support from healthcare professionals, as the reason for the planned TOP may have been lack of support or inability to disclose information about the pregnancy to anyone else.

Healthcare professionals are responsible for ensuring that they adopt a non-judgemental approach to all women who experience miscarriage and address their psychological needs without presumption and with compassion.

The woman receiving news of a miscarriage within the EPAU setting will often need practical information about the management of the miscarriage; options should be discussed, as appropriate. On occasions the patient may be too upset to approach these decisions and it is important that the option be given to call back and discuss the options at a later time. Written literature is very useful in this instance and should be supplied for all women, including information about emotional responses to miscarriage and details of local and national support groups.

The woman and her partner will almost always ask why this has happened to them and it is important to be honest, you must approach any possible causes factually and practically, with advice and management planning, as appropriate. Frequently the patient or her partner will believe it is a result of their actions and it is extremely important to allow them time to voice any concerns that you can then address and, in most cases, dispel.

Women can be referred to either the Ectopic Trust or to the Miscarriage Association for help, support, and factual information.

Chapter 16

Care of the woman in emergency gynaecology units

Heavy vaginal bleeding

Within gynaecology, heavy vaginal bleeding is one of the most common reasons a woman will attend as an emergency. Some hospitals have emergency gynaecology units; in others, patients will be seen in A&E or within the ward environment. Pregnancy, and therefore miscarriage, should always be ruled out as a cause of heavy bleeding (📖 see Chapter 15, p.415).

Possible causes outside pregnancy

Common

- Idiopathic.
- Fibroids.
- Adenomyosis.
- Endometriosis.
- Trauma.
- Haematoma formation after surgery.

Less common

(More likely to present with IMB as opposed to heavy bleeding.)

- IUD
- Endometrial polyps.
- Infection.
- Malignancy.
- Ineffective hormone therapy.
- Systemic—liver diseases, renal, coagulation disorders, anticoagulant therapy.

Assessment

⚠ It is first important to ensure that the patient is stable; therefore, the level of bleeding and whether the patient is haemodynamically compromised should be determined before all else.

Frequently a patient will present with heavy vaginal bleeding, which, on assessment, is not clinically 'heavy'. The bleeding may be heavy relative to the patient's expected menstrual flow and, therefore, deemed as an emergency by the patient for this reason. It is important to confirm that the bleeding is vaginal and not from the urinary tract or the rectum.

Begin by taking a thorough history from the patient, with specific reference to the nature of the bleeding, flow, duration, and any related symptoms, such as offensive discharge or abdominal pain.

History taking should also include a thorough exploration of any recent or previous gynaecological problems or surgery, or other medical problems or drug intake. Any other symptoms being experienced should be noted, whether considered relevant by the patient or not.

A sexual history should be taken with investigation as to possible recent trauma or exposure to an STI.

Examination should achieve an overall assessment of the patient's condition:

- BP, pulse, temperature, respiratory rate, and oxygen saturation level to assess if they are decompensating.
- Urinalysis to exclude infection and a pregnancy test.
- Assess bleeding, flow, consistency, colour, presence, and type of clots.
- Visual assessment of the vulva and vagina.
- Assessment of pain, if any.
- Abdominal examination to identify any previous surgical scars, distension, visible masses.
- Gentle abdominal palpation to assess and localize any pain, guarding, rebound, or palpable masses.
- Vaginal speculum examination to fully assess bleeding, identify site of bleeding, identify any discharge, and take swabs, as needed; assess the cervix and identify any visible polyps.
- Bimanual examination should be performed to assess the uterus and adnexa and assess for cervical excitation.

Investigations

- FBC and Group and Save.
- Consider clotting studies.
- HVS and endocervical swabs.
- USS preferably once bleeding stopped to allow appropriate and accurate assessment of the endometrium.
- Consider hysteroscopy and endometrial biopsy, again to be performed once bleeding controlled.
- Urgent examination under anaesthesia may become necessary.

Management

The priority should be to stabilize the patient and minimize the bleeding. IV access should be obtained on arrival in the department in case of deterioration. Observations should be monitored closely and recorded if bleeding is heavy.

The patient must be stabilized, then managed either as an inpatient or an outpatient.

Treatment will depend on the history, assessment, and diagnosis.

If history and investigations indicate that pharmacological treatment (either hormonal or non-hormonal) is appropriate, then consider the following as outpatient therapies:

- Tranexamic acid, mefenamic acid, or COCP.
- Progestogen therapy, e.g. norethisterone 5mg tds.
- GnRH analogues may be used in selected cases and, sometimes, within the acute setting if the bleeding is very heavy.
- Mirena® intra-uterine system, which can be inserted after the acute episode either in outpatients or in the community.

Once stabilized, refer the patient to GP or outpatient clinic for ongoing management and further investigations, as necessary.

Acute pain

Acute pain is the second problem where women will attend as an emergency. Pregnancy should always be ruled out as a cause. (📖 see Chapter 15, p.415).

Non-pregnancy related causes for acute pain may pose a diagnostic challenge, so a thorough history, examination, and assessment is needed to establish a diagnosis and formulate a management plan. With pain, it is important to remember that it may not be related to gynaecology, and the patient may need to be referred to other specialties.

Possible causes

- Ovarian cyst complication.
- Ovarian torsion.
- Ovulation pain (mittelschmerz).
- Acute PID with salpingitis, pyosalpinx.
- Fibroid degeneration.
- Torsion of a pedunculated subserous fibroid.
- Trauma.
- Endometriomas/endometriosis.
- Misplaced or recently inserted IUS/IUD.
- Post-operative complication.
- Surgical cause.
- Bowel related—IBS, constipation, diverticular disease.
- Urinary tract related—UTI, cystitis, renal colic.

Assessment

Begin by taking a thorough history, with specific reference to the nature of the pain, site, duration, and any exacerbating factors.

History taking should also include a thorough exploration of any previous gynaecological problems or other medical problems, also any other symptoms being experienced should be noted, whether considered relevant by the patient or not.

Examination should obtain an overall assessment of the patient's condition:

- BP, pulse, temperature, respiratory rate, and oxygen saturation level, if indicated.
- Urinalysis to exclude pregnancy and infection.
- Assessment of response to pain.
- Visual assessment of the abdomen to identify any previous surgical scars.
- Gentle abdominal palpation to assess and localize pain, guarding, rebound, or masses.
- Bimanual examination should be performed to assess the uterus and adnexa further and also to assess for cervical excitation. This is elicited by moving the cervix from side to side, which disturbs the adnexal organs and overlying peritoneum, resulting in acute sharp pain.
- Speculum assessment should be performed to allow assessment of any vaginal discharge and/or bleeding, and enable swab taking.

Investigations

After the initial observations, as outlined above, investigations should include:

- High vaginal and endocervical swabs and/or complete infection screen.
- Pregnancy test.
- MSU to exclude UTI.
- FBC and CRP.
- Transvaginal ultrasound scan.

Management

Management will depend on the diagnosis. However, in all cases of presentation with acute pain, pain should be controlled as quickly as possible, IV access should be obtained in case of deterioration, and the patient should remain nil-by-mouth (NBM) until stabilized.

Post-operative problems

Post-operative problems present in a variety of ways, specific to the procedure itself. The most helpful method of obtaining a speedy diagnosis is to obtain the theatre notes to identify the exact procedure undertaken. However, there are some common problems such as:

- Pain, e.g. haematoma, infection, bowel complication.
- Excessive or erratic bleeding, e.g. secondary haemorrhage.
- Wound breakdown/dehiscence.
- Suspected infection.
- Collection or haematoma.
- Non-resolution of the original problem.
- Urinary retention.
- Chest infection.
- DVT/PE.
- UTI.
- Suture problems.

Investigations should be related to the symptoms and procedure. The management of the problem will depend on the diagnosis.

🕮 See Post-operative complications, p.332.

Chapter 17

Fertility and subfertility

Preconceptual care

Before planning a pregnancy, couples should assess their lifestyle, health, and fitness. Factors such as unhealthy diet, smoking, drug abuse, and lack of exercise can cause harm to an unborn child. An emphasis should be made for both male and female partners to improve their general well-being.

Body weight

Couples are advised to maintain a well-balanced diet with regular exercise. Couples should aim to have an acceptable body mass index (BMI).

$$\text{BMI} = \frac{\text{Body weight (kg)}}{\text{Height x Height (m)}}$$

An individual is considered to be obese if BMI >30. Obese women should seek dietetic advice prior to conceiving, as being overweight may cause obstetric complications (📖 see Chapter 20, p.525).

Underweight women may experience amenorrhoea and anovulatory cycles. Women with low BMI are at risk of miscarriage and premature delivery.

Smoking

It is advisable to stop smoking prior to conceiving, as smoking is toxic to sperm function and egg quality. Women who smoke are at risk of miscarriage, premature delivery, and low birth-weight babies (📖 see Chapter 20, p.525).

Alcohol

Couples are advised to stop alcohol consumption prior to conceiving. Alcohol, especially binge-drinking, has a profound effect on sperm function and may cause sexual dysfunction, including impotence. In women, alcoholism may cause ovulatory disorders and amenorrhoea. Heavy drinking is associated with low birth-weight, serious birth defects, and is the main cause of foetal alcohol syndrome (📖 see Chapter 20, p.525).

Recreational drugs

Recreational drugs can inhibit ovulation, affect tubal function, and semen quality. These drugs also endanger the baby's health, may cause miscarriage, and premature delivery.

Folic acid

Women are advised to take folic acid prior to conception and continue up to 12 weeks gestation, as this reduces the risk of having a baby with neural tube defects (NTD). The daily requirement is 0.4mg. A higher dose (5mg) is advised if women are in a high risk group e.g. on anti-epileptic medication, have had a previous pregnancy affected by NTD, coeliac disease, diabetes, or sickle cell anaemia.

Rubella

Women are advised to have vaccination against rubella (German measles) prior to conceiving. They are advised to see their GP for rubella screening to ensure they are immune. Non-immune women are advised to use contraception for 1 month post-vaccination, due to a small theoretical teratogenic risk as it is a live vaccine.

Cervical screening

Women are advised to have cervical cytology in accordance with the national screening programme guidance. Abnormal smears can cause delay in starting fertility treatment.

Inherited disorders

Couples should be offered screening for inherited disorders, such as sickle cell anaemia and thalassaemia.

Age

Female fecundity rapidly declines with advancing age. This is primarily related to diminished ovarian reserve.

Resources

Department of Health (2002) *Alcohol and health. Drinking sensibly.* Food Standards Agency Publications.

Psychological effects and counselling for subfertility

Subfertility, the investigations, and the treatments can cause psychological stress, anxiety, and depression.

Stress in male and female partners:
- has an impact on the relationship;
- may reduce libido and hence frequency of intercourse.

Inability to conceive can be a traumatic experience. Accepting childlessness is emotionally and psychologically very difficult, especially for some couples from certain backgrounds, as there is pressure to procreate.

Couples need support from each other, family, and friends to cope with their subfertility and childlessness.

Couples should be given information on fertility support groups and offered counselling.

Counselling

The Warnock Report (1984) recognized the need for provision of counselling for couples undergoing fertility treatments.

The need for counselling is stated in the HFEA Code of Practice (1991). This specifies the types of counselling available to patients:
- Implications counselling: aims to help the person to understand how the implications of the proposed treatment will affect them individually, as a couple, their family, and any child born as a result of the treatment.
- Support counselling: aims to give emotional support at any time, particularly post-failed treatment.
- Therapeutic counselling: aims to enable patients to cope with the consequences of subfertility, focusing to resolve the effects of subfertility.

The British Infertility Counselling Association defines counselling as:

'A process through which individuals and couples are given an opportunity to explore themselves. Given this opportunity, couples will often change their perspectives, become less stressed, and be in a better position to make more informed decisions for the future. The counselling should assist the patient to learn and grow from the past, to live in the present and be better equipped to deal with the future.'

The counsellor should 'demonstrate a capacity for offering support, non-judgemental acceptance and unconditional respect within a confidential relationship.'

Resources

British Subfertility Counselling Association (1990) *Counselling: guidelines for practice*. BICA, London.
Human Fertilization and Embryology Act (1991) Code of Practice. HFEA, London.
Warnock Report (1984) *Report of the committee of inquiry into fertilization and embryology*. HMSO, London.

Useful support groups for patients:
Donor conception network: www.dcnetwork.org
Daisy network: www.daisynetwork.org.uk
Human fertilization and embryology authority: www.hfea.gov.uk
www.subfertilitynetworkuk.com

Male and female factors affecting subfertility

1:6 couples in the UK are estimated to experience difficulty in conceiving.

Definitions

Subfertility: inability to conceive within 1 year of regular unprotected intercourse.

Primary subfertility: couples who have never conceived.

Secondary subfertility: couples who have previously conceived, regardless of pregnancy outcome.

Main causative factors

Male factors

- Causes of male subfertility may be idiopathic, congenital, iatrogenic, or genetic (📖 see p.456).

Female factors

- Anovulation (📖 see p.454).
- Tubal disease/damage.
- Endometriosis (📖 see p.136):
  - Associated with subfertility and pelvic pain. Endometriosis can also contribute to tubal damage.
  - Mild degree considered equivalent to unexplained subfertility.
  - If the patient is symptomatic with pelvic pain, treat endometiosis medically or surgically, prior to embarking on fertility treatment.
  - Ablation of endometriosis and removal of endometriotic cysts is recommended prior to fertility treatments.
- Uterine abnormalities:
  - Subfertility is associated with the presence of endometrial polyps, submucous fibroids, intra-uterine adhesions and uterine septae.
  - The management of the above is with hysteroscopic surgery (📖 see p.128).
- Unexplained subfertility (📖 see p.466).

Resources

Hull, MG, Glazener, CM, Kelly, NJ, Conway, DI, Foster, PA, Hinton, RA *et al.* (1985) Population study of causes, treatment, and outcome of subfertility. *British Medical Journal* **291**: 1693–1697.

Royal College of Obstetricians and Gynaecologists (RCOG) (1992) *Subfertility: guidelines for practice*. RCOG Press, London.

Anovulation

- Ovulatory disorders account for 30% of subfertility in women.
- Women present with amenorrhoea (absence of periods) or infrequent periods (oligomenorrhoea).

The cause of anovulation determines the treatment. Some causes are unsuitable for ovulation induction.

Causes

- Hypothalamic–pituitary failure and dysfunction.
- Ovarian failure (see Chapter 6, p.99).
- Hyperprolactinaemia.
- Hypothyroidism.

Hypothalamic-pituitary failure/dysfunction

- Hypogonadotrophic hypogonadism: women experience amenorrhoea, with low levels of gonadotrophins. It accounts for 10% of ovulatory disorders and the commonest causes are excessive exercise (exercise-related amenorrhoea), being underweight (weight-related amenorrhoea), and stress.
- Kallman's syndrome: X-linked, congenital lack of gonadotrophin-releasing hormone. Women present with amenorrhoea and anosmia (loss of sense of smell).
- Idiopathic.
- Sheehan's syndrome: hypopituitarism and hypogonadotrophic hypogonadism caused by infarction of anterior pituitary, usually after severe post-partum haemorrhage.
- Cerebral radiotherapy: for tumours affecting the pituitary or hypothalamus.
- Craniopharyngioma (cerebral tumour arising in the craniopharyngeal pouch).
- Hypophysectomy (excision of pituitary gland).

Ovarian causes

- Women often present with amenorrhoea or oligomenorrhoea.
- Commonest cause is polycystic ovarian syndrome (PCOS), which accounts for 70% of anovulatory subfertility. Women present with hirsutism, acne, and infrequent menses. It is associated with an excess of androgen production within the ovaries. Some women with PCOS are obese. Women have normal follicule stimulating hormone (FSH), may have raised leuteinizing hormone (LH) or testosterone (see Chapter 6, p.99).
- Premature ovarian failure, also known as premature menopause. The condition is irreversible. Women have raised FSH and low oestradiol levels and hence may experience menopausal symptoms. The only treatment option available is IVF treatment with egg donation. (See Chapter 6, p.99.)
- Can be idiopathic.
- Radiotherapy or chemotherapy to the ovaries can also result in ovarian failure.
- Surgical removal of the ovaries.

- Chromosomal abnormalities: the commonest genetic abnormality is Turner's syndrome.
- Androgen-insensitivity syndrome, previously known as testicular feminization.

⚠ Women in this group are unsuitable for ovulation-induction treatment, except women with PCOS.

Hyperprolactinaemia

- Women present with amenorrhoea or oligomenorrhoea. Some experience galactorrhoea.
- Have raised prolactin levels.
- Commonest cause is pituitary adenoma. Micro- or macro-adenoma, depending on the size of the tumour. They are invariably benign tumours that are detected by MRI. Macro-adenomas impinge on optic chiasma and hence some patients experience visual disturbances. These patients must have a visual field study.
- Medication: psychiatric drugs may induce raised prolactin levels.

Hypothyroidism

An insufficiency of thyroid secretion.

Investigations for anovulation

- Check body mass index (BMI).
- Endocrine profile of LH, FSH, oestradiol, testosterone, thyroid stimulating hormone (TSH), prolactin, and progesterone.
- Pelvic ultrasound scan.
- Karyotype.
- MRI of pituitary.

Management of anovulation

Only specific causes can be treated.

Hypothyroidism Corrected by thyroxine replacement. Ovulation may occur spontaneously once TSH is normalized.

Ideal BMI

- Overweight women (BMI >30) with PCOS should be advised on weight loss. A dietetic referral may be helpful.
- Underweight women (BMI <20) should be advised on weight gain. Fertility treatment should not be initiated until BMI is within the normal range.

Hyperprolactinaemia Treated with bromocriptine or cabergoline. Prolactin levels should be checked. Once prolactin levels normalized, regular menstrual cycles and ovulation occurs in 70–80% of women.

Ovulation induction treatment (📖 see p.468).

Resources

Rowe, PJ, Comhaire, FH, Hargreave, TB and Mellows, HJ (1997) *WHO manual for the standardized investigation and diagnosis of the infertile couple.* Cambridge University Press, Cambridge.

Male subfertility

Affects approximately 30% of subfertile couples.

Causes of male subfertility

May be idiopathic, congenital, iatrogenic, or genetic. Occupational and environmental factors also affect sperm function.

Sexual dysfunction

Erectile dysfuction can be caused by beta blockers, thiazide diuretics, and metoclopramide. Men with erectile failure are usually treated with sildenafil.

Occupational factors

Exposure to heat, radiation, and chemicals (herbicides, pesticides) can damage sperm production.

Drugs—medical and recreational

Alcohol and cigarette smoking, as well as marijuana, cocaine, and anabolic steroid abuse have a deleterious effect on sperm function. Impaired spermatogenesis can be caused by sulfasalazine, methotrexate, and nitrofurantoin.

Semen analysis terminology

- Normozoospermia: normal semen parameters.
- Aspermia (anejaculation): no ejaculate.
- Asthenozoospermia: reduced sperm motility.
- Azoospermia: absence of sperm in seminal fluid.
- Necrozoospermia: non-viable or non-motile sperm.
- Oligozoospermia: reduced sperm count:
  - Mild–moderate oligozoospermia: 5–20 million/ml of sperm.
  - Severe oligozoospermia: <5 million/ml of sperm.
- Oligoasthenoteratozoospermia: reduced count, reduced motility, and increased abnormal sperm.
- Teratozoospermia: increased abnormal sperms.

Azoospermia

- Caused by testicular failure, hypogonadotrophic hypogonadism, or testicular obstruction.
- Hypogonadotrophic hypogonadism:
  - identified by low LH, FSH, and testosterone levels;
  - treated with gonadotrophin-releasing hormone (GnRH) pump or gonadotrophin injections.
- Obstructive azoospermia:
  - Men have normal spermatogenesis (process by which sperm are produced), normal size testes, and normal hormone profile.
  - On examination, if neither of the vas deferens are palpable, diagnosis of congenital bilateral absence of vas deferens (CBAVD) is made.
  - Majority of men with CBAVD carry cystic fibrosis mutation.
  - Epididymal obstruction can be caused by sexually transmitted infections such as *chlamydia trachomatis* or gonorrhoea. Blockages may also be due to tuberculosis.

- Non-obstructive azoospermia:
  - Majority cases of non-obstructive azoospermia are idiopathic.
  - Chemotherapy or radiotherapy.
  - Crypto-orchidism (undescended testes).
  - Klinefelter's syndrome (47, XXY karyotype).
  - Y-chromosome microdeletions.

Men should have testicular exploration or surgical sperm retrieval. Sperm retrieved can be frozen for use in *in vitro* fertilization (IVF) treatment with intra-cytoplasmic sperm injection (ICSI). Surgical sperm retrieval should only take place in centres that have a sperm-freezing facility.

The options for men with no sperm are donor insemination or adoption.

- Severe oligoasthenoteratozoospermia:
  - Main cause idiopathic.
  - Can also be caused by chronic prostatitis.
  - Occasionally due to genetic abnormality.

The treatment option is IVF with ICSI.

Resources

Hirsh, AV (1999) Investigation and therapeutic options for the infertile men presenting in assisted conception units. In: Brinsden, PR (ed.) *In-vitro fertilization and assisted reproduction* (2nd edn). Parthenon, London.

Rowe, PJ, Comhaire, FH, Hargreave, TB and Mahmoud AMA (2000) *WHO manual for the standard investigations, diagnosis and management of the infertile male.* Cambridge University Press, Cambridge.

Tubal factor

Tubal disease accounts for 20–35 % of subfertility.

Causes of tubal damage

Pelvic infection

This is the main cause of tubal damage. Can be caused by sexually transmitted diseases, especially *chlamydia trachomatis* and gonorrhoea, termination of pregnancy, puerperal sepsis, insertion of intra-uterine contraceptive device, and pelvic tuberculosis.

Chlamydia trachomatis

📖 See Chapter 8, p.167.

- Accounts for almost 50% of acute pelvic inflammatory disease (PID).
- Most common sexually transmitted infection (STI) in UK.
- Often undiagnosed as patients are asymptomatic.
- Can cause salpingitis and consequently tubal damage and peritubal adhesions.
- Can cause pelvic pain, ectopic pregnancy, and subfertility.

Gonorrhoea

In 30–50% of women both chlamydia and gonorrhoea can co-exist.

Pelvic tuberculosis

Can cause tubal blockage, tubo-ovarian abscesses, or frozen pelvis.

Endometriosis

Can cause pelvic adhesions and may affect fimbrial mobility.

Surgery

- Previous laparotomy may contribute to tubal damage.
- Post-sterilization: some women wish to conceive after this, especially if they enter a new relationship.

Diagnosis of tubal disorders

Hysterosalpingo-contrast sonography (HyCosy)

A simple outpatient procedure using ultrasonography, which is tolerated well by women. An echocontrast fluid is introduced into the uterine cavity using a catheter. The patency of the fallopian tubes and ovarian morphology can be assessed. The use of transvaginal ultrasonography avoids radiation exposure. Sonography can also occasionally aid in detecting hydrosalpinges. HyCosy is unsuitable for women who have a history of sexually transmitted infections, pelvic inflammatory disease, past ectopic pregnancy or termination of pregnancy, and previous gynaecological surgery.

Hysterosalpingogram

An outpatient procedure, performed in the X-ray department to assess the uterine cavity and tubal patency.

Selective salpingography

A relatively new technique. It is diagnostic and can be therapeutic. Can be useful in patients with proximal tubal damage. A guided wire and catheter is passed along the tube to overcome obstruction. This procedure is not helpful for patients with distal tubal damage.

Laparoscopy and dye test

A day-surgery procedure performed under general anaesthesia. It enables assessment of the pelvic cavity, tubal status, and can also detect endometriosis. It is the 'gold standard' test. Laparoscopy is suitable for women who are experiencing gynaecological symptoms, such as pelvic pain or dysmenorrhoea, and can be combined with hysteroscopy. Laparoscopy can also be used in the treatment of conditions such as endometriosis.

Laparoscopy and dye test is an injection of methylene blue (methylthioninium chloride) through the cervix to assess whether the dye reaches the peritoneal cavity indicating tubal patency. It also allows assessment for conditions such as endometriosis.

Prevention of tubal damage

The patients should be screened for chlamydia before carrying out invasive procedures.

Management

- A small % of women with tubal damage may conceive naturally, but may have an increased risk of ectopic pregnancy.
- The suitability of tubal surgery depends on the extent of tubal damage.
- If tubal damage is mild—tubal microsurgery, e.g. laparoscopic adhesionolysis can be performed.
- For extensive tubal damage—IVF treatment is the best option.
- If hydrosalpinges is present, this compromises IVF treatment outcome and hence salpingectomy is recommended.
- IVF treatment is superior to tubal surgery, as it is associated with better pregnancy outcome.

Resources

Hull, MGR and Fleming CF (1995) Tubal surgery versus assisted reproduction: assessing their role in subfertility therapy. *Current Opinion in Obstetrics and Gynaecology* **7**: 160–167.

Tests and investigations: female partner

Clinical assessment

Factors to consider:

- Menstrual cycle history: amenorrhoea or oligomenorrhoea? ovulatory?
- Age of patient and partner.
- Duration of infertility, subfertility.
- History of pelvic inflammatory disease or previous STIs.
- Previous ectopic pregnancy.
- Previous pelvic or tubal surgery.
- Gynaecological symptoms; dyspareunia, dysmenorrhoea.
- Body mass index.

Blood tests

Baseline gonadotrophin profile:

- Luteinizing hormone (LH).
- Follicle stimulating hormone (FSH).
- Oestradiol.
- LH:
  - Performed in early follicular phase (days 2–4 of menstrual cycle).
  - Result: a normal LH level should be similar to the level of FSH (this is normally <10mIU/l).
  - LH>FSH may be indicative of polycystic ovarian syndrome.
- FSH:
  - Performed in early follicular phase (days 2–4 of menstrual cycle).
  - Result: >10mIU/l indicates reduced ovarian reserve—counsel women accordingly.
  - >15mIU/l indicates ovarian failure—advise IVF treatment with egg donation.
  - <5mIU/l indicates hypothalamic/pituitary problems.
- Progesterone:
  - Performed in mid-luteal phase of cycle (day 21 of 28-day cycle).
  - Result: >30nmol/l confirms ovulation; <30nmol/l confirms anovulation.

⚠ Test not indicated if history of amenorrhoea or oligomenorrhoea.

- Testosterone:
  - Performed randomly.
  - Result: >2.5nmol/l indicates polycystic ovaries; >5nmol/l indicates congenital adrenal hyperplasia.
- Prolactin:
  - Performed randomly.
  - Result: >1000mIU/l repeat assay to confirm hyperprolactinaemia, pituitary adenoma; may need MRI.

⚠ Test not indicated if regular menstrual cycles.

- Thyroid stimulating hormone (TSH):
  - Performed randomly.
  - Result: ↑TSH indicates hypothyroidism.

⚠ Test not indicated if regular menstrual cycles.

- Rubella screen:
  - Result: if non-immune, advise immunization and contraception for 1 month post-vaccine.

Further investigations

Chlamydia trachomatis screening

If positive:

- treat with antibiotics;
- screen male partner and treat accordingly;
- refer to GUM.

Transvaginal pelvic ultrasound scan

- Confirms polycystic ovaries.
- Presence of endometrial polyp.
- Presence of fibroids.
- Congenital abnormalities.

CT pituitary/MRI

If ↑ prolactin confirms pituitary adenomas.

Karyotype

- Indication: primary amenorrhoea.
- Confirms chromosomal abnormalities:
  - Turner's syndrome (45, X).
  - Androgen-insensitivity syndrome (46, XY).

Tubal patency tests

- HyCosy.
- HSG.
- Laparoscopy.

📖 See Tubal factors, p.458.

Resources

Balen, AH and Jacobs, HS (2003) *Infertility in practice* (2nd edn). Churchill Livingstone, London.
Royal College of Obstetricians and Gynaecologists (1998) Evidence based clinical guidelines. Initial investigations and management of the subfertile couple. RCOG Press, London.

Tests and investigations: male partner

Male partner should be assessed by a clinician specializing in reproductive medicine or an andrologist.

Clinical assessment

History taking

- Coital frequency.
- Erectile or ejaculatory problems.
- Past illnesses.
- Testicular maldescent, torsion, or orchidopexy.
- Previous urogenital surgery.
- History of sexually transmitted infections.
- Chemotherapy or radiotherapy.
- Family history of cystic fibrosis, genetic conditions.
- Occupation details.
- Drug history (medical and recreational).
- Recreational habits (alcohol intake).

Physical examination

- Facial and body hair distribution.
- Testicular size: length and volume measured by orchimeter.
- Check for undescended testes, check for presence/absence of vas deferens.

Normal semen analysis

- Volume: 2–5ml.
- Sperm concentration: >20 million/ml.
- Motility: >50% should be motile, grades a) rapid and b) slow.
- Morphology: >15% normal forms.

Semen sample should be produced by masturbation. Recommend abstainence from coitus for 2–3 days prior to submitting sample. If initial sample abnormal, repeat after 6 weeks.

Further tests

- Hormone profile: LH, FSH, testosterone, and prolactin.
- Atrophic testes, elevated FSH levels, and low testosterone levels indicate testicular failure.
- For men with non-obstructive azoospermia or severe oligozoospermia, arrange chromosome analysis (karyotype) to diagnose Klinefelter's syndrome or Y-chromosome microdeletions.
- For men with CBAVD, arrange cystic fibrosis screen. Female partner should also have a CF screen as they may carry a cystic fibrosis mutation.
- Scrotal ultrasound scan.
- Testicular biopsy.

General advice for men

- Reduce alcohol intake. Avoid binge-drinking.
- Stop smoking. Avoid use of recreational drugs.
- Regular intercourse (x 2–3 per week).
- Avoid chemicals (herbicides, pesticides), radiation, and heat at work.
- Wear boxer shorts. Avoid tight trousers.
- Avoid hot baths.

Resources

Hirsh, AV (1999) Investigation and therapeutic options for the infertile men presenting in assisted conception units. In: Brinsden, PR (ed.) *In-vitro fertilization and assisted reproduction* (2nd edn). Parthenon, London.

Rowe, PJ, Comhaire, FH, Hargreave, TB and Mahmoud AMA (2000) *WHO manual for the standard investigations, diagnosis and management of the infertile male.* Cambridge University Press, Cambridge.

Role of the fertility nurse specialist

A fertility nurse specialist is a qualified nurse or midwife who provides a holistic approach to fertility investigation, treatment, and, where appropriate, early pregnancy through compassionate, informed, and evidence-based practice, of which research plays a fundamental part. Fertility nurse specialists work as part of a multi-professional team consisting of doctors, nurses, embryologists, counsellors, administrative staff, and others, who combine to deliver a high standard of care.

Investigations and causes of subfertility

- Use knowledge of the reproductive system to identify normal and abnormal structure and function.
- Use knowledge of a wide range of possible causes of male and female subfertility to undertake appropriate investigations and discuss treatment options. These include: tubal damage, endometriosis, polycystic ovarian syndrome (PCOS), ovarian failure, uterine abnormalities such as bicornuate uterus, and male factor subfertility.
- Support client and partner through appropriate investigations and discussion of treatment options.
- Establish and maintain systems for privacy and confidentiality at all times with clients and their partners.
- Provide clients with information regarding the range of fertility investigations available. These include:
  - women: hormone blood tests checking FSH, LH, testosterone, prolactin, thyroid function, laparoscopy, and dye/hysterosalpingogram, antral follicle count;
  - men: semen analysis and, where appropriate, the above endocrine profiles.
- Enable clients to make an informed choice.
- Perform vaginal ultrasound scan to undertake uterine assessment; ovarian position and description; identify anatomical landmarks; normal and abnormal pathology.

Treatments

- Undertake a range of treatments including ovulation induction (OI), donor insemination (DI), intra-uterine insemination (IUI), and *in vitro* fertilization (IVF).
- Manage treatment cycle and monitor progress under supervision.
- Manage post-operative care and follow-up.
- Ensure best practice in relation to handling of gametes and embryos.
- Explain to clients the rationale behind choice of drugs and treatment process, and educate with regards to safe injection technique.
- Undertake aspects of clinical role, including: patient consultation and consent completion, performing baseline scans, follicular tracking, early pregnancy scanning, assisting at oocyte retrieval, performing donor insemination, intra-uterine insemination, and embryo transfer.
- Manage follow-up procedure post-insemination for DI, IUI, or IVF.
- Provide appropriate care based on an awareness of aetiology of ovarian hyperstimulation syndrome (OHSS), its causes, and treatment.

Guidelines and counselling

- Ensure policies and procedures reflect the requirements of Human Fertilization and Embryology Authority (HFEA), and other relevant bodies.
- Understanding and implementation of RCOG guidelines; HFEA regulations; and Healthcare Commission National Standards.
- Maintenance of accurate documentation.
- Provide basic emotional support for client(s), appropriate to their needs and care.
- Use basic counselling skills, from an informed knowledge-base, with patients/clients.
- Recognize situations where referral to independent counselling services may be appropriate.
- Use knowledge of basic embryology, implantation rates, psychological effects of treatment failure, miscarriage, ectopic pregnancy, etc., to appropriately support the individual when providing information and implication counselling.
- Demonstrate knowledge of consenting procedures and legislation relating to specific consent for investigation/treatments.
- Awareness of range of pharmaceutical products used in the management of subfertility.
- Advise clients in an appropriate manner demonstrating an understanding of the legislation in relation to surrogacy and adoption.

Unexplained subfertility

- Couples should be referred for subfertility investigations after trying to conceive for 1 year.
- Couples are usually diagnosed to have 'unexplained subfertility' after excluding tubal, male, and ovulatory factors, and no other abnormality has been found.
- Accounts for 25–28% of couples referred for investigations.

On completion of investigations, treatment options are discussed with couples. Some options are influenced by age of female partner and conception delay.

Options

1. Await spontaneous conception: this is usually expectant management and couples find this very frustrating.
2. Ovulation induction treatment (📖 see p.469) using clomiphene citrate; 3–6 cycles are offered.
3. Super-ovulation and intra-uterine insemination treatment (📖 see Intra-uterine insemination, p.472).

Options 2 and 3 are usually used as intermediate options.

4. IVF treatment (📖 see *In vitro* fertilization, p.474).

IVF treatment, first option if female partner >35 years or history of subfertility of >3 years.

Resources

Hull, MG, Glazener, CM, Kelly, NJ, Conway, DI, Foster, PA, Hinton, RA *et al.* (1985) Population study of causes, treatment, and outcome of subfertility. *British Medical Journal* **291**: 1693–1697.

Ovulation induction

Ovulation-induction treatment options are based on the cause of anovulation. The aims are to achieve ovulation and to increase the chance of conception. Before initiating treatment ensure:

- women have BMI 20–30;
- women have had a tubal patency test;
- male partners have had a semen analysis.

Medical treatments

Pulsatile gonadotrophin-releasing hormone (GnRH).

- Recommended for women with hypogonadotrophic hypogonadism.
- GnRH is administered subcutaneously through an infusion pump; a bolus dose of GnRH released at 90-minute intervals.
- Patients are monitored by follicle tracking (serial transvaginal pelvic ultrasound scans).
- Treatment usually leads to unifollicular ovulation.
- Conception rate 20–30% per cycle.

Clomifene citrate

- Used mainly for women with PCOS.
- Anti-oestrogen treatment, acts by blocking oestrogen receptors, inducing release of FSH, stimulating the ovary to develop a few follicles.
- Patients are monitored by follicle tracking or serum progesterone assay.
- Dosage: 50mg orally taken daily from day 2 to day 6 of menstrual cycle (spontaneous or induced cycle). If cycle ovulatory, continue with same dose for three cycles.
- If anovulatory, increase dose to 100mg.
- 70% of women with PCOS will ovulate.
- 40–60% conception rate at 6 months.
- Side-effects of clomifene are hot flushes, mood swings, abdominal distension, visual disturbances, ovarian hyperstimulation.
- Incidence of twins is approximately 10%, triplets 1%.
- Recommend total of 6 cycles.

Metformin

- Many studies have reported that metformin improves menstrual regularity and restores ovulation in women with anovulatory PCOS.
- Metformin reduces insulin and free testosterone.
- Metformin can be used in conjunction with clomifene.
- Dosage: initiate at 500mg daily for a week, then twice daily for a week, then three times daily.
- Patients warned of risk gastro-intestinal side-effects.

⚠ Metformin is unlicensed for ovulation induction treatment.

Gonadotrophin injections

- Treatment with follicle-stimulating hormone.
- Indicated for women with hypothalamic-pituitary causes of anovulation and women with PCOS who are clomifene-resistant.
- Injections administered subcuatneously, of recombinant FSH starting on day 2 or 3 of the menstrual cycle (spontaneous or induced cycle).
- Women monitored by follicle tracking.
- Dosage is incremental subject to follicular response.

⚠ Patients should be warned of ovarian hyper-stimulation syndrome (OHSS) and multiple pregnancy.

With GnRH pump, clomifene, or gonadotrophin-injection treatment, HCG injection to induce ovulation can be administered when a lead follicle measuring 18–20mm is seen.

Surgical induction—laparoscopic ovarian drilling

- Laparoscopic ovarian drilling has replaced ovarian wedge resection in women with PCOS.
- Indicated for anovulatory PCOS in women who are clomifene-resistant.
- At laparoscopy, 4–6 punctures are made in each ovary.
- 80% of women achieve ovulation, 56% achieve pregnancy within 1 year post-operatively.
- Post-operative complications: small risk of pelvic adhesion formation, risk of ovarian tissue destruction if many punctures are made.
- Reduces risk of OHSS and multiple pregnancy.

Resources

Balen, AH and Jacobs, HS (1994) A prospective study comparing unilateral and bilateral laparoscopic ovarian diathermy in women with the polycystic ovary syndrome. *Fertility & Sterility* **62**: 921–925.

Hamilton-Fairley, D, Kiddy, D, Watson, H, Sagle, and, Franks, S (1991) Low dose gonadotrophin therapy for induction of ovulation in 100 women with polycystic ovary syndrome. *Human Reproduction* **6**: 1095–1099.

Homburg, R, Armar, NA, Eshel, A, Adams, and, Jacobs, HS (1998) Influence of serum luteinising hormone concentration on ovulation, conception and early pregnancy loss in polycystic ovary syndrome. *British Medical Journal* **297**: 1024–1026.

Assisted conception

Assisted conception is a term used to describe the methods available to help subfertile couples to become pregnant when they are having difficulty in conceiving. Subfertility is failure to conceive after 1 year of unprotected regular intercourse. Within the NICE guidelines,[1] subfertility is defined as failure to conceive after regular unprotected sexual intercourse for 2 years in the absence of known reproductive pathology.

NICE guidelines recommend that people who have not conceived after 1 year of regular unprotected sexual intercourse, should be offered further clinical investigations.

For pregnancy to occur, each month, a woman develops an egg in one of the ovaries in a small sac of fluid called a follicle. The egg is released from the ovary and passed down one of the fallopian tubes, which are attached to the uterus (womb). For pregnancy to occur, sperm, which has been deposited in the vagina during intercourse, has to swim towards the egg in the fallopian tube. This is when fertilization occurs.

The fertilized egg (embryo) begins to develop as it travels through the fallopian tube towards the uterus. After about 5 days, the embryo hatches out of its outer coating (zona pellucida) and buries itself (implants) in the lining of the uterus, where it begins to grow. This is the beginning of the pregnancy.

One in six couples take longer than a year of regular, unprotected sexual intercourse to become pregnant. Assisted conception may be needed if:
- the woman's ovaries do not produce an egg each month;
- there is a blockage in the fallopian tubes; or
- there are problems with the sperm.

Assisted conception—types
- IUI: intra-uterine insemination.
- IVF: *in vitro* fertilization.
- ICSI: intra-cytoplasmic sperm injection.

1. NICE (2004). Fertility: assessment and treatment for people with fertility problems. Clinical Guideline ☞ www.nice.org.uk (Accessed April 2009.)

Intra-uterine insemination (IUI)

This type of treatment is offered to a couple if there is evidence that the female partner's fallopian tubes are patent and:

- there is unexplained fertility;
- the female partner does not regularly release an egg—called anovulation—often due to polycystic ovarian syndrome (PCOS);
- there are very mild abnormalities of the sperm;
- retrograde ejaculation;
- ejaculatory failure.

In the absence of sperm from the male partner, donor sperm may be used. If the couple opt to use donor sperm, they are required by law to have received counselling about the implications. Under the regulations of the HEFA, only 10 pregnancies can result from one donor.

If the female partner does not normally ovulate, clomifene tablets or follicle-stimulating hormone injections are used to stimulate the ovaries to produce one or two follicles (📖 see Ovulation induction, p.468). However, the injections may produce more than two follicles.

For women with normal ovulation, the use of ovulation-stimulating medication may be an option; this may improve the chances of becoming pregnant.

The woman is monitored regularly with a vaginal ultrasound scan to count and measure follicles. The aim is to get 1–3 follicles, with a lead follicle measuring more than 17mm in order to make a decision as to whether to go ahead with the IUI procedure.

⚠ If the patient over-responds and produces 4 or more follicles, the cycle will be cancelled.

When the lead follicle is identified, an injection of chorionic gonodotrophin (human chorionic gonadotrophin, HCG) is given to mature these follicles, so that the eggs are released. The IUI is timed 24–36h after administering the chorionic gonadotrophin (human chorionic gonadotrophin, HCG) injection.

The male partner will be advised when to bring his sperm sample to the lab, where it is prepared and the sperm is separated from the seminal fluid. Motile sperm is used for this procedure.

The procedure will be explained fully to the couple with written and verbal information and consent forms signed. During the procedure, a thorough identification check is performed in the presence of the patient and medical staff. The aim is to confirm the patient's identity to ensure these match with the sperm sample and the signature.

The procedure

- This is a clean procedure in a sterile environment.
- The patient is assisted into the dorsal lithotomy position.
- The speculum is inserted and the cervix cleansed with normal saline.
- Sperm is loaded in the syringe.
- The catheter is inserted into the cervical os and advanced.

- The syringe with the sperm is attached to the catheter and the sperm are expelled slowly depressing the syringe plunger fully.
- After this procedure, the catheter is removed slowly after waiting 30–60 seconds.

Women need to be aware that:

- The risk of multiple pregnancies is 5–10%.
- There is a small risk of infection at the time of the procedure.
- There is no guarantee that a pregnancy will result.
- Should a pregnancy be established (as in natural conception), there is a small risk of miscarriage, ectopic pregnancy, and foetal abnormality.

In vitro fertilization (IVF) and intracytoplasmic sperm injection (ICSI) treatment

In vitro fertilization is sometimes called 'test-tube baby' treatment. During IVF, sperm and eggs are placed together in a culture dish to allow fertilization to occur in the laboratory. Not every egg will fertilize when mixed with the sperm, so in order to increase the chances of success, hormones have to be used to stimulate the ovaries.

In an ICSI cycle, an individual sperm is injected into a mature egg then placed in the dish to allow fertilization to occur.

Indications for IVF

- Blocked tubes: where the female partner has blocked fallopian tubes, the eggs and sperm may not be able to meet to allow fertilization. The fertilized egg cannot make its way into the uterus.
- Anouvulation: where the woman is not producing hormones to release eggs.
- Endometriosis: the migration and implantation of endometrial tissue, which forms the lining of the uterus in other parts of the body. This may affect the pelvic region, ovaries, fallopian tubes, uterine muscle, colon, and bladder.
- Unexplained fertility: where no cause has been found for being able to unable to conceive, especially in couples who have been trying for more than three years.
- Sperm defects: IVF can be used where the number of sperm is low, sperm do not move well, or there are high numbers of abnormal sperm.

Indications for ICSI treatment

- Abnormal sperm, decreased numbers, reduced movement, or increased number of sperm with an abnormal appearance.
- A man has no sperm from his ejaculate, but sperm can be obtained from the testicles, using surgical sperm retrieval.
- The male produces high levels of antibodies against his own sperm—this can affect the ability of the sperm to bind to the egg.
- Previous history of IVF treatment with an unexplained failure of the eggs to fertilize.
- The male has retrograde ejaculation—the sperm passes backwards into the bladder and can be found in the urine.

IVF protocols

There are two main protocols often used in IVF treatment: the long protocol and the short protocol.

- The long protocol is preferred for women whose hormones are functioning normally and have regular cycles.
- The short protocol is for those who have increased follicle stimulating hormone (FSH) levels or who have responded poorly to ovarian stimulation in the past. This is best carried out in tertiary centres.

Short protocol

This protocol is known as the boots or flare-up regime. It takes advantage of the natural flare in FSH and LH levels in a woman's cycle around day 2 or 3 of the cycle, which stimulates follicles to develop. A suppression drug, which comes as nasal sprays or subcutaneous injections, is administered from day 2 or 3 of the cycle to prevent premature ovulation. FSH injections will commence on day 2 or 3 after a baseline vaginal ultrasound scan. In contrast to the long protocol, which waits for 14 days to allow down-regulation before starting stimulation drugs, the short protocol prescribes FSH injections the next day. From then the two protocols are the same.

Long protocol

- Down-regulation: the woman's natural hormone production of FSH and LH is temporarily switched off, using medication. The down-regulation can be commenced from day 2 or day 21 of the menstrual cycle. The female partner uses the suppression medication for at least 2 weeks. The suppression drugs are administered either by injections or nasal spray. This allows control of when eggs should be produced and released.
- Down-regulation scan: after 2 weeks of using suppression drugs, the woman is scheduled for a scan to check and confirm suppression. A vaginal ultrasound scan is performed to assess the ovaries for cysts and the lining of the uterus, which should be very thin. If the scan confirms down-regulation, the woman's ovaries are stimulated with FSH hormone injections to produce eggs, and down-regulation continues.
- Monitoring scan: after 9 days of the female partner administering the FSH injections, a vaginal ultrasound scan is preformed to measure how the follicles are developing. The follicles are measured and counted. When there are at least 3 follicles measuring more than 18mm in diameter, the woman is ready to be triggered for an egg collection.
- Egg maturation: when the woman is ready for egg collection, chorionic gonadotrophin (human chorionic gonadotrophin, hCG) is administered and timed 34–36h before egg collection to allow for egg maturation.
- Egg collection: this procedure is performed under mild anaesthetic drugs, hence nothing to eat or drink 6h prior to the procedure. This procedure is preformed under ultrasound guidance. A vaginal probe is placed in the female vagina and a fine needle is passed alongside within a protective cover. The needle is gently passed through the vaginal wall into the nearest follicle in the ovary. The needle is passed from one follicle to the next until all the follicles in one ovary are drained. The needle is then removed and the procedure is repeated in the other ovary.
- Fertilization: the embryologist will examine the fluid from each follicle under the microscope and check for any eggs. As each egg is found, it is placed in special fluid in an incubator. The semen sample is prepared by separating the normal and moving sperm from the ejaculated sample. In an IVF cycle, the prepared sperm sample and eggs are placed together in a dish and left overnight to allow fertilization. In an ICSI cycle, a single sperm is injected into each mature egg, then placed in a dish and left overnight to allow fertilization to occur.

Embryo transfer

The sperm and eggs are examined the next morning to see if fertilization has occurred. A fertilized egg becomes an embryo and embryo development begins with cell division.
- 2 days after fertilization, the embryos should have 2–4 cells.
- 3 days after fertilization, the embryo should have 6–8 cells.

Embryo transfer happens between day 2 and 5 after fertilization. The embryologist will select the best embryos for transfer and discuss this fully with the patient.
- A speculum is inserted into the vagina to clearly see the cervix. It is important to clean any mucous from the cervical canal.
- The embryologist will load the embryos into a small, flexible catheter that will be inserted through the vagina and cervix into the uterus. No more than 2 embryos should be transferred during any one cycle of IVF treatment (NICE guidelines 2004).[1]

► A full bladder makes the procedure technically easier. The bladder lies in front of the uterus, filling up the bladder straightens out the uterus and makes it easier to direct a soft catheter, which contains embryos.
- Once the catheter is inserted in the uterus and is in the best position, the embryos are gently injected.
- The catheter is then removed and checked to make sure the embryo(s) have been replaced.
- The woman is advised to do a pregnancy test sixteen days after egg collection.

Cryo-preservation

NICE recommends that women preparing for chemotherapy or radiotherapy, which is likely to render them infertile, should be advised that preservation of ovarian tissue is still in an early stage of development and oocyte cryo-preservation has limited success. Couples will need extensive counselling to help cope with the stress of the treatment and psychological impact for themselves.

If cryo-storage is undertaken, it should occur before such treatment is started.

Problems associated with assisted conception

Ovarian hyper-stimulation syndrome and ectopic pregnancy are the main problems though sometimes ethical considerations can be paramount

OHSS

Can occur more when gonadotrophin-releasing hormone analogues are used and the woman's ovaries are stimulated such that a large number of follicles are produced. It can occur early after chorionic gonadotrophin (human chorionic gonadotrophin, hCG) administration or late—up to 2 weeks after embryo transfer. Women complain of nausea, vomiting, abdominal pain, distension, leg oedema. In cases of severe OHSS ascites, pleural effusion, and arterial and venous thrombosis can occur.

1. NICE (2004). Fertility: assessment and treatment for people with fertility problems. Clinical Guideline: www.nice.org.uk. (Accessed April, 2009)

In mild cases, increasing fluid intake helps. In moderate cases, hospitalization and thromboprophylaxis should be considered with monitoring of LFTs, FBC, clotting screen, and renal function tests. Severe cases need intensive monitoring with strict fluid-balance recording and drainage of effusions.

Ectopic pregnancies

Following IVF, 4% of pregnancies will be ectopic. It can be picked up early, as ultrasound monitoring is the norm in IVF pregnancies.

Pre-implantation genetic diagnosis (PGD) and ovum donation

PGD

Pre-implantation genetic diagnosis is specialized treatment for couples who carry an inherited genetic defect that could cause serious health risks for their children, such as cystic fibrosis, sickle cell disease, or Huntington's disease.

PGD is used to test embryos for genetic disorders; only embryos without abnormalities can be transferred in PGD IVF/ICSI cycles. On day 3, embryos have divided into 6–8 cells. A single cell can be removed from each embryo to test if the disease affects that embryo. Only unaffected embryos will be replaced in the uterus.

Ovum donation resources

This is performed when a couple wishes to have a child, but the woman's ovaries are no longer able to produce eggs. This is usually due to:

- an early menopause;
- surgical removal of the ovaries;
- radiation treatment or chemotherapy after the diagnosis of cancer in women of child-bearing age;
- gonadal dysgenesis due to Turner's syndrome; or
- simply a result of age.

The donor can be known or anonymous to the recipient. Ideally, she should be under 35 years of age to reduce the likelihood of foetal abnormalities and should have had children. All donors are screened for infectious diseases and genetic disorders before treatment is started. There should be no financial gain to the person donating eggs.

- The egg donor must undergo drug treatment to stimulate her ovaries to produce more follicles, aiming to collect as many eggs as possible on the day of egg collection (📖 see IVF, p.474).
- At the same time, the woman who is to receive the eggs (recipient) must undergo drug treatment to prepare the lining of the uterus to receive embryos.
- The eggs that are collected from the donor are fertilized with the sperm of the partner of the woman who is to receive the eggs (recipient).
- Once the fertilized eggs have developed into an embryo, they are assessed for quality as they grow; and then returned to the recipient.
- Implication: counselling is a must and the donor and recipient must be registered with the Human Fertilization and Embryology Authority (HFEA).

Resources

Balen, AH and Jacobs I (1997) *Subfertility in practice*. Churchill Livingstone.

West, Z (2003) *Fertility and conception the complete guide to getting pregnant*. Dorling Kindersley Limited.

Khalaf Y, Grace Y, Braude P. *The ACU patient information booklet*. Guy's and St Thomas's NHS Foundation Trust.

Adoption and surrogacy

Adoption

Providing a family to children who cannot be raised by their birth parents. This is a legal procedure in England, Wales, and Northern Ireland. Scotland has its own legal proceedings.

Adoption must be through a local or voluntary agency. Agencies must comply with key provisions stated in Adoption and Children Act (2002). The welfare of the child is paramount in all decisions pertaining to adoption.

- Adopters should be over 21 years, there is no upper age-limit as long as adopters have the physical and mental energy to raise children and provide a 'loving home'.
- Applicants will undergo a medical examination.
- Record of offences checked.
- Prospective parents can be from any ethnic background and religion. Agencies make efforts to find a family to match a child's identity.
- Single people, unmarried or married couples, and lesbian or gay couples can also adopt.
- Adopters need to be assessed by social workers. The process can take up to 6 months.
- Adopters need to provide personal references.
- Adopters' applications are considered by the agency's independent adoption panel and informed if approved or not.
- If applications are approved, the agency finds a suitable match for children and adopters.

Adoption agencies advocate open adoption—that adopted children should be brought up with the knowledge that they were adopted.

At age 18 years, adopted children have the right to see their original birth certificate.

Surrogacy

Surrogacy involves a woman carrying a baby for another woman.

Indications for surrogacy:

- Women without a uterus: this could be due to a congenital absence of uterus or due to hysterectomy.
- Women with a history of recurrent miscarriage, who are unable to carry a child to term.
- Women with medical conditions for whom a pregnancy may be life-threatening.

Two forms of surrogacy exist: straight or host.

Straight surrogacy

- Also known as traditional surrogacy.
- Pregnancy is achieved by using surrogate's egg fertilized with intended father's sperm.
- Intended father's sperm is artificially inseminated.
- Some fertility clinics provide help with this.

Host surrogacy

- Also known as gestational surrogacy.
- Pregnancy is conceived through IVF treatment, using intended parents' gametes.

Surrogacy is legal in the UK. The surrogate should not be paid for her services other than 'reasonable expenses'.

Surrogacy is not a legally binding contract. Six weeks post-delivery, intended parents can apply for Parental Order, which enables the couple to have full parental rights over the child and only then does the surrogate lose her rights over the child.

Resources

Adoption and Children's Act (2002): www.opsi.gov.uk

British Association for Adoption and Fostering (BAAF): www.baaf.org.uk

Appleton, T (1994) *Surrogacy—a guide for patients.* Subfertility Support Counselling Presentations, Cambridge.

Voluntary surrogacy organisation in the UK: www.surrogacy.org.uk.

Fertility preservation

Introduction

Nurse specialists working within both gynae-oncology nursing and fertility nursing have witnessed many advances in medical technology that have directly impacted upon the success of treatments offered to patient groups. Fertility preservation is a challenging issue faced by professionals and patients, and creates many ethical and moral dilemmas. Many do not view the potential to preserve fertility as a priority at the time of investigation, diagnosis, and prognosis. This time is stressful, not only for patients but also for professionals, for whom the topic may cause embarrassment to some who do not feel confident in raising the issue with distressed patients.

New developments: gonadal preservation

New developments within gynae-oncology have contributed to increased survival rates for patients. Gonadal-preservation treatments are being improved and introduced into treatment programmes. These include combinations of radiotherapy and/or chemotherapy, which commonly cause gonadal and endocrine disturbances that historically, cause ovarian failure and premature menopause in women, and testicular failure in men. Radiotherapy may also cause gonadal failure both from direct exposure from pelvic or low abdominal treatment, and from the scatter effect, even if the ovaries are outside the field of radiation.

Men may be referred to fertility units to freeze sperm prior to oncology treatments and surgery. Frequently, due to the nature of their illness, the sperm quality is poor and once they have recovered and wish to start a family, they will require IVF with intra-cytoplasmic sperm injection (ICSI) to aid fertilization of eggs. Freezing gametes is more complex for women than men—they are required to undertake IVF treatment in order to freeze embryos or eggs.

IVF

IVF treatment is primarily managed in two key ways, either a short or long protocol, the latter being the more commonly used method in the UK. Unfortunately when treating cancer patients, the speed of diagnosis of malignant disease and the urgency to commence treatment, means that the long-protocol approach is not an option.

IVF combines:

- Super-ovulation.
- Transvaginal ultrasound guided oocyte retrieval.
- Insemination of sperm with an oocyte in the laboratory.
- Fertilization.
- Replacement of embryos.

Super-ovulation

This is achieved with the administration of FSH injections (dosages range from 50 to 350 units), which recruits a cohort of follicles and promotes development and maturation. Purified preparations are delivered subcutaneously via auto-injector by the woman or her partner.

To ensure maturation of the follicles and oocytes, administration of chorionic gonodotrophin (human chorionic gonadotrophin, hCG) is required 35h prior to oocyte retrieval. To establish appropriate management of super-ovulation, and to avoid premature ovulation due to the LH surge, many units incorporate GnRH agonists or antagonists to prevent ovulation. These drugs bind to GnRH receptors on the pituitary gonadotrophins and desensitize the pituitary. The agonists initiate a 'flare response', which will cause a withdrawal bleed in the woman. The antagonists lead to immediate suppression and can be used for a much shorter time-frame. These drugs are administered either by subcutaneous injection or by nasal sniffs.

This process occurs in the first-half of the cycle designed to use stored FSH, which occurs after using a GnRH agonist, which is started on day 2. Then exogenous FSH is started on day 3 of the cycle.

Transvaginal ultrasound guided oocyte retrieval

Women are monitored with transvaginal ultrasound to measure the size of the follicles, which should be approximately 18mm in size, prior to administration of chorionic gonodotrophin (human chorionic gonadotrophin, hCG) and then oocyte retrieval. Generally, lower doses of gonadotrophins are used and the time period is more patient-friendly. These drugs are used to prevent the LH surge and are administered within the first-half of the cycle, following several days of FSH administration. The drug is injected daily from day 5 of the cycle, along with the gonadotrophin. This process provides a shorter treatment time and fewer injections for the woman.

Fertility preservation: alternative treatments

Cryo-preservation of oocytes

This has been researched as a treatment option for fertility preservation. There have been few reported successful treatments with data showing a live-birth rate of 1% per thawed oocyte. Researchers have confirmed that transplanted ovarian tissue may initiate cyclical function after transplantation without vascular anastomosis. Although researchers have demonstrated the possibility of transplantation of frozen thawed ovarian tissue, the survival rates are limited.

Transplantation techniques

Include following approaches. First, orthotopic transplants, where strips are grafted near the infundibulopelvic ligaments or, occasionally, on a post-menopausal ovary. A key component to potential success with transplantation surgery is the vascularization of the site, as decreased blood supply will lead to ischaemia and failure of the graft to function.

Gynaecologists have developed new laparoscopic techniques involving lifting the ovaries higher in the abdominal cavity to reduce the scatter effect of the radiation. Transposition of the ovaries enables surgeons to reposition these organs away from the target site. The non-surgical approach includes concomitant treatment with GnRH analogues (GnRHa). This induces ovarian shutdown and may help to prevent the follicles from reaching a chemotherapy-sensitive stage via suppression of the granulosa cells.

Other alternative treatments

Include donor oocyte programmes, adoption, or surrogacy. They have immense emotional and ethical implications, and require significant counselling, implications counselling, and knowledge of the Human and Fertilization Authority (HFEA) legislation. Surrogacy also provides an alternative method of achieving a family if gonadal function is destroyed by oncology treatment. Adoption provides another option for the woman and her partner if they are unable to achieve a pregnancy with her own eggs following recovery from cancer. All adoptions in the UK have to be managed by an adoption agency, which may either be a local authority agency or voluntary body. Professionals provide implications counselling as they are difficult decisions for people to make.

The Human Fertilization and Embryology Authority (HFEA)

The HFEA is the government body in the United Kingdom which monitors the handling of all gametes and regulates clinics performing treatments using human sperm, eggs, and embryos. The HFEA was created in 1990 by the passage into law of the Human Fertilization and Embryology Act. This was established in response to deep public concern about the implications that new technologies for assisted reproduction might have for the perception and valuing of human life and family relationships. All licensed clinics require a 'person responsible' who has specific responsibilities to insure the condition of the license are carried out.

The role of the HFEA

- Publishes and maintains a code of practice for centres in the United Kingdom carrying out licensed treatment. Any changes in treatment or any reviews and amendments to the code of practice must be communicated and adhered to promptly within individual centres.
- Inspects licences and regulates clinics offering fertility treatment.
- Gives advicse and information to patients, clinics, and doctors.
- Publishes patient information such as *Patients' Guide to IVF Clinics.* Many other booklets are available.

The HFEA code of practice guidelines

- Staff: the code sets out minimum qualifications for staff involved in clinical, scientific, nursing, and counselling services.
- Facilities: it gives a broad guideline on the quality of clinical, laboratory, and counselling facilities that should be available.
- Assessing patients and donors: It gives guidelines on the confidentiality, consideration of the welfare of the child who may be born as a result of the treatment, and any other children who may be affected by the birth.
- Screening of donors.
- Consents: written consents are required for centres to store gametes, to use them for patients' own treatment, or the treatment of other women. The HFEA has issued standard forms for consent both to treatment and to the use of sperm, eggs, and embryos.
- Counselling: must be offered to all patients and donors. This is an HFEA obligation. However, patients are under no obligation to accept it. Donors and recipients must be offered implication counselling prior to treatment.
- Use of gamete and embryos: the code limits the number of embryos that can be transferred in a single IVF/ICSI treatment—it prohibits the transfer of more than three embryos in women under the age 40.
- Storage of gametes and embryos: the code gives guidance on security and safety of storage of gametes and embryos.
- Research: all research on embryos must be licensed by the HFEA and a licence will only be granted if the research is designed to promote advances in the treatment of infertility/subfertility.

- Records: the HFEA must by law keep a confidential register about patients undergoing licensed treatments and about donors. The register was set up in 1991 and has information about children conceived from licensed treatment since that date.
- Complaints: the HFEA requires that all clinics have a procedure for dealing with complaints

Resources

Human Fertilization and Embryology Authority (2007) *Code of practice* (7th edition). Human and Fertilization and Embryology Authority, London.
Balen, AH and Jacobs, I (1997) *Subfertility in practice*. Churchill Livingstone, London.

Chapter 18

Colposcopy

The NHS cervical screening programme (NHS CSP)

The NHS CSP was set up in 1988 when the Department of Health instructed all health authorities to introduce computerized cervical screening call and recall systems and to meet certain quality standards. It invites women who are registered with a GP, although any woman can have a cervical screening test.

Aim

The programme aims to reduce the incidence and mortality rate of cervical cancer by regularly screening all women at risk, so that conditions that might otherwise develop into invasive cancer can be identified and treated. It saves around 4500 lives every year in England.

Who is eligible for screening?

The national recommendations are shown in Table 18.1.

Table 18.1 National recommendations for cervical screening

Age group (years)	Frequency of screening
25	First invitation
25–49	3 yearly
50–64	5 yearly
65+	Only screen those who have not been screened since aged 50 or who have had abnormal tests

Cervical cancer is very rare in women under 25. However, some argue that screening women under the age of 25 may reduce morbidity and allow fertility-preserving treatment.

If a woman has never been sexually active with a man, research evidence shows that her chance of developing cervical cancer is very low. In these circumstances, a woman might choose to decline the invitation for cervical screening.

Coverage and cost

The programme screens almost 4 million women in England each year. Cervical screening, including the cost of treating cervical abnormalities, has been estimated to cost around £157 million a year. The cost per woman screened equates to £37.50.

Cervical screening is funded through the global sum paid to each GP practice monthly in advance and further funding is available for delivering a quality service.

Barriers to uptake of screening

The barriers to uptake of screening include: anxiety related to testing, lack of awareness, mobile populations, fear of loss of privacy and confidentiality, negative coverage in the media, issues of consent in women with severe learning difficulties, and women from ethnic minority groups.

Incidence and mortality rate of cervical cancer

On a worldwide basis it is the second commonest female cancer acknowledging the fact that Third World countries have no screening programme. Half a million women worldwide die of cervical cancer each year. Cervical cancer is the eleventh most common cause of cancer deaths in women in the UK and accounts for 2% of all female cancers.

Is cervical screening effective?

Whilst cervical screening cannot be 100% effective, cervical screening programmes have been shown to reduce the incidence of cancer in a population of women. For the first time ever, death rates from cervical cancer have fallen below 1000, with a recorded 927 deaths registered in 2002. It prevents about 3700 cases of invasive cervical cancer every year in the UK. The effectiveness of the programme can also be judged by coverage of the target population.

Resources

NHS cervical screening programme (2004) *Cervical screening: a pocket guide.*

Sample taking

Liquid-based cytology (LBC)

Liquid-based cytology (LBC) is a new way of preparing cervical cell samples for examination in the laboratory. This has replaced the conventional smear test and there are two different systems used:

- Thin prep: the brush with a green handle is rinsed in the vial and discarded.
- Sure path: the brush with a blue handle is detached and left in the vial.

Steps in taking LBC sample

- The patient is given an explanation of the procedure.
- Prepare all equipment before starting the procedure.
- Note expiry date on the collection vial and do not use expired vial.
- Ensure plastic seal is removed from the lid.
- Complete patient details on the request form and the vial.
- Remove the lid from the vial.
- Use a small amount of K-Y® Jelly and avoid placing the lubricant at the tip of the speculum.
- Insert the central bristles of the cervex brush into the endo-cervical canal and rotate the brush 5 times in a clockwise direction (📖 see Fig. 18.2).
- If using thin prep, rinse the brush by agitating it in the bottom of the vial 10 times forcing the bristles apart. Do not leave the head of the brush in the vial. If using sure path, detach the brush and leave in the vial.
- Tighten the cap so that the black torque line on the cap passes the black torque line on the vial.
- Place the vial and the form in a specimen bag for transportation to the laboratory.

The transformation zone

- Cervical sample is taken from the transformation zone of the cervix.
- Transformation zone is defined as the area enclosed between the original squamocolumnar junction at its outermost margin and the new squamocolumnar junction at its innermost aspect (📖 see Fig. 18.1).
- Colposcopic features of the transformation zone are dependent upon both age and hormonal status.
- Prior to puberty, eversion of the cervix is minimal.
- During pregnancy and oral contraceptive use, greater eversion occurs.

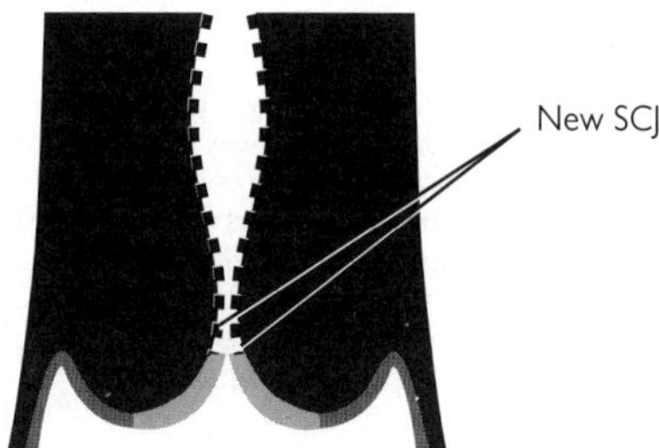

Fig. 18.1 The transformation zone. Adapted with kind permission of BSCCP.

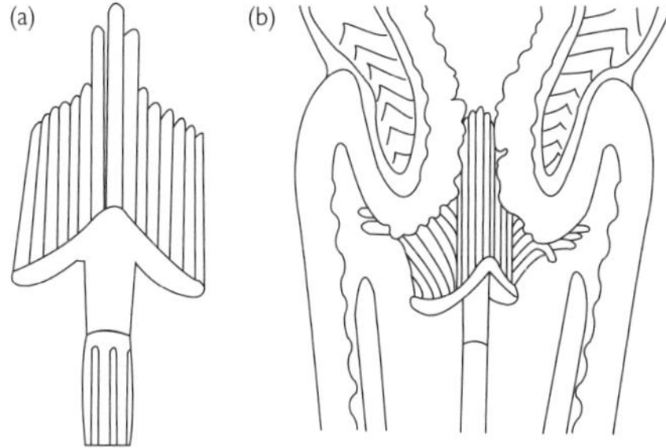

Fig. 18.2 LBC sample taking. (a) The end of a typical Cervex brush,® (b) representation of how to use a typical Cervex brush®. Reproduced from Thomas J and Monaghan T (2007). *Oxford Handbook of Clinical Examination and Practical Skills*, with permission from Oxford University Press.

Colposcopy

Colposcopy is an examination of the cervix using a colposcope. A colposcope is a microscope mounted on a freely movable stand that allows both magnification and illumination of the cervix (📖 see Fig. 18.3). The magnification range is usually between 6- and 40-fold. It allows assessment of the cervix to establish the extent and severity of any cervical abnormality, to determine appropriate treatment, and to allow biopsy for histological diagnosis and/or treatment, as required. It was first described by a German gynaecologist called Hans Hinselmann in 1925.

Informed consent

A woman is given informed choice/consent prior to the procedure. Informed consent involves understanding the nature and purpose of the intervention; intended and unintended side-effects; risks, harms, and hoped for benefits, and reasonable alternatives,

The procedure

History taking is important with particular attention to a history of:

- regular smears; a past smear abnormality and/or colposcopy or treatment to the cervix for abnormal cells;
- inter-menstrual and/or post-coital bleeding.

The patient is placed in a modified lithotomy position in a colposcopy couch, with her dignity and privacy maintained at all times. She is kept warm and encouraged to keep relaxed, whenever possible.

The cervix is exposed using a bivalve speculum. A repeat smear may be taken at this stage. Acetic acid 5% is applied to the cervix and left *in situ* for about 10 seconds.

The acetic acid aids identification of both normal and abnormal epithelium. Metaplastic changes between normal squamous and columnar epithelium will show as faint white. Columnar epithelium also shows a faint white change. Abnormal skin changes will show as a more pronounced and well-demarcated aceto-white area on the cervix. There may also be evidence of abnormal vascular patterns associated with pre-cancer of the cervix (mosaic pattern and punctation), cervical intra-epithelial neoplasia (CIN).

Lugol's iodine can be used to outline atypical epithelium, particularly prior to excision treatments, as dysplastic epithelium contains little or no glycogen and will not readily take up the stain, as will normal columnar epithelium. Normal squamous epithelium is well-glycogenated and will readily take up the stain, turning a very dark brown colour. This is called Schiller's test.

Some colposcopists will perform a saline colposcopy initially before the application of acetic acid. When used in conjunction with the green filter on the colposcope, it is particularly useful in identifying abnormal blood-vessel patterns, such as mosaicism and punctation.

A cervical punch biopsy is taken for histological diagnosis. Bleeding is arrested either by application of Monsel's solution (ferric subsulphate solution) or silver nitrate. Treatment may be performed if high-grade abnormality is suspected following a smear suggesting high-grade dyskaryosis or if the examination is deemed unsatisfactory.

The colposcopy findings are detailed in hand-drawn documentation using standard terminology. It is important to indicate if the squamo-columnar junction has been visualized or not seen in its entirety, and any areas of abnormality are carefully drawn. A digital image can be taken and saved in the patients records. Results of cytology and histology are communicated to the patient and the GP or referrer by letter.

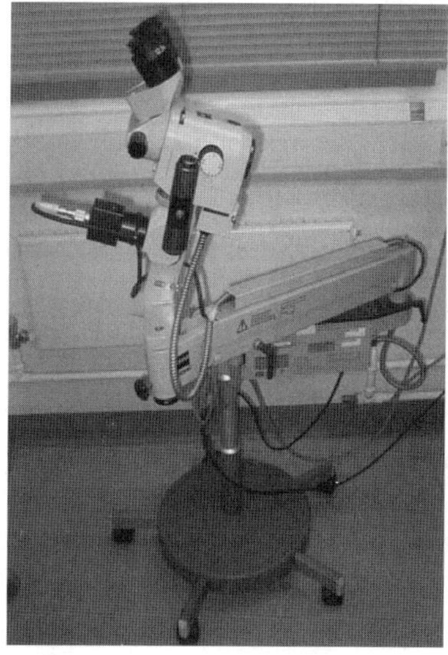

Fig. 18.3 A colposcope.

Indications for referral

- 3 x succesive inadequate samples.
- Borderline changes in:
  - squamous cells;
  - endo-cervical cells;
  - abnormal results of any grade;
  - mild dyskaryosis x 1 result;
  - moderate dyskaryosis;
  - severe dyskaryosis;
  - possible invasion;
  - glandular neoplasia.

► Dyskaryosis means an abnormal maturation seen in exfoliated cells that have normal cytoplasm but hyperchromatic nuclei.

- Suspicious looking cervix:
  - cervical warts—these should be referred to GUM clinic;
  - cystic lesion;
  - a nabothian follicle or retention cyst is a cyst resulting from some obstruction of cervical glands—this is a variant of a normal cervix and does not need referral to colposcopy (see Fig. 18.5);
  - ulcerated cervix—urgent referral;
  - white plaque.
- Suspicious symptoms—some of these women may be referred to gynaecology clinics:
  - post-coital bleeding—refer to gynaecology after genital swabs;
  - inter-menstrual bleeding, only if associated with other symptoms or abnormal smear—refer to gynaecology after colposcopy and swabs;
  - contact bleeding on smear taking does not warrant colposcopy referral.

Waiting times for colposcopy

- At least 90% of women with an abnormal test result should be seen in a colposcopy clinic within 8 weeks of referral.[1]
- At least 90% of women with test result of moderate or severe dyskaryosis should be seen in a colposcopy clinic within 4 weeks of referral.[1]

1. Luesley, D and Leeson, S (2004) Colposcopy and programme management guidelines for the NHS cervical screening programme. Publication no. 20. **4**(11): 14.

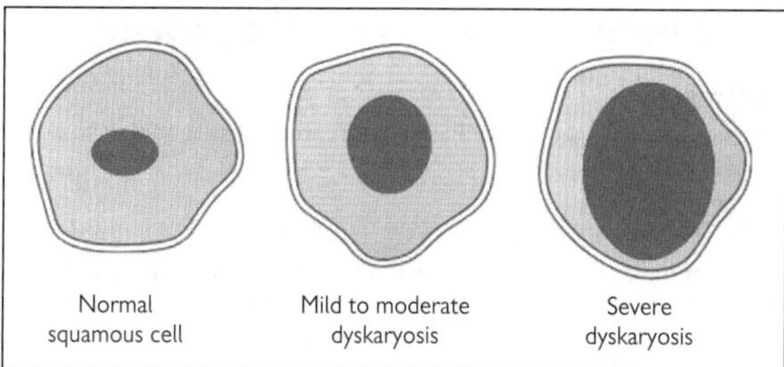

Fig. 18.4 Dyskaryotic cells demonstrating an increased nuclear/cytoplasmic ratio. Produced by Stephanie Jokhan.

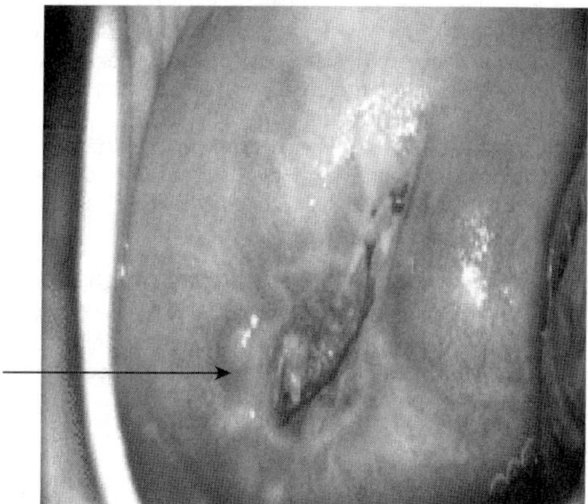

Fig. 18.5 Nabothian follicles. Reproduced with kind permission of BSCCP.

Treatments/see and treat/follow-up

Treatments

Conservative management entails colposcopic surveillance after discussion with the patient:

- In low-grade CIN.
- If the patient is immuno-suppressed (HIV-positive, transplant patients).

Treatment methods aim to destroy the transformation zone by either:

- Ablative or destructive method by cold coagulation. Here a probe is applied to the cervix and the tissue is destroyed by heat (100–120°C).
- Excisional method using an electrified loop wire known as large loop excision of the transformation zone (LLETZ).
- Cold coagulation and LLETZ procedures are performed under local anaesthetic on an outpatient basis. There are some concerns around association of LLETZ with pre-term labour, but more work is required in this field.
- Surgical knife cone biopsy involves deeper excision of the endo-cervical canal and this is performed under general anaesthetic. The main complications include haemorrhage and post-operative cervical stenosis, depending on the length of the cone involved. Stenosis makes cytological and colposcopic follow-up more difficult.
- Hysterectomy may be needed in a woman with persistent high-grade CIN and other gynaecological pathology, such as fibroids, menorrhagia, or prolapse. There is a 0.3–0.4% incidence of invasive cancer following these procedures.

Management of abnormal smears during pregnancy

Difficulties can sometimes arise in the management of pregnant patients with abnormal smears. NHSCP's policy is to do an initial colposcopic assessment and exclude invasive disease. If this is excluded, the patient can be followed-up during pregnancy and after childbirth.

See and treat

The colposcopist aims to 'see and treat' women at first visit only, when there is reasonable suspicion of high-grade disease on colposcopic appearances, following a high-grade cytology referral. Clinics undertaking treatment at first visit must audit the proportion of cases with CIN (target >90%).

Follow-up

Women treated with high-grade disease (CIN 2 and CIN 3) require 6- and 12-month follow-up cytology and annual cytology for the subsequent 9 years at least, before returning to screening at the routine interval.

Women treated for low-grade disease (CIN I) require 6-, 12- and 24-months follow-up cytology. If all results are negative, then women may be returned to screening at the routine interval.

Resources

Luesley, D and Leeson, S (2004) Colposcopy and programme management guidelines for the NHS cervical screening programme. Publication no. 20 **8**(5): 32.

The role of the nurse in cervical screening in primary care

- Ensure informed consent is obtained from the women to enable them to make an informed choice about whether or not to participate in cervical screening.
- Provide health education/lifestyle advice on the prevention of cervical cancer.
- Encouraging non-responders to use the service to increase coverage.
- Provide a private, warm, secure, and comfortable environment for sample taking.
- Ensure appropriate equipment and instruments are prepared for the procedure.
- Answer questions and concerns that women may have regarding test results.
- Follow-up and treatment.
- Ensure the patient receives notification of her test results.
- Refer patients for further investigation, if necessary.
- Co-operate with laboratory failsafe enquiries.
- Undertake continuous audit which may include:
  - the number and rate of inadequate samples;
  - percentage of abnormal results;
  - monitoring population uptake and coverage.
- Attend cytology training update.

Nurse colposcopists: overview

The first idea of nurse colposcopist was developed in 1999 as part of a drive to improve quality across the whole colposcopy service. This has gained acceptance and where it had been tried at that time, nurses, consultants, and patients were enthusiastic about it and now it has become the norm in colposcopy.

Why do we need nurse colposcopists?

- Because of increased workload.
- To reduce waiting times.
- Lack of trained staff (Calman, fewer specialist registrars).
- To provide continuity of care.
- To ensure patient's choice.

Entry requirements

- Membership of the British Society for Colposcopy and Cervical pathology.
- Recognized nursing or medical qualification.
- Attendance at a BSCCP accredited basic colposcopy course.

The diagnostic training programme

This involves:

- Direct supervision of 50 colposcopy cases.
- Indirect supervision of 100 cases.
- Completion of the log-book.
- Histo-pathological and cytological sessions.
- Objective Structured Clinical Examinations (OSCEs).

Average duration of training is 18 months and this leads to the award of the BSCCP Certificate in Diagnostic Colposcopy. Optional treatment module leads to the award of Certificate in Therapeutic Colposcopy.

The trainee will be considered trained in local treatment if he/she:

- Has witnessed at least 10 cases of treatment.
- Has performed, under supervision, at least 10 cases of local treatment.
- Has performed, under supervision, at least 5 cases of conization.

3-yearly re-accreditation involves:

- Evidence of work-load and audit.
- Evidence of continued medical education.

Conclusions drawn from studies on nurse colposcopist performance

- Increasing workload would have caused a crisis with existing manpower were it not for nurse colposcopists.
- Women prefer to see a female nurse.
- Nurses are skilled colposcopists.[1]
- Nurses are better at keeping accurate records.[1]
- Introduction of nurse colposcopists has:
  - reduced waiting times for new referral without compromising standard;
  - added credibility to colposcopy accreditation.

1. Todd RW, Wilson S, Etherington I, Luesley D (2002) Effects of nurse colposcopists on a hospital based service. *Br J of Hosp Med.* **63**(4): 218–223.

HPV/testing/vaccines

Human papilloma virus (HPV)

- Plays a major role in the aetiology of CIN and cancer of the cervix. 99.7% of all cancers are high-risk HPV-positive.
- A highly sexually transmitted virus with up to 80% lifetime risk of exposure.
- Peak incidence is up to age 30 and prevalence in this group is 30–40%.
- Most infections are transient. Approximately 90–95% will be cleared within a year by the immune system.
- There are more than 100 different types.
- Subdivided into 'high-' and 'low-risk' types. Low-risk types are not associated with cancer, can cause skin warts, verrucas, and genital warts (HPV 6). High-risk types are 16 (accounts for 60–85% of high-grade CIN and cervical cancer), 18, 31, and 33. (📖 See Figs. 18.6 and 18.7.)
- There is a need for the development of consistent and clear information about HPV, and to identify a role for GPs and other clinicians in providing women with this information.

HPV testing

Carrying out an HPV test at the same time as a woman has a cervical test may help to decide how to manage the patient if her test shows minor abnormalities; it could also avoid referral to colposcopy with its associated anxiety. This will help improve accuracy for referral to colposcopy.

The LBC national pilot looked at using HPV testing to triage low-grade abnormalities to reduce referral to colposcopy, and to provide clear evidence on the costs, medical effects.

Studies suggest that there is a role for HPV DNA testing after treatment of CIN as a 'test of cure'. The test has the potential to enhance the detection of persistent/recurrent disease.

HPV vaccines

The HPV vaccine is highly effective in preventing HPV. It gives almost 100% protection. There are two HPV vaccines:

- Gardasil®
  - Quadrivalent—protects against HPV 6, 11, 16, and 18.
  - Given at 0, 2, 6 months (three doses).
  - A national vaccination campaign started in September 2008 as part of immunization programme for girls aged 12–13 years with catch-up programme for up to 18 years olds.
- Cervarix®
  - Bivalent—protects against HPV 16 and 18.
  - Given at 0, 1, 6 months.
  - Licensed for use in 9–26 year olds.

In studies of Gardasil®, no serious side-effects were reported. Minor side-effects reported that are common with many vaccinations were:

- pain at the site of injection;
- redness at the site of injection;
- fever;
- nausea;
- dizziness.

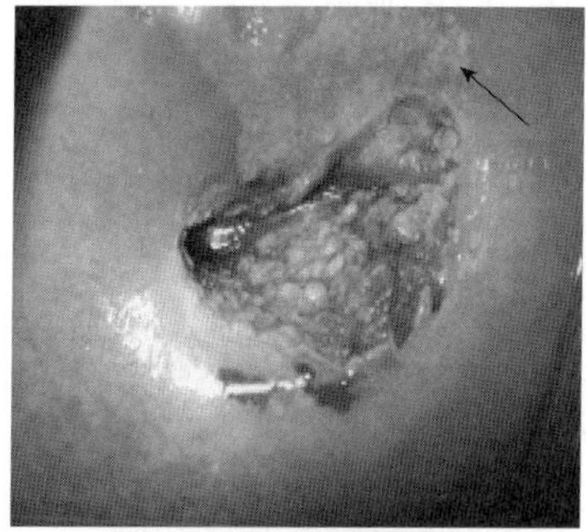

Fig. 18.6 Human papilloma virus—appearance of the cervix after application of acetic acid. Reproduced with the kind permission of the BSCCP.

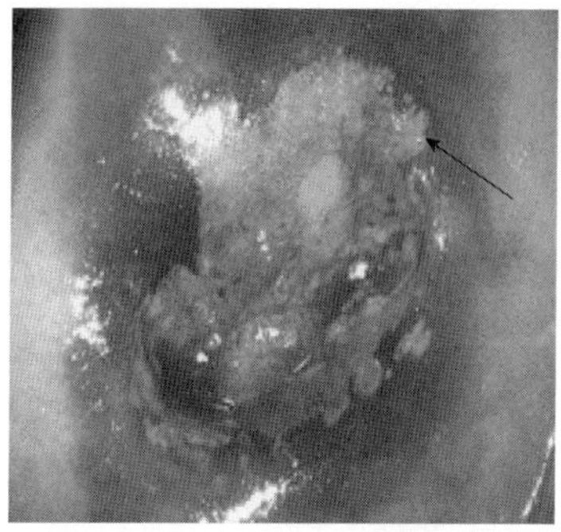

Fig. 18.7 Human papilloma virus—appearance of the cervix after application of iodine. Reproduced with the kind permission of the BSCCP.

Resources

Wallboomers, JM, Jacobs, MV, Manos, MM, Bosh, FX, Kumar, JA, Shah, KV *et al.* (1999) Human papillomavirus is a necessary cause of invasive cervical cancer worldwide. *Journal of Pathology* **189**: 12–19.

Waller, J, McCafferty, K, Nazroo, J, Wandle, J (2005) Making sense of information about HPV in cervical screening: a qualitative study. *British Journal of Cancer* **92**(2): 265–270.

Future developments

Liquid-based cytology (LBC)

LBC has now been accepted as the way forward and by 2008 all laboratories in the UK will be converted. LBC has brought about a decline in laboratory backlogs, which should not be seen again. Women are receiving their results faster and inadequate rates have dropped, reducing anxiety and uncertainty. LBC also facilitates HPV testing using the same sample.

HPV testing

Evidence for the clinical utility of HPV testing has increased over the years and has now become very convincing. Some potential uses of HPV testing include:

- Triage of women with borderline and mild-grade dyskaryosis and related management strategies.
- As a test of cure post-treatment.
- Most importantly, as an adjunct to cytology in routine cervical disease screening programmes in women over the age of 30.

HPV vaccines

Because there is a 10–20-year gap between HPV infection and development of cervical cancer, it will take some years for the HPV vaccine to have a major effect on the number of cases of cervical cancer (📖 see Fig. 18.8). However, the development of the vaccines has given us a fantastic opportunity to prevent the development of the majority of cases of cervical cancer, and, in turn, to reduce the number of deaths from the disease.

Technological innovation

Computer-assisted detection of cervical abnormalities is a possibility for the future.

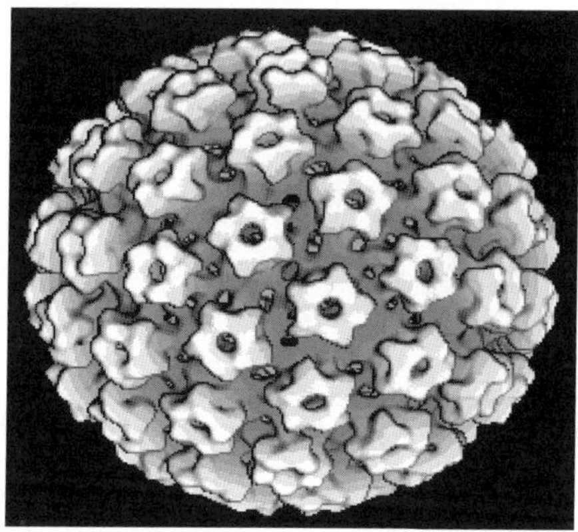

Fig. 18.8 Human papilloma virus. Produced by Stephen Harrison.

Cervical polyps

Cervical polyps occur in 2–5% of adult women and almost invariably arise from endo-cervical columnar epithelium (📖 see Figs. 18.9 and 18.10).

Symptoms

Most are symptomless but may present with:

- Vaginal discharge.
- Post-coital bleeding.
- Inter-menstrual bleeding.
- Menstrual irregularities.

Clinical features

- At its onset, the polyp is covered by columnar epithelium and may only be discovered during colposcopic assessment of the endo-cervical canal.
- As the polyp continues to grow, it will protrude beyond the external os. The origin of the polyp, i.e. the point at which the stalk begins, must be determined, as removal of the tip but not the stalk will simply result in regrowth. Occasionally, endometrial polyps will present at the external os.
- Sometimes a necrotic polyp may lead to a false diagnosis of cervical carcinoma.
- Malignancy in a cervical polyp is very uncommon but should always be considered.

Management

- All women with cytological abnormality and cervical polyps should be referred to the colposcopy clinic.

► Women with cervical polyps and normal cytology should be managed within gynaecology clinics.

- Provided the smear is normal, and if the base of the polyp is clearly visible and accessible, the polyp is avulsed and sent for histological confirmation; otherwise the endo-cervical canal should be assessed.
- The polyp and its stalk are removed and the base of the stalk is treated by silver nitrate and/or diathermy.
- Hysteroscopy, endometrial biopsy, and/or ultrasound scan will prove useful in symptomatic women and asymptomatic post-menopausal women with polyps.
- A high vaginal swab, chlamydia, and gonorrhoea tests may be taken in pre-menopausal women.

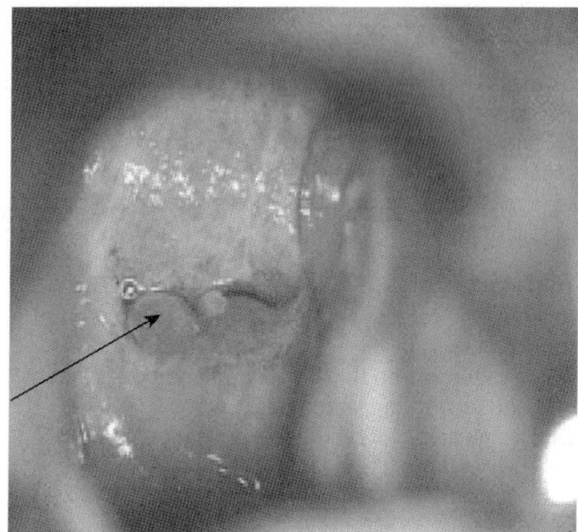

Fig. 18.9 Endo-cervical polyp under low magnification range. Reproduced with kind permission of the BSCCP.

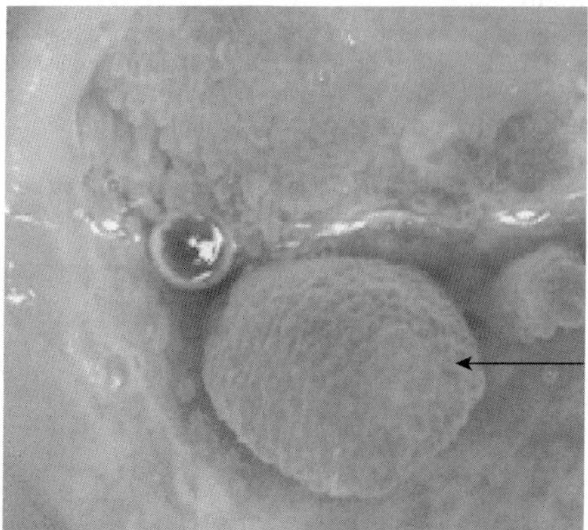

Fig. 18.10 Endo-cervical polyp under high magnification range. Reproduced with kind permission of the BSCCP.

Resources

Aaron, LA, Jacobson, J and Soule, EH (1963) Endo-cervical polyps. *Obstetrics and Gynaecology* **21**: 659.

Cervical ectropion

- Describes the presence of everted endo-cervical columnar epithelium on the ectocervix.
- Often clinically referred to as an ectopy or erosion.
- It is influenced by oestrogen and common in teenagers.
- Frequently develops in women taking combined oral contraceptive pills and during pregnancy.

Clinical features

- It appears as a large reddish area and a firmly taken cervical smear will often produce bleeding.
- Usually more extensive on the anterior lip and posterior lips of the ecto-cervix and less on the lateral lips.
- Diagnosis is confirmed by speculum examination giving an appearance of a red ring around the os.

Symptoms

- Most women are asymptomatic except for some mucoid discharge.
- An ectropion is not painful and does not cause dyspareunia.
- Some women may present with contact bleeding or post-coital bleeding or vaginal discharge.

Management

- An ectropion is not an abnormal finding but a normal physiological occurrence and, therefore, does not require treatment unless it is causing symptoms such as post-coital bleeding or excessive vaginal discharge.
- Cryo-cautery to the cervix or cold coagulation may be performed in symptomatic patients.
- It is important to explain the finding so that the patient can be reassured, and so that unnecessary referral to colposcopy can be avoided.

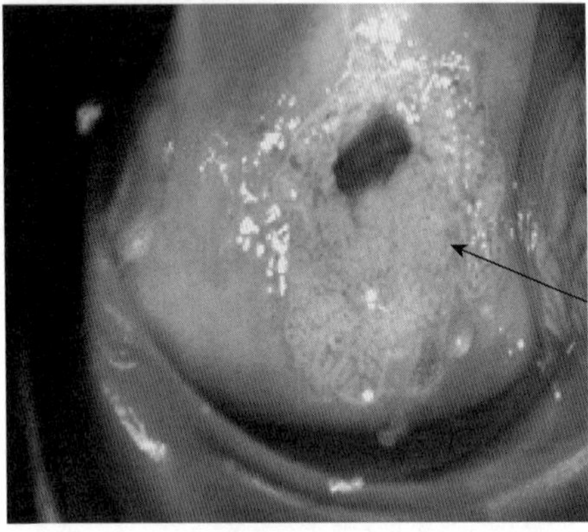

Fig. 18.11 Cervical ectropion under low magnification range. Reproduced with kind permission of the BSCCP.

Chapter 19

Breast

Breast introduction

Although breast care and surgery is not undertaken by Gynaecologists in the UK, many women will discuss breast problems when they see nurses, practice nurses, reproductive health staff, and gynaecology staff. In some areas in the UK, breast surgery is mixed with gynaecology surgery in the same ward.

In response to nurses' anxiety, the RCN published guidance in 2007 for the role of the nurse, outside of specialist roles. It states that nurses should not undertake routine palpation. They suggest that nurses' role should include:

- Encouraging breast awareness and back up with verbal and written information.
- Being aware of common problems and their management.
- Ability to refer, if needed.
- Encourage screening through national screening programme.

Breast pain: mastalgia

Mastalgia is a common complaint accounting for a quarter of breast clinic referrals. 70% of women complain of breast pain at some stage in their lives, two-thirds of which are cyclical/intermittent and one-third non-cylical/constant.

Causes

- Hormonal: likely to be cyclical, seen in early months after initiation of hormonal contraception. Oestrogenic pills are more likely to cause breast tension/engorgement and heaviness. Progestogens are more likely to cause true mastalgia.
- Muscular: anterior chest wall pain or referred pain from any part of the thoracic cage. Sources could be:
  - Cervical spine: spondylosis.
  - Gall bladder: cholecystitis, gall stones.
  - Rib cage: costochondritis—so called Tietze's syndrome.
  - Hiatus hernia.
  - Muscles: fibromyalgia.
- Infective: 📖 see p.515.
- Breast cysts may present as small cystic lumps.
- Breast cancer: pain is the presenting symptom in less than 10% of cases. However, breast cancer patients often experience pain after treatment.

Principles of management

- Take a good history. To illustrate cyclicity, a pain chart/calendar is useful to gain insight into the pain triggers.

► Physiological or menstrual-related mastalgia is diffuse and bilateral.

► Pain from actual breast disease is constant and localized and can be reproduced during examination. However, a cyst may cause premenstrual pain.

- Breast examination to exclude organic disease backed by mammography, if appropriate.
- If the cause is benign, reassurance and simple lifestyle advice is all that is required.

Reassurance and lifestyle advice

- The use of the right size bra.
- Losing weight.
- Posture.
- Position in bed.
- The option of wearing a bra in bed.
- Simple occasional analgesia, if required.
- Advice on relaxation and exercise.
- Advise premenstrual salt restriction for cyclical mastalgia.

Treatment

- When the association is with pill use, switching to a pill with lower or different progestogen may help. Using ultra-low dose pills may also relieve cyclical pain. Using the pill in an extended regimen, omitting the hormone-free interval, reduces menstrual mastalgia.
- Evening primrose oil/gamma-linolenic acid was used extensively for mastalgia. Some women respond well to what is perceived as a natural product. The dose is 240–320mg gamma-linolenic acid per day for 3 months. As the therapeutic effect is mediated through manipulation of hormone receptors, symptom relief can take as long as 3 months to happen. Improvement in severity of cyclical and non-cyclical mastalgia is 58 and 38%, respectively.
- Bromocriptine: this dopamine agonist inhibits prolactin production, thereby reducing the glandular breast tissue response. The dose is increased gradually from a starting dose of 1.25mg to a maximum of 5mg a day. With maximum dose, relief is of the order of 54% in cyclical mastalgia and 33% in non-cyclical mastalgia.

⚠ Side-effects, such as nausea, constipation, and postural hypotension are common and need to be discussed with the patient.

- Other agents used include:
    - Danazol: limited by side-effects but low doses of 100 per day.
    - Tamoxifen: ⚠unlicensed use.
    - Cabergoline: as for bromocriptine.
- For musculo-skeletal pain, simple analgesia, NSAIDs, physiotherapy, or local anaesthetic and steroid injections (for costochondritis) have all been used. In severe cases, referral to a pain clinic may be warranted.

Resources

Pollit, J, Twine, C, Gately, CA (2006) Benign breast disease. *Women's Health Medicine* **3**(1): 1–4.
www.breastcancercare.org.uk. (Accessed January 2009)

Benign breast conditions

While breast cancer is more common in post-menopausal women, benign breast conditions are mostly hormonal driven and occur in younger women. The majority of presenting breast problems are benign and fall under 4 categories:

- Breast lumps/cysts—these are a source of worry for the patient but only 10% are cancerous.
- Nipple discharge.
- Mastalgia.
- Mastitis.

Fibro-adenoma

Description and symptoms

- The classically described breast mouse is a firm mobile nodule. They are usually seen at a young age.
- The majority will cause no symptoms and do not change. 5% increase in size and 20% regress.

Cause

Fibro-adenomas are oestrogen-sensitive and will generally regress at the menopause. Sometimes calcified fibro-adenomas are seen on mammograms.

Referral and treatment

- A lump in a woman >30mm size requires referral for investigations.
- Surgery is indicated when the adenoma is large (>3cm) or causes symptoms. Large fibro-adenomas may be phylodes and some women may develop multiple fibro-adenomas.

Breast cysts

Description

These are more common in the peri-menopause, tend to be bigger, and may cause pain. They can vary in number and frequency and normally stop formation in the menopause.

Symptoms and cause

- Pain and lump within breast.
- Cause may be hormonal.

Referral and treatment

- Ultrasound is the investigation of choice.
- If symptomatic, they can be needle-aspirated under ultrasound control. Fine-needle aspiration can also be used in a diagnostic capacity if there is doubt about a cyst.

Fibrocystic disease

Breast nodularity in pre-menopausal women is defined as fibrocystic disease. It can present as a palpable breast mass. This should be managed as for any breast mass.

Nipple discharge

Types include:

- Physiological: this tends to be spontaneous, intermittent, thin, small volume discharge. It may be clear or cloudy. Women who then express their breasts will reproduce the discharge. Management is reassurance.
- Gestational discharge: this can occur anytime from the 2nd trimester of pregnancy. It tends to be milky in colour. Examination to exclude organic problems and reassurance is all that is required. Follow-up at the conclusion of the pregnancy and breast feeding aims to confirm resolution.
- Blood stained/serosanguinous discharge can occur in the gestational period but is more likely to be associated with breast epithelial hyperplasia and ductal papilloma (most common cause of unilateral single duct discharge). Discharge in breast cancer cases is uncommon but tends to be associated with a lump. Treatment of intraductal papilloma is surgical excision.
- Galactorrhoea: the discharge of galactorrhoea is milk-like, copious, and bilateral. There is no associated breast abnormality. (See Box for causes.)
- Pituitary adenoma: there is associated hyperprolactinaemia. Micro-adenomas cause no other symptoms but larger tumours are associated with visual disturbances (homonymous hemianopia), menstrual irregularity, and, in some, GI symptoms.

Diagnosis is based on raised prolactin and imaging the pituitary fossa. Treatment is medical with dopamine agonists, such as bromocriptine and cabergoline. Surgery is indicated if there are pressure symptoms.

Causes of galactorrhoea

- Drugs: dopamine agonists commonest cause.
- Pituitary tumours: adenomas, functional.
- Cushings's disease: rare.
- Hypothyroidism.

Mastitis

Infections of the breast have become less common in the UK. Breast infections are divided into lactational and non-lactational. Lactational are related to lactation and caused by staphylococci and respond to penicillin. Non-lactational infections—periductal mastitis affects young women 90% of whom smoke cigarettes, Tuberculosis and viral infections are rare causes. Antibiotic therapy should be started early and the patient reviewed every 3 days to assess response to antibiotics. If it is not responding to antibiotics, the patient should be referred to a breast unit for review and management, where ultrasound guided aspiration/microscopy culture and sensitivity (MC+S) is an option. Abscess formation is managed by immediate drainage.

Resources

Pollit, J, Twine, C, Gately, CA (2006) Breast infections. *Women's Health Medicine* **3**(1):4–6.

Breast history and examination

In addition to the usual history of the complaint, the clinician needs to enquire about menstruation including last menstrual period, obstetric history, family history, past or recent mammography, and the use of hormones.

Breast examination must be done in a relaxed setting, ensuring privacy and dignity. Inspection and palpation while comparing the two breasts looking for asymmetry, puckering of the skin, dilated vessels, and visible lumps. The breast is examined in upright position with hands on the hips and with the hands behind the head, then again reclining at a 45-degree angle. 📖 See Figs 19.1–19.3.

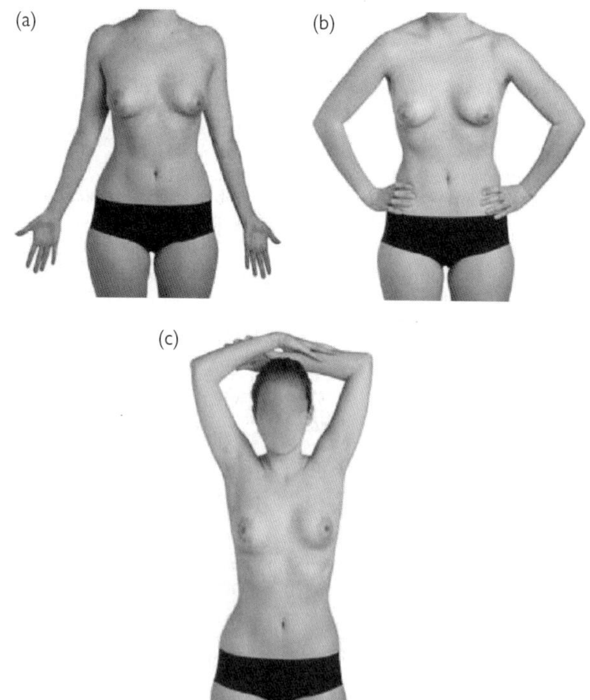

Fig. 19.1 Manoeuvres for breast inspection: (a) anatomical position; (b) hands on hips; (c) arms crossed above the head. Reproduced from Thomas J and Monaghan T (2007). *Oxford Handbook of Clinical Examination and Practical Skills*, with permission from Oxford University Press.

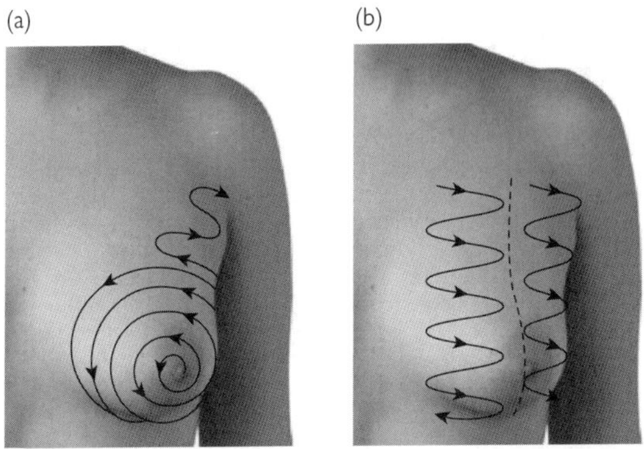

Fig. 19.2 Two methods for the systematic palpation of the breast: (a) work circumferentially from the areola; (b) examine each half at a time, working from top to bottom. Reproduced from Thomas, J and Monaghan T (2007). *Oxford Handbook of Clinical Examination and Practical Skills*, with permission from Oxford University Press.

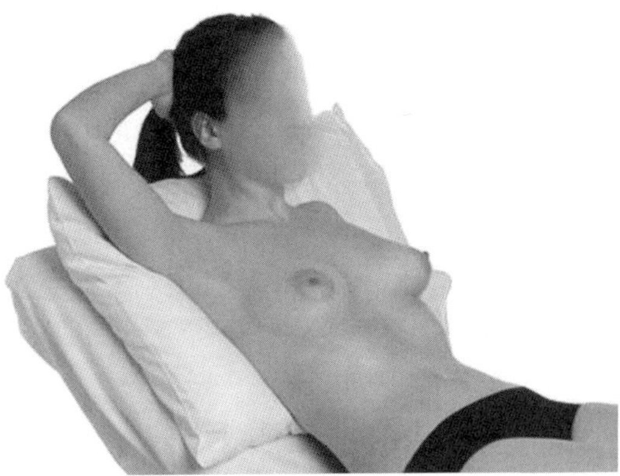

Fig. 19.3 Correct position of the patient for examination of the breast. Reproduced from Thomas J and Monaghan,T (2007). *Oxford Handbook of Clinical Examination and Practical Skills*, with permission from Oxford University Press.

Breast disease: screening and investigation

Mammography

The NHS breast screening programme (NHSBSP), established in the mid-80s in the UK, has been a great success. It is based on 3-yearly single-view (now double-view) mammography, starting at age 50 until the age of 70, after which patients may self-refer. It is estimated that breast cancer mortality has been reduced by 24%. The age band has recently been extended and is now offered to women between 47 and 73 years of age.

Survival in breast cancer is improving and the single most important factor is early diagnosis before metastatic disease sets in. Mammography has stood the test of time as a screening test. Sensitivity (fewer false-positives) is as high as 90% and specificity (fewer false-negative) is 95%. Breast density, use of HRT, and technical radiology factors affect the performance of mammography.

Women are invited in a 3-year cycle, starting at 47. If the basic screen suggests an abnormality (clustered microcalcification, lumps, or asymmetry), the woman is invited back to attend a multidisciplinary team assessment.

Many units may have a breast care nurse who is central to this follow-up assessment, offering explanation and support, and being a resource to answer questions.

Women may be referred to a breast clinic for further investigations such as mammograms, ultrasound, CBE, aspiration, core biopsy, or vacuum-assisted biopsy.

Only 10–30% of those recalled will have malignant changes; they are referred to specialist units for further management.

What do women need to know?

- The breast screening programme has built-in quality assurance. Films are double 'read'. Units are required to submit performance indicators.
- The radiation to which the breast is exposed is small and the risk of inducing malignant change is 1: 100,000, which is miniscule compared to the prevalent risk of breast cancer.
- The majority of recalls (up to 90%) are for benign or no disease.
- Screening is never 100%, so women who get interval symptoms should report these to their GP.
- Breast awareness should be encouraged but not forced on women. Women should be encouraged to get familiar with the look and feel of their breasts when they are dressing or in the bath.

Other imaging techniques

- All are secondary to mammography.
- Ultrasound can be used as a primary investigation for clinically suspected benign conditions such as breast cysts. The main use for ultrasound is to differentiate a solid from a cystic mass, and to assist in the aspiration of a cyst, especially when the aspiration is deemed incomplete.
- Doppler ultrasound is used to improve the diagnostic capability.
- MRI is being investigated as an adjunct or replacement to mammography

Screening high-risk groups: women with a family history of breast cancer

5% of breast cancer has significant genetic basis mainly BRCA 1 and 2 mutations. Such women, and their immediate family, should be referred to family history clinics. Their life-time risk of breast cancer is as high as 80%. They tend to be offered early screening: mammograms. CBE and MRI can be used as surveillance tools in high-risk cases. See NICE for referral guidance[1].

Fine-needle aspiration

This is a component of the diagnostic workup of breast disease. It is used for solid and cystic tumours to obtain the aspirate.

Core-needle biopsy (Trucut biopsy)

A method of histological sampling where no lump is palpable. It is done under local anaesthetic and ultrasound guidance.

Other investigations

- Nipple cytology is only suitable for single-duct nipple discharge.
- If there is an abscess, then aspiration/MC+S.
- Punch biopsy is needed for skin or nipple problems.

Resources

Reddy, M, Given-Wilson R (2006) Screening for breast cancer. *Women's Health Medicine* **3**(1): 22–26. www.NICE.org.uk

1. NICE (2006) National collaborating centre for primary care. Familial breast cancer, *Clinical guidelines* CG41: www.nice.org.uk (Accessed January 2009)

Breast cancer: clinical picture and management options

Breast cancer is a disease of Western societies, though the incidence is rising worldwide as lifestyle changes modify risks. In 2002, the incidence in Europe was over 80 per 100,000 and the death rate was just over 20 per 100,000.

Classification

- Pre-invasive/carcinoma *in situ*.
- Invasive cancer.
- Metastatic disease.

Principles of management

- Multidisciplinary approach with the breast cancer team including the surgeon, medical oncologist, clinical oncologist/radiotherapist, radiologist, breast care nurse, chemotherapy nurse, histo/cytopathologist, and radiographers.
- If a lump is found, the initial investigation is triple assessment with clinical examination, mammography, and ultrasound followed by pathology.
- Core biopsy is more sensitive than needle biopsy aspiration.
- MRI can give additional information, such as the extent of the disease.
- The patient is closely involved in shaping her treatment plan.
- Surgery remains the primary treatment aiming to remove the tumour and any involved lymph nodes. This can be conservation surgery or mastectomy and node clearance. There are also many reconstruction techniques.
- Radiotherapy is usually used with conservation treatment.
- Chemotherapy is systemic and can be combined with any of the above.
- Other systemic treatments include hormone therapy (tamoxifen, goserelin) or aromatase inhibitors (anastrozole, letrozole or exemestane) and trastuzumab (Herceptin®).
- Breast reconstruction is offered after a mastectomy and can be done at the time of the operation or later.

Surgery could be:

- Lumpectomy.
- Wide local excision: lump + limited excision of surrounding breast tissue—ideal for *in situ* tumours and tend to be combined with radiotherapy.
- Quadrantectomy: as much as a quarter of the breast is removed; wide local excision and lumpectomy aim at conservation of the breast.
- Simple total mastectomy: the breast is removed including the nipple—this is recommended for central tumours, where local excision will distort the anatomy of a small breast, multi-focal disease, or at patient's request.
- Modified radical mastectomy: in addition to the breast, chest wall muscles may be removed.

- Lymph node clearance can be combined with the above. Lymphoedema is a potential complication and can occur any time after surgery. Avoidance of cuts and scratches to the arm in question reduces the risk.
- Sentinel lymph node biopsy is a technique where radioactive material is injected into the breast to identify the 1st node into which the tumour drains. This node is biopsied and, if clear, then all the other nodes should be clear. An alternative route uses axillary ultrasound and needle biopsy.

Adjuvant treatments

- Radiotherapy: tends to be combined with local excision and is started a few weeks after surgery. A course can be up to 6 weeks. If lymph nodes are not removed, radiotherapy of the axillary nodes may be offered. Lymphoedema is a post-treatment risk.
- Chemotherapy (anthracyclines and taxanes) is offered for large tumours, if lymph nodes are involved, and for certain types of tumour. It usually, but not always, follows radiotherapy. Chemotherapy given prior to surgery to help shrink or control a tumour is called neo-adjuvant therapy.
- Hormone therapy: oestrogen antagonists that bind and block the oestrogen receptors are used post-surgery of oestrogen-receptor positive cancers. Several agents are in use, tamoxifen being the prototype usually used for 5 years.
- Aromatase inhibitors, such as anastrozole: these were endorsed by NICE as 1st line adjuvant therapies for receptor-positive early breast cancer. They are more effective than tamoxifen in preventing recurrences. The risk of fractures is higher than tamoxifen but VTE risk is lower.
- Trastuzumab (Herceptin®) is a monoclonal antibody against the human epidermal growth factor receptor 2 present in 23% of breast cancers and found to improve survival rates in HER2-positive cases when given alone or with chemotherapy.

Follow-up

- Annual mammograms for 5 years.
- Follow-up within breast units will vary but is usually 2+ years.
- Psychological follow-up and counselling, if needed. in relation to altered body image and reduction in fertility with some modalities of treatment.

Other issues include:

- Prosthetics.
- Lymphoedema.
- Chest wall tenderness.
- Psychological.
- Fatigue.
- Altered body image.
- Menopausal symptoms (📖 see Chapter 9, p.221).
- Sexual problems.

Breast cancer: risk factors and prevention

Prevalence

Breast cancer is the most prevalent cancer in developed countries and the second most common malignancy globally responsible for over 400,000 deaths annually. 37,000 cancers were recorded in the UK in 2004. 80% of cancers occur in the post-menopause.

Risk factors for breast cancer

- Age: there is a 2.8% year-on-year increase in risk
- Geographical: women living in developed societies have 5 times the risk of less developed countries, probably reflecting lifestyle differences.
- Early menarche (<11) and late menopause (>54).
- Delaying 1st term pregnancy over age 35. Having a termination of pregnancy is not a risk factor.
- Family history assessment can depend on the age of diagnosis and the number of family members affected, generally an affected 1st degree relative doubles the baseline risk (see cancer referral guidelines and NICE).
- Lifestyle factors:
    - Obesity in post-menopause only.
    - High-fat diet poses a relative risk of 1.5.
    - High alcohol intake: it is estimated that an extra 2000 cases a year are due to heavy drinking. There is a 7% increase in risk for every 10g additional alcohol consumed per day.
- Oral contraception: traditional teaching is that there is a small risk (odds ratio of 1.24) only in women <35, but recent evidence shows no overall increase in risk.
- HRT: the risk is linked to duration of use, but, disappears after 10 years of discontinuation.
    - In the million women study, relative risk for oestrogen-only HRT is 1.3, (excess cases 5/1000 at 10 years), for combined HRT is 2 (excess risk 19/1000 at 10 years), and for tibolone it is 1.45.
    - In the Women's Health Initiative study, the overall relative risk for combined HRT was lower at 1.26 and for oestrogen only HRT, a reduced risk of 0.77.
- Parity is protective, especially if it occurs early in the reproductive years.

Factors with less clear association

Several factors are suspected to protect or predispose to breast cancer but consensus is not universal. These include:

- Smoking: likely to increase the risk modestly.
- Breastfeeding: likely to be protective.
- Exercise is protective.
- Red meat may pose a small increased risk.
- Exposure to moderate or high-dose ionizing radiation is acknowledged as a rare risk factor.

Prevention strategies

- Avoidance of the risk factors.
- Regular mammography from age 47. In the UK, women over 73 need to proactively request a mammogram.
- Where there are genetic factors (BRCA mutation), specialist advice on risk profiling and consideration of prophylactic mastectomy.

Resources

For patients:

- www.breastcancer.org.uk
- www.cancerscreening.nhs.uk
- www.cancerbacup.org.uk
- www.NICE.org

For professionals:

Cassidy J, Bissett, D, Spence, R, Payne, M (2006) *Oxford Handbook of Oncology*. Oxford: Oxford University Press.

Tadman M, Roberts, D (2006) *Oxford Handbook of Cancer Nursing*. Oxford: Oxford University Press.

Chapter 20

Lifestyle issues

Diet and women's health

Healthy eating is eating a low-fat, low-sugar, high-carbohydrate, high-fibre, and a low-salt diet.

The advice given to women in any healthcare interventions should be to:

- Eat lots of bread, pasta, rice, and other starch-based food, as they stabilize blood sugar and provide soluble fibre.
- Eat foods rich in vitamin B6, such as potatoes, bananas, and oatmeal, and try and get 100mg of vitamin B6 a day.
- Magnesium should come from beans, tofu, and peanuts. Good for PMS sufferers.
- Eating oily fish twice a week (tuna, mackerel, sardines, salmon, herrings) is thought to be beneficial. Oily fish fats can help prevent heart disease and arthritis.
- Avoid biscuits, cakes, and chocolates.
- Try to avoid frying and cooking with lard and butter or ghee, use polyunsaturated oils instead.
- Keeping well hydrated is important.

Role of fruit and vegetables

The role remains poorly understood. The evidence that five fruits and vegetables a day can prevent certain cancers, lower heart disease, and prevent some forms of arthritis is scanty. The average consumption in Britain is three fruits and vegetables a day.

Red and processed meat

The World Cancer Research Fund (WCRF) second report (2007) indicates that red and processed meats convincingly cause colorectal cancer. There appears to be a 30% higher risk in women who eat more red meat, compared to those who eat the least. The WCRF recommend that the intake of red meat should be no more than 300g a week. Limiting high-fat foods, particularly red meat, full-fat dairy products, and hard cheese, lowers heart disease. Lean meat, chicken, and turkey are considered better, compared to beef and pork.

Alcohol

Alcohol can increase the risk for cancers of the mouth, pharynx, larynx, oesophagus, colon, rectum, and breast. It can predispose to cirrhosis of the liver and liver cancer. Current advice in Britain is to drink no more than 2–3 units a day.

Nutritional supplements

Most women eating a well-balanced diet will not need additional multivitamins or multi-minerals.

A woman's diet should include the following.

- The requirement for calcium in pre-menopausal women can vary between 700–1000mg daily. This can come from milk, tofu, salmon, and broccoli.
- Antioxidants such as folates, vitamin E and C.
- Women attempting to conceive should take 400µg of folic acid daily to prevent spina bifida in the baby.
- Benefits of supplements like ginseng, aloe vera juice, and starflower are questionable.

Impact of diet

Extreme nutritional deprivation can result in anorexia. This can lead to long-term health problems, such as amenorrhoea and osteoporosis.

Over-eating can be associated with obesity, which is discussed later in this chapter.

Smoking and women's health

Smoking is the single biggest preventable cause of premature death in women: it kills half a million women each year. Fewer women and men smoke now than was the case in the 1970s, but, whereas most smokers used to be men, now there are more women smokers. Younger women are more likely to smoke compared to men and they often start early, around age 12 and 13. Women may smoke as a response to stress.

Cardiovascular effects

- Smokers have higher blood pressure, pulse rate, and blood viscosity.
- There is an altered lipid profile with increase in low density lipoprotein (LDL) cholesterol.
- Smoking is a risk factor for coronary spasm and myocardial infarction in young women.
- Cigarette smokers are four times more likely to develop a subarachnoid haemorrhage compared to non-smokers.
- New evidence suggests increased risk of VTE.

Cancer risks

- Relative risk (RR) of cervical cancer is 2–3 times higher in smokers.
- RR of lung cancer is higher in women who smoke.
- RR of lung cancer associated with having a husband who smokes under one pack is 2.4 and 3.4 for husbands smoking more than one pack a day.
- Active exposure to smoking is a risk factor for rectal cancer (relative risk 1.95).
- No relationship between smoking and epithelial ovarian cancer and breast cancer.
- Smoking is not a risk factor for colon cancer.

Reproductive risks

- Smoking reduces fertility by 25%. It affects sperm count and function.
- Smoking in pregnancy increases risk of miscarriage, premature rupture of membranes, pre-term labour, low birth-weight babies, and congenital defects, e.g. cleft palate.
- There is a mean difference of 200g in birth-weight of smoking and non-smoking women. The negative effect of maternal smoking increases with age.
- Menopause is accelerated by 1.7 years.
- Smoking is a risk factor for osteoporosis.
- Smokers are more likely to have breakthrough bleeding on the pill.

Other risks

- Life-expectancy is reduced in women who smoke.
- Bronchitis and emphysema can be associated with smoking and result in long-term health problems and premature death.
- Heavy smoking and smoking cessation correlate with higher body weight.
- Young children who breathe in cigarette smoke are more prone to ear and chest infections.

- Because of passive smoking at an early age, children of smokers are more likely to become smokers at an early age, compared to children of non-smokers.
- There is a 45% higher risk of developing age-related macular degeneration compared to non smokers.
- There is a strong association between smoking and glaucoma, cataract and Grave's opthalmopathy.

Interventions

- A sensitive approach is required.
- Self-help groups can prove useful.

The role of the practice nurse

The practice nurse is vital in that she can provide help, support, and encouragement in quitting. Healthcare professionals should offer smoking-cessation advice more often. A smoker's chance of quitting increases after receiving smoking-cessation information and support from healthcare professionals. It should be acknowledged that it can be very hard to give up smoking as tobacco is addictive, though success can be achieved with persistence. Encouragement should be offered to set up a quit date and women need to be made aware that half of all smokers are killed by their habit and it could lead to early death.

Nicotine replacement therapy (NRT)

Can be offered to women with a target stop date in the form of patches, gums, gels, or nasal sprays for 6 months in the first instance and continued for 3 months after cessation of smoking. It can minimize withdrawal symptoms. Side-effects of NRT include dreams, dry mouth, and gastrointestinal disturbances.

Bupropion

This is an atypical anti-depressant and can be used as an alternative to NRT.

Varenicline

This is used less frequently.

Cognitive behavioural therapy

This is the basis for most smoking-cessation counselling programmes.

Other interventions that some patients find helpful include hypnotherapy and acupressure/acupuncture. Animal studies on nicotine vaccine show good results and human studies in relation to safety, efficacy, and dosage are underway.

Resources

For health professionals:

National Institute for Health and Clinical Excellence. Brief interventions and referral for smoking cessation. Public health guidance. (March 2006) 🔗 www.nice.org.uk (Accessed April 2009.)

For women:

🔗 www.gosmokefree.co.uk

NHS smoking helpline: Tel: 0800 169 0169

Obesity: risk factors, assessment, prevention, and treatment

The National Institute of Health and World Health Organization (WHO) define obesity as a body mass index (BMI) >/= 30kg/m^2. BMI is calculated by dividing weight by height squared.

BMI

Underweight	<18.4kg/m^2
Normal	18.5–24.9kg/m^2
Overweight	25–29kg/m^2
Obesity 1	30–34.9kg/m^2
Obesity 11	35–39.9kg/m^2
Obesity 111	>40kg/m^2

The prevalence of obesity has increased dramatically both in the UK and the US, and is a major public health concern. 23% of women in the UK are obese (The NHS Information Centre 2005).[1]

Risk factors

- Genes may play a role. Family history significant, if one or both parents are obese.
- Sex: women more likely to be obese compared to men.
- Inactivity can promote weight gain.
- Regular consumption of high calorie foods is a risk.
- Quitting smoking: partly due to nicotine's ability to raise the rate at which the body burns calories.
- Pregnancy.
- Certain medications: steroids and tricyclic anti-depressants.
- Medical conditions: hypothyroidism, Cushing's syndrome.

Assessment of obesity

- Assess medical history including diabetes, high blood pressure.
- Assess social history: lifestyle, physical exercise, diet, smoking, alcohol.
- Measure height, weight, and calculate BMI.
- Measure waist circumference.
- Take BP using large cuff.

Prevention

Daily 30-minute consistent physical activity is effective in reducing body weight compared to no treatment at 12 months (NICE 2006).[2]

Enjoying healthy meals and snacks, with a particular focus on fruits and vegetables and whole grains. Keep saturated fat low. Know and avoid the food traps that precipitate eating and monitor weight regularly; being consistent helps.

1. The NHS information Centre: www.ic.nhs.uk/statistics-and-data-collection (Accessed April 2009)
2. National Institute for Health and Clinical Excellence (NICE) Obesity: the prevention, identification, assessment and management of overweight and obesity in adults and children. Clinical guidelines CG43. December 2006. www.nice.org.uk (Accessed April 2009)

Treatment

- Lowering total calorie intake will achieve a healthy weight (NICE 2006).[2]
- Dietary habit changes are the cornerstone of success.
- Increasing physical activity. A 30-minute brisk walk every day can help to burn calories regularly.
- Setting realistic goals and plans on weight-reduction is important.
- Behaviour-modification programmes led by a psychologist, therapist, or other trained professional can help.

Weight-loss medication

If BMI is >30 and other methods of weight loss have not worked, orlistat can be used but only continued beyond 3 months if weight loss exceeds 5%. It is contraindicated in chronic malabsorption syndrome. Side-effects include flatulence with rectal discharge.

Sibutramine can be used in chronic malabsorption.

Weight-loss surgery (gastric bypass surgery)

Indicated or considered if BMI>40. This surgery is often not without complications.

Coping skills

Help as emotional suffering and self-blame can make obese people feel it is a moral failing not a personal choice.

Implications of obesity

Obesity is linked to many health problems which can increase morbidity and mortality.

Type 2 diabetes mellitus

Associated with central obesity. Normally insulin is necessary for transport of blood glucose into muscle and fat cells. By transporting glucose into cells, insulin keeps the blood glucose levels within normal range. When the effectiveness of this transport mechanism is diminished, the pancreas initially responds by increasing the output of insulin. If the pancreas continues to produce more insulin, the insulin-resistant state can last for years. When the pancreas can no longer keep up with producing more insulin, blood glucose levels begin to rise resulting in type II diabetes.

Hypertension

Reduction in capacity of blood vessels to transport blood can cause high blood pressure.

Dyslipidemias

Obesity is associated with low levels of HDL cholesterol (HDL cholesterol protects the heart) and high levels of triglycerides. As obesity is linked to diets high in saturated fats, the bad cholesterol (LDL) levels rise.

Arthritis

Extra weight appears to increase the risk of osteoarthritis by placing extra pressure on joints and wearing away the cartilage that normally protects them.

Gall stones

The risk of gall stones is higher in obese women because they have more cholesterol that can be deposited in the gall bladder.

Coronary heart disease

Women with a BMI >30 run a higher risk of developing high blood pressure and a 3-fold risk of developing coronary heart disease. For every 1kg increase in body weight, the risk of dying from coronary heart disease increases by 1%.

Stroke

Obesity is associated with atherosclerosis—build up of fatty deposits in arteries throughout the body including arteries in the brain. If a blood clot forms in a narrowed artery in the brain, it can block blood flow to an area of the brain.

Fatty disease of the liver

Fat accumulation in the liver can lead to inflammation and scarring of the liver, which can lead to cirrhosis.

Cancers

5% of all cancers in post-menopausal women are attributable to being overweight or obese.

- Breast cancer: BMI has a varying effect in pre-menopausal and post-menopausal women. In pre-menopausal women the risk decreases with increasing BMI, except in Asia Pacific populations. In post-menopausal women, the risk increases with high BMI in women who have never used HRT.
- Endometrial cancer. There is an increased risk of endometrial cancer with increasing BMI.
- Cancer of the gall bladder can be associated with high BMI.
- Cancer of the colon. Relationship differs in pre-menopausal and postmenopausal women and studies lack consistency in results.
- With high BMI, there is an increase in risk of adenocarcinoma of the oesophagus, kidney, and pancreatic cancer.
- There is scanty data if any on the relationship between BMI and haematopoeitic cancers.

Fertility and pregnancy risks

- Obesity and PCOS co-exist.
- Obesity can increase the risk of spontaneous miscarriage during infertility treatment and lower the chances of success.
- Pregnancy: gestational diabetes can occur during pregnancy and may increase the risk of birth defects. Obesity has a statistically significant association with gestational hypertension, pregnancy-induced hypertension, high birth-weight babies, failed induction, chorio-amnionitis, and an increase in the rate of Caesarean deliveries.

Resources

For health professionals:

Reeves, GK, Prie, K, Beral, V *et al.* (2007) Cancer incidence and mortality in relation to BMI in the million women study: a cohort study. *British Medical Journal* **335**: 1134–1138.

National Institute for Health and Clinical Excellence (NICE) CG43 Obesity: the prevention, identification, assessment and management of overweight and obesity in adults and children December 2006. ☞ www.nice.org.uk (Accessed April 2009.)

For women:

Your weight, your health booklet: ☞ www.dh.gov.uk

Appendix: resources

The following sections contain website information for both women and health professionals. There are some that are of use to both.

Resources for professionals

B

- www.bashh.org
- www.britishfertilitysociety.org.uk
- www.brook.org.uk
- www.bsccp.org.uk
- www.bsge.org.uk

C

- www.cancerhelp.org.uk
- www.cancerbackup.org.uk

D

- www.daisynetwork.org.uk

E

- www.earlymenopauseuk.co.uk
- www.ectopic.org.uk
- www.endometriosis-uk.org

F

- www.figo.org
- www.fpa.org.uk
- www.fsrh.org

G

- www.gynaeonc.net

H

- www.hfea.gov.uk
- www.hysterectomy-association.org.uk

I

- www.infertilitynetworkuk.com

J

- www.jotrust.co.uk

L

- www.library.nhs.uk

M

- www.miscarriageassociation.org.uk
- www.menopausematters.co.uk
- www.menopause.org

N

- www.nhsdirect.nhs.uk
- www.nice.org.uk
- www.nmc-uk.org
- www.nos.org.uk
- www.npc.co.uk

P

- www.patient.co.uk
- www.pms.org.uk
- www.prodigy.nhs.uk

R

- www.rcog.org.uk
- www.rcog.org.uk/bsug
- www.rcn.org.uk

T

- www.thebms.co.uk

V

- www.verity-pcos.org.uk

W

- www.wellbeingofwomen.org.uk
- www.womens-health-concern.org
- www.womenshealthlondon.org.uk

Resources for women

A

www.acupuncture.org.uk

www.althysterectomy.org

B

www.bcma.co.uk

www.bladderandbowelfoundation.org

www.bupa.co.uk

C

www.cancerbacup.org.uk

www.cancerscreening.nhs.uk/cervical

www.CenterForEndo.com

www.child.org.uk

www.colposcopy.org.uk

www.continence-foundation.org.uk

D

www.daisynetwork.org.uk

E

www.earlymenopause.com

www.ectopic.org

www.endometriosis.org.uk

www.endometriosispaintreatment.com

www.endo.org.uk

F

www.fibroids.co.uk

H

www.healthywomen.org

www.hmole-chorio.org.uk

www.homeopathy-soh.org

www.hysterectomy-association.org.uk

I

www.issue.co.uk

L

www.lichensclerosus.org

M

www.medicines.org.uk

www.menopausematters.co.uk

www.miscarriageassociation.org.uk

N

www.naturopathy.org.uk

www.ncbi.nlm.nih.gov/pubmed

www.nimh.org.uk

www.nlm.nih.gov/medlineplus

www.nos.org.uk

O

www.osteofound.org

www.ovacome.org.uk

P

www.pcosupport.org

www.pelvicpain.org

www.pms.org.uk

www.pofsupport.org

R

www.rchm.co.uk

S

www.shetrust.org.uk

T

www.thrushadvice.org

www.trusthomeopathy.org

V

www.verity-pcos.org.uk

www.vulvalpainsociety.org

W

www.wellbeing.org.uk

www.womens-health-concern.org

www.womens-health.co.uk

www.womenshealthlondon.org.uk

Index

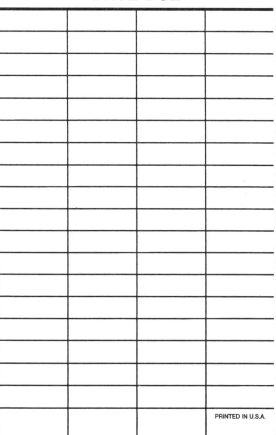